Technology in Diabetes

Editor

GRAZIA ALEPPO

ENDOCRINOLOGY AND METABOLISM CLINICS OF NORTH AMERICA

www.endo.theclinics.com

Consulting Editor
ADRIANA G. IOACHIMESCU

March 2020 • Volume 49 • Number 1

ELSEVIER

1600 John F. Kennedy Boulevard • Suite 1800 • Philadelphia, Pennsylvania, 19103-2899

http://www.theclinics.com

ENDOCRINOLOGY AND METABOLISM CLINICS OF NORTH AMERICA Volume 49, Number 1 March 2020 ISSN 0889-8529, ISBN 13: 978-0-323-69761-3

Editor: Katerina Heidhausen
Developmental Editor: Nicole Congleton

Endocrinology and Metabolism Clinics of North America (ISSN 0889-8529) is published quarterly by Elsevier Inc., 360 Park Avenue South, New York, NY 10010-1710. Months of issue are March, June, September, and December. Periodicals postage paid at New York, NY and additional mailing offices. Subscription prices are USD 375.00 per year for US individuals, USD 799.00 per year for US institutions, USD 100.00 per year for US students and residents, USD 454.00 per year for Canadian individuals, USD 988.00 per year for Canadian institutions, USD 497.00 per year for international individuals, USD 988.00 per year for international institutions, USD 100.00 per year for Canadian students/residents, and USD 245.00 per year for international students/residents. To receive student/resident rate, orders must be accompanied by name of affiliated institution, date of term, and the signature of program/residency coordinator on institution letterhead. Orders will be billed at individual rate until proof of status is received. Foreign air speed delivery is included in all *Clinics* subscription prices. All prices are subject to change without notice. **POSTMASTER:** Send address changes to *Endocrinology and Metabolism Clinics of North America*, Elsevier Health Sciences Division, Subscription Customer Service, 3251 Riverport Lane, Maryland Heights, MO 63043. **Customer Service: Telephone: 1-800-654-2452** (U.S. and Canada); **1-314-447-8871** (outside U.S. and Canada). **Fax: 1-314-447-8029. E-mail: journalscustomerservice-usa@elsevier.com (for print support)**; **journalsonlinesupport-usa@elsevier.com (for online support)**.

Reprints. For copies of 100 or more, of articles in this publication, please contact the Commercial Rights Department, Elsevier Inc., 360 Park Avenue South, New York, NY 10010-1710; phone: +1-212-633-3874; fax: +1-212-633-3820; E-mail: reprints@elsevier.com.

Endocrinology and Metabolism Clinics of North America is covered in *MEDLINE/PubMed (Index Medicus), EMBASE/Excerpta Medica, Current Contents/Clinical Medicine, Current Contents/Life Sciences, Science Citation Index, ISI/BIOMED, BIOSIS,* and *Chemical Abstracts*.

Contributors

CONSULTING EDITOR

ADRIANA G. IOACHIMESCU, MD, PhD, FACE
Professor of Medicine (Endocrinology) and Neurosurgery, Emory University School of Medicine, Atlanta, Georgia, USA

EDITOR

GRAZIA ALEPPO, MD, FACE, FACP
Professor of Medicine, Division of Endocrinology, Metabolism and Molecular Medicine, Feinberg School of Medicine, Northwestern University, Chicago, Illinois, USA

AUTHORS

GRAZIA ALEPPO, MD, FACE, FACP
Professor of Medicine, Division of Endocrinology, Metabolism and Molecular Medicine, Feinberg School of Medicine, Northwestern University, Chicago, Illinois, USA

LINDSAY M. ANDERSON, PhD
Pritzker Department of Psychiatry and Behavioral Health, Ann & Robert H. Lurie Children's Hospital of Chicago, Chicago, Illinois, USA

TADEJ BATTELINO, MD, PhD
Professor, Department of Paediatric Endocrinology, Diabetes and Metabolic Diseases, UMC - University Children's Hospital, University Medical Centre Ljubljana, Faculty of Medicine, University of Ljubljana, Ljubljana, Slovenia

RICHARD M. BERGENSTAL, MD
International Diabetes Center, Minneapolis, Minnesota, USA

CHARLOTTE K. BOUGHTON, MRCP, PhD
University of Cambridge Metabolic Research Laboratories, Wellcome Trust-MRC Institute of Metabolic Science, Addenbrooke's Hospital, Cambridge, United Kingdom

ANDERS L. CARLSON, MD
International Diabetes Center & Health Partners, Minneapolis, Minnesota, USA

JESSICA R. CASTLE, MD
Associate Professor, Division of Endocrinology, Diabetes and Clinical Nutrition, Oregon Health & Science University, Harold Schnitzer Diabetes Health Center, Portland, Oregon, USA

EDA CENGIZ, MD, MHS, FAAP
Associate Professor, Yale School of Medicine, New Haven, Connecticut, USA; Visiting Professor, Bahçeşehir Üniversitesi, Istanbul, Turkey

AMY B. CRIEGO, MD, MS
International Diabetes Center, Park Nicollet Clinic Pediatric Endocrinology, Minneapolis, Minnesota, USA

GEORGIA M. DAVIS, MD
Department of Medicine, Emory University, Atlanta, Georgia, USA

HANNAH R. DESROCHERS, MSN, RN, CPNP
Pediatric Nurse Practitioner, Section on Clinical, Behavioral, and Outcomes Research, Pediatric, Adolescent, and Young Adult Section, Joslin Diabetes Center, Harvard Medical School, Boston, Massachusetts, USA

KLEMEN DOVC, MD, PhD
Assistant Professor, Department of Paediatric Endocrinology, Diabetes and Metabolic Diseases, UMC - University Children's Hospital, University Medical Centre Ljubljana, Faculty of Medicine, University of Ljubljana, Ljubljana, Slovenia

MEREDYTH EVANS, PhD
Assistant Professor, Pritzker Department of Psychiatry and Behavioral Health, Ann & Robert H. Lurie Children's Hospital of Chicago, Department of Psychiatry and Behavioral Sciences, Feinberg School of Medicine, Northwestern University, Chicago, Illinois, USA

MARISSA A. FELDMAN, PhD
Child Development and Rehabilitation Center, Johns Hopkins All Children's Hospital, Saint Petersburg, Florida, USA

FEDERICO Y. FONTANA, PhD
Department of Neurosciences, Biomedicine and Movement Sciences, University of Verona, Verona, Italy; Team Novo Nordisk Professional Cycling Team, Atlanta, Georgia, USA

RODOLFO J. GALINDO, MD, FACE
Department of Medicine, Emory University, Atlanta, Georgia, USA

KIMBERLY GARZA, MPH
Department of Anthropology, The University of Illinois at Chicago, Chicago, Illinois, USA

ROMAN HOVORKA, PhD, FMedSci
Professor of Metabolic Technology, University of Cambridge Metabolic Research Laboratories, Wellcome Trust-MRC Institute of Metabolic Science, Addenbrooke's Hospital, Cambridge, United Kingdom

PETER G. JACOBS, PhD
Associate Professor, Department of Biomedical Engineering, Oregon Health & Science University, Portland, Oregon, USA

JELENA KRAVARUSIC, MD, PhD
Assistant Professor of Medicine, Division of Endocrinology, Metabolism and Molecular Medicine, Feinberg School of Medicine, Northwestern University, Chicago, Illinois, USA

LORI M. LAFFEL, MD, MPH
Senior Investigator, Head, Section on Clinical, Behavioral, and Outcomes Research, Chief, Pediatric, Adolescent, and Young Adult Section, Joslin Diabetes Center, Professor of Pediatrics, Harvard Medical School, Boston, Massachusetts, USA

DANA M. LEWIS, BA
Founder and Independent Researcher, OpenAPS, Seattle, Washington, USA

THOMAS W. MARTENS, MD
International Diabetes Center, Minneapolis, Minnesota, USA

ALEXANDRA L. MIGDAL, MD
Department of Medicine, Emory University, Atlanta, Georgia, USA

MEDHA N. MUNSHI, MD
Director of Joslin Geriatric Diabetes Programs, Joslin Diabetes Center, United States, Associate Professor of Medicine, Harvard Medical School, Beth Israel Deaconess Medical Center, Boston, Massachusetts, USA

JACLYN LENNON PAPADAKIS, PhD
Pritzker Department of Psychiatry and Behavioral Health, Ann & Robert H. Lurie Children's Hospital of Chicago, Chicago, Illinois, USA

ANNE L. PETERS, MD
Professor of Clinical Medicine, Keck School of Medicine of USC, Los Angeles, California, USA

WILLIAM H. POLONSKY, PhD
Behavioral Diabetes Institute, University of California, San Diego, San Diego, California, USA

RUBIN POONI, MSc
School of Kinesiology and Health Science, York University, Toronto, Ontario, Canada; York University, North York, Ontario, Canada

MICHAEL C. RIDDELL, PhD
Professor, School of Kinesiology and Health Science, York University, LMC Diabetes & Endocrinology, Toronto, Ontario, Canada; York University, North York, Ontario, Canada

ALAN T. SCHULTZ, MSN, RN, CPNP
Pediatric Nurse Practitioner, Emergency Department, Montefiore Medical Center, The Bronx, New York, USA

SAM N. SCOTT, PhD
Team Novo Nordisk Professional Cycling Team, Atlanta, Georgia, USA; Department of Diabetes, Endocrinology, Nutritional Medicine and Metabolism, Bern University Hospital, University of Bern, Bern, Switzerland

JENNA B. SHAPIRO, PhD
Pritzker Department of Psychiatry and Behavioral Health, Ann & Robert H. Lurie Children's Hospital of Chicago, Chicago, Illinois, USA

LAURIE GAYES THOMPSON, PhD
Assistant Professor, Pritzker Department of Psychiatry and Behavioral Health, Ann & Robert H. Lurie Children's Hospital of Chicago, Department of Psychiatry and Behavioral Sciences, Feinberg School of Medicine, Northwestern University, Chicago, Illinois, USA

ELENA TOSCHI, MD
Staff Physician, Joslin Diabetes Center, United States, Instructor of Medicine, Harvard Medical School, Boston, Massachusetts, USA

GUILLERMO E. UMPIERREZ, MD, CDE, FACP, FACE
Department of Medicine, Emory University, Atlanta, Georgia, USA

JILL WEISSBERG-BENCHELL, PhD, CDE
Professor, Pritzker Department of Psychiatry and Behavioral Health, Ann & Robert H. Lurie Children's Hospital of Chicago, Department of Psychiatry and Behavioral Sciences, Feinberg School of Medicine, Northwestern University, Chicago, Illinois, USA

LEAH M. WILSON, MD
Assistant Professor, Division of Endocrinology, Diabetes and Clinical Nutrition, Oregon Health & Science University, Harold Schnitzer Diabetes Health Center, Portland, Oregon, USA

Contents

Foreword: Technological Advances in Management of Diabetes Mellitus xiii

Adriana G. Ioachimescu

Preface: Technology in Diabetes: The Future Is Today xv

Grazia Aleppo

Evolution of Diabetes Technology 1

Klemen Dovc and Tadej Battelino

Technological innovations have fundamentally changed diabetes care. Insulin pump use and continuous glucose monitoring are associated with improved glycemic control along with a better quality of life; automated insulin-dosing advisors facilitate and improve decision making. Glucose-responsive automated insulin delivery enables the highest targets for time in range, lowest rate and duration of hypoglycemia, and favorable quality of life. Clear targets for time in ranges and a standard visualization of the data will help the diabetes technology to be used more efficiently. Decision support systems within and integrated cloud environment will further simplify, unify, and improve modern routine diabetes care.

Use of Diabetes Technology in Children: Role of Structured Education for Young People with Diabetes and Families 19

Hannah R. Desrochers, Alan T. Schultz, and Lori M. Laffel

The current era has generated a surge of advanced diabetes technologies. Young people with diabetes and their families require detailed, structured diabetes education in order to optimize device use. There is need for youth and their families to participate in both the selection of particular devices for personal use, and comprehensive education regarding the safe and effective implementation of such technologies. The education process can efficiently ensure that youth and their families receive realistic expectations of the role that advanced technologies play in diabetes management while avoiding disappointment, sub-optimal outcomes, and the premature discontinuation of such systems.

Diabetes Technology Use in Adults with Type 1 and Type 2 Diabetes 37

Jelena Kravarusic and Grazia Aleppo

In the last 2 decades, diabetes technology has emerged as a branch of diabetes management thanks to the advent of continuous glucose monitoring (CGM) and increased availability of continuous subcutaneous insulin infusion systems, or insulin pumps. These tools have progressed from rudimentary instruments to sophisticated therapeutic options for advanced diabetes management. This article discusses the available CGM and insulin pump systems and the clinical benefits of their use in adults with type 1 diabetes, intensively insulin-treated type 2 diabetes, and pregnant patients with preexisting diabetes.

Benefits and Challenges of Diabetes Technology Use in Older Adults 57

Elena Toschi and Medha N. Munshi

With successful aging of adults with type 1 diabetes, there is an increased opportunity to use technology for diabetes management. Technology can ease the burden of self-care and provide a sense of security. However, age-related cognitive and physical decline can make technology use difficult. Guidelines using technology in the aging population are urgently needed, along with educational material for the clinicians and caregivers. In this article, we review the evidence supporting the use of diabetes-related technologies in the older population and discuss recommendations based on current data and the authors' clinical knowledge and experience.

Integration of Diabetes Technology in Clinical Practice 69

Anne L. Peters

This article attempts to aid clinicians in using diabetes devices in their clinical practice. It reviews device selection, initiation, and follow-up. It discusses work flow in an office and provides tips on billing. It stresses the need for patient choice, education, and on-going support through downloading and interpretation of data to optimize care.

Diabetes Technology in the Inpatient Setting for Management of Hyperglycemia 79

Georgia M. Davis, Rodolfo J. Galindo, Alexandra L. Migdal, and Guillermo E. Umpierrez

In past decades, a rapid evolution of diabetes technology led to increased popularity and use of continuous glucose monitoring (CGM) and continuous subcutaneous insulin infusion (CSII) in the ambulatory setting for diabetes management, and recently, the artificial pancreas became available. Efforts to translate this technology to the hospital setting have shown accuracy and reliability of CGM, safety of CSII in appropriate populations, improvement of inpatient glycemic control with computerized glycemic management systems, and feasibility of inpatient CGM-CSII closed-loop systems. Several ongoing studies are focusing on continued translation of this technology to improve glycemic control and outcomes in hospitalized patients.

HbA_{1c}: The Glucose Management Indicator, Time in Range, and Standardization of Continuous Glucose Monitoring Reports in Clinical Practice 95

Anders L. Carlson, Amy B. Criego, Thomas W. Martens, and Richard M. Bergenstal

Continuous glucose monitoring (CGM) use is growing rapidly among people with diabetes and beginning to be standard of care for managing glucose levels in insulin therapy. With this increased use, there is a need to standardize CGM data. CGM standardization has been set forth by expert panels. The Glucose Management Indicator is a concept using the CGM-derived mean glucose to provide a value that can be understood similarly to hemoglobin A_{1c}. The times an individual spends in various glucose ranges is emerging as an important set of metrics. Metrics derived from patient CGM data are changing the way diabetes is managed.

Diabetes Technology and Exercise 109

Michael C. Riddell, Rubin Pooni, Federico Y. Fontana, and Sam N. Scott

Advances in technologies such as glucose monitors, exercise wearables, closed-loop systems, and various smartphone applications are helping many people with diabetes to be more physically active. These technologies are designed to overcome the challenges associated with exercise duration, mode, relative intensity, and absolute intensity, all of which affect glucose homeostasis in people living with diabetes. At present, optimal use of these technologies depends largely on motivation, competence, and adherence to daily diabetes care requirements. This article discusses recent technologies designed to help patients with diabetes to be more physically active, while also trying to improve glucose control around exercise.

Psychosocial Aspects of Diabetes Technology Use: The Child and Family Perspective 127

Jaclyn Lennon Papadakis, Lindsay M. Anderson, Kimberly Garza, Marissa A. Feldman, Jenna B. Shapiro, Meredyth Evans, Laurie Gayes Thompson, and Jill Weissberg-Benchell

This article offers a systematic review of the literature on psychosocial aspects of technology use in children and adolescents with type 1 diabetes and their families, searching for relevant articles published the past 5 years. Topics included continuous subcutaneous insulin infusion, continuous glucose monitoring, predictive low-glucose suspend, and artificial pancreas systems. The review indicates there are positive and negative psychosocial aspects to diabetes technology use among youth and their families. Although consistent findings were revealed, contradictions exist. Discussed are recommendations for future research and implications for how health care providers can collaborate with families to discuss and manage diabetes technology.

Psychosocial Aspects of Diabetes Technology: Adult Perspective 143

William H. Polonsky

The success of diabetes technologies depends on the attitudes and behavior of the individuals who choose to adopt them. Real-time continuous glucose monitoring, continuous subcutaneous insulin infusion, and sensor-augmented pump systems may positively affect diabetes-related quality of life (QOL), although the influence on QOL outcomes seems to be modest and the results from randomized controlled trials are limited and controversial. In contrast, more consistently positive QOL-related responses are apparent from observational data. The newer generations of devices hold the promise for more strongly enhancing diabetes-related QOL. Appropriate training and ongoing support are likely to be the key to successful uptake.

Automated Insulin Delivery in Children with Type 1 Diabetes 157

Eda Cengiz

The advent of insulin pump therapy marked an important milestone in diabetes treatment in the past few decades and has become the tipping point for the development of automated insulin delivery systems (AID).

Standalone insulin pump systems have evolved over the course of years and have been replaced by modern high-technology insulin pumps with continuous glucose monitor interface allowing real-time insulin dose adjustment to optimize treatment. This review summarizes evidence from AID studies conducted in children with type 1 diabetes and discusses the outlook for future generation AID systems from a pediatric treatment perspective.

Automated Insulin Delivery in Adults **167**

Charlotte K. Boughton and Roman Hovorka

Hybrid closed-loop (artificial pancreas) systems have recently been introduced into clinical practice for adults with type 1 diabetes. This reflects successful translation from research studies in highly supervised settings to evaluation of the technology in free-living home settings. We review the different closed-loop approaches and the key clinical evidence supporting adoption of hybrid closed-loop systems for adults with type 1 diabetes. We also discuss the growing evidence for automated insulin delivery in pregnant women and in hospitalized patients with hyperglycemia. We consider the psychosocial impact of closed-loop systems and the challenges and potential future advancements for automated insulin delivery.

Role of Glucagon in Automated Insulin Delivery **179**

Leah M. Wilson, Peter G. Jacobs, and Jessica R. Castle

Treatment of type 1 diabetes with exogenous insulin often results in unpredictable daily glucose variability and hypoglycemia, which can be dangerous. Automated insulin delivery systems can improve glucose control while reducing burden for people with diabetes. One approach to improve treatment outcomes is to incorporate the counter-regulatory hormone glucagon into the automated delivery system to help prevent the hypoglycemia that can be induced by the slow pharmacodynamics of insulin action. This article explores the advantages and disadvantages of incorporating glucagon into dual-hormone automated hormone delivery systems.

Do-It-Yourself Artificial Pancreas System and the OpenAPS Movement **203**

Dana M. Lewis

People with diabetes have been experimenting with and modifying their own diabetes devices and technologies for many decades in order to achieve the best possible quality of life and improving their long-term outcomes, including do-it-yourself (DIY) closed loop systems. Thousands of individuals use DIY closed loop systems globally, which work similarly to commercial systems by automatically adjusting and controlling insulin dosing, but are different in terms of transparency, access, customization, and usability. Initial outcomes seen by the DIY artificial pancreas system community are positive, and randomized controlled trials are forthcoming on various elements of DIYAPS technology.

ENDOCRINOLOGY AND METABOLISM CLINICS OF NORTH AMERICA

FORTHCOMING ISSUES

June 2020
Obesity
Michael D. Jensen, *Editor*

September 2020
Pituitary Disorders
Niki Karavitaki, *Editor*

December 2020
Pediatric Endocrinology
Andrea Kelly, *Editor*

RECENT ISSUES

December 2019
Endocrine Hypertension
Amir H. Hamrahian, *Editor*

September 2019
Pregnancy and Endocrine Disorders
Mark E. Molitch, *Editor*

June 2019
Transgender Medicine
Vin Tangpricha, *Editor*

SERIES OF RELATED INTEREST
Medical Clinics
https://www.medical.theclinics.com

VISIT THE CLINICS ONLINE!
Access your subscription at:
www.theclinics.com

Foreword
Technological Advances in Management of Diabetes Mellitus

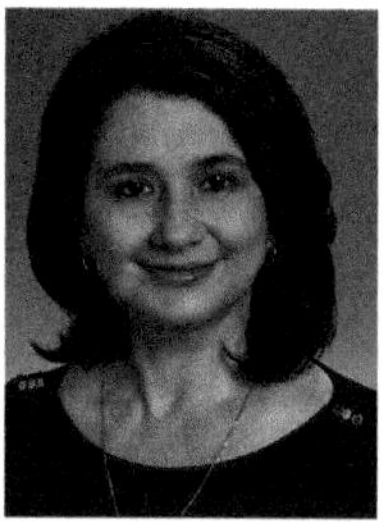

Adriana G. Ioachimescu, MD, PhD, FACE
Consulting Editor

The "Technology in Diabetes" issue of the *Endocrinology and Metabolism Clinics of North America* offers updated information on a topic that has progressed significantly in the last decade. The guest editor is Dr Grazia Aleppo, Professor of Medicine at Feinberg School of Medicine, Northwestern University, Chicago, Illinois. Dr Aleppo's primary clinical and research interests consist of applications of the insulin pump therapy and real-time continuous glucose (CGM) sensor therapy in diabetes. Dr Aleppo was involved in the Endocrine Society working panel of experts that released recommendations on optimizing postprandial glucose management in insulin-requiring diabetes mellitus patients.

A lot of progress has been made with regard to CGM systems, new insulin pumps, as well as their combination for automated insulin delivery. Endocrinologists are at the forefront of medical care for insulin-requiring diabetes patients. In recent years, several clinical trials evaluated the efficacy and safety of new generations of CGM and insulin pump systems. The current issue tackles the application of technology in several categories of patients, including type 1 and type 2 diabetes, children and older adults, as well as hospitalized and outpatient settings. This field has enjoyed the public's attention, with patients and families having become more engaged in the translation of research results to clinical care.

Our hope is that physicians in training, practicing endocrinologists, and other health care professionals who interact with patients with diabetes will greatly benefit from this collection of articles illustrating the successful intersection between medicine and bioengineering.

Endocrinol Metab Clin N Am 49 (2020) xiii–xiv
https://doi.org/10.1016/j.ecl.2019.11.004

I thank Dr Aleppo for guest-editing this important issue and the authors for their excellent contributions. I would also like to acknowledge the Elsevier editorial staff for their support.

Adriana G. Ioachimescu, MD, PhD, FACE
Emory University School of Medicine
1365 B Clifton Road
Northeast, B6209
Atlanta, GA 30322, USA

E-mail address:
aioachi@emory.edu

Preface

Technology in Diabetes: The Future Is Today

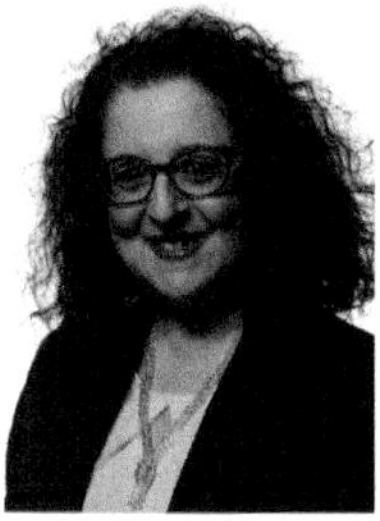

Grazia Aleppo, MD, FACE, FACP
Editor

Knowledge in the field of diabetes is expanding at a rapid rate. This is especially true for the field of diabetes technology. More accurate, easier-to-use factory-calibrated continuous glucose monitoring (CGM) systems, sophisticated insulin pumps systems, and their combination for automated insulin delivery models are developing at an increasingly faster pace. Therefore, having another issue of the *Endocrinology and Metabolism Clinics of North America* dedicated to the use of technology in diabetes is most appropriate at this time.

In previous years, issues of the *Endocrinology and Metabolism Clinics of North America* contained just 1 or 2 articles dedicated to the use of technology within the management of diabetes topics. Just a few years later, with several clinical trials studying the effects of CGM and insulin pump therapy in patients with type 1 and type 2 diabetes, from childhood to the aging adult, a wealth of data has been generated addressing multiple aspects of this therapy. Several generations of CGM and insulin pumps systems have been launched in the market in just a few years, and reports of standardization as well as glucometrics for interpretation of CGM data and outcomes have been established very recently. Clinical trials describing the benefits and challenges of diabetes technology use have been reported, many of these with results specific to various populations and age groups. Among these, there are emerging fields, such as the use of diabetes and technology in older adults since the coverage of CGM therapy by the Centers for Medicare and Medicaid Services in 2017, and the use of technology in pregnancy with diabetes, which has already shown promising results, even though not yet approved by the Food and Drug Administration at the time of this writing.

In addition, the use of technology in diabetes has created the need for additional research fields, such as the study of the psychosocial aspects of this therapy for adults as well as for children and their families. Technology in diabetes has enhanced

Endocrinol Metab Clin N Am 49 (2020) xv–xvi
https://doi.org/10.1016/j.ecl.2019.11.003
0889-8529/20/© 2019 Published by Elsevier Inc.

biomedical engineering and medicine multidisciplinary collaborations for the development of automated insulin delivery models whether with single hormone or dual hormone. It has also sparked a growing movement of publicly available algorithms for "do-it-yourself" artificial pancreas models for those who "are not waiting."

Finally, the use of insulin pump and CGM therapy has provided people with diabetes a better understanding of exercise and its effects on glucose levels as well as the opportunity to modulate insulin delivery to allow safer physical activity routines and decrease hypoglycemia risk. With all of these developments, it is no surprise that the discussion of technology in diabetes today requires a stand-alone, fully dedicated issue to explore the multiple facets of this growing field.

The enclosed comprehensive and interdisciplinary articles beautifully illustrate the various aspects of the use of technology in diabetes. I am privileged to have contributions from colleagues who are experts in their fields, with insightful, stimulating, and state-of-the-art reviews of topics that have seen the most advances in very recent years.

I have learned a lot while editing this issue and hope that the readers will have a similarly enlightening experience of this continuously changing field.

Grazia Aleppo, MD, FACE, FACP
Division of Endocrinology, Metabolism and Molecular Medicine
Feinberg School of Medicine
Northwestern University
645 North Michigan Avenue
Suite 530
Chicago, IL 60611, USA

E-mail address:
aleppo@northwestern.edu

Evolution of Diabetes Technology

Klemen Dovc, MD, PhD[a,b], Tadej Battelino, MD, PhD[a,b,*]

KEYWORDS

- Artificial pancreas • Type 1 diabetes • Continuous glucose monitoring
- Insulin pump • Technology • Closed loop • Self-monitoring of blood glucose
- Multiple daily injections

KEY POINTS

- Diabetes technology is rapidly changing traditional care; safety, efficacy, and cost-effectiveness are driving reimbursement and adoption.
- Insulin pump use is associated with improved metabolic control, less glucose variability, less hypoglycemia, and improved quality of life.
- Continuous glucose monitoring is strongly associated with improved metabolic control, more time in range, less time in hypoglycemia, reduced anxiety, and improved quality of life; insulin-dosing advisors improve decision making.
- Glucose-responsive automated insulin delivery, currently at the hybrid closed-loop stage, achieves the highest time in range, lowest hypoglycemia, and favorable quality of life.
- Achievable targets for time in range and standard visualization of the continuous glucose monitoring data will help professionals and individuals with diabetes improve long-term outcomes with less disease burden; integrated decision support systems will further improve routine diabetes care.

INTRODUCTION

Type 1 diabetes is characterized by autoimmune destruction of insulin-secreting pancreatic β cells leading to disturbed glucose regulation and overt hyperglycemia.[1] Consequently, individuals with type 1 diabetes have a lifelong dependency on insulin replacement therapy. For more than 30 years, since the results of the landmark Diabetes Control and Complications Trial (DCCT) and the Epidemiology of Diabetes Interventions and Complications (EDIC) follow-up study of the DCCT cohort, individuals

[a] Department of Paediatric Endocrinology, Diabetes and Metabolic Diseases, UMC - University Children's Hospital, University Medical Centre Ljubljana, Bohoriceva 20, Ljubljana SI–1000, Slovenia; [b] Faculty of Medicine, University of Ljubljana, Ljubljana, Slovenia
* Corresponding author. Department of Paediatric Endocrinology, Diabetes and Metabolic Diseases, UMC - University Children's Hospital, University Medical Centre Ljubljana, Bohoriceva 20, Ljubljana SI–1000, Slovenia.
E-mail address: tadej.battelino@mf.uni-lj.si

Endocrinol Metab Clin N Am 49 (2020) 1–18
https://doi.org/10.1016/j.ecl.2019.10.009 endo.theclinics.com
0889-8529/20/

with type 1 diabetes have been treated intensively, mimicking physiologic insulin secretion to achieve glucose levels as close to normal as possible and as early as possible in the course of the disease to prevent or delay the late microvascular and macrovascular disease complications.[1–8] Current guidelines for adult and pediatric type 1 diabetes populations suggest that hemoglobin A1c (HbA1c) level, identified decades ago as the primary marker of long-term average glucose control and the gold standard assay that reflects average glycaemia, should be less than 53 mmol/mol (7%).[9,10] However, the attainment of precise glucose control is complicated by the individual variability in insulin requirements, even more pronounced in young children, and may be difficult to overcome with established treatment options.[11] In addition to this, fear of hypoglycemia is an important hurdle for treatment optimization, especially in pediatric populations, being also a major source of stress and anxiety for families and caregivers, affecting the quality of life (QOL) and psychological well-being of the youth and their families.[12–14] At present, only a minority of individuals with type 1 diabetes, especially among adolescents and young adults, meet recommended glycemic targets.[15,16]

The continuing emergence of innovations and novel treatment modalities has reshaped the management of diabetes and offered the potential to optimize glycemic control, improve QOL, and reduce the burden of type 1 diabetes. Although most participants in clinical studies regarding diabetes technology are individuals with type 1 diabetes and this is also the focus of this article, there are numerous reports also including individuals with type 2 diabetes.[17–21] This article summarizes the evolution of technology intended for diabetes care up to currently available and almost available products, focusing on insulin delivery, glucose monitoring, glucose-responsive automated insulin delivery, and data management and interpretation tools.

INSULIN DELIVERY

Progress in the pharmacokinetics and pharmacodynamics of insulin analogues and the technology for insulin delivery diversified insulin replacement designs to resemble the secretion of the endogenous insulin as closely as possible.

Insulin Pens

Insulin pens contain insulin in a cartridge that is administered into subcutaneous tissue through a fine, replaceable needle. Introduced in 1981 as convenient, easy-to-use injection devices, pens are widely used as a part of multiple daily injection (MDI) therapy to deliver insulin and are continuously developing. Insulin pens, allowing push-button injections, come as disposable pens with prefilled cartridges or reusable insulin pens with replaceable insulin cartridges. In 2017, the first smart pen with built-in Bluetooth connectivity received regulatory approval in the United States (InPen, Companion Medical, California, USA). Smart pens can record the amount and timing of each insulin dose, display the last dose and insulin onboard, and wirelessly transmit the information via Bluetooth to a dedicated mobile app. This associated smartphone application also makes dosing recommendations and transfers data automatically on the cloud for sharing with health care professionals.[22] Similarly, NovoPen 6 and NovoPen Echo Plus reusable insulin pens equipped with near-field communication technology (Novo Nordisk, Gentofte, Denmark) were approved in the European Union. In addition, Insulclock (Insulcloud, Madrid, Spain) is a device capable of tracking dosing, timing, and missing insulin injections from 7 different conventional insulin pens.[23] Globally, administering insulin with a syringe or pen remains the treatment modality used by most individuals with diabetes.

Continuous Subcutaneous Insulin Infusion

The administration of insulin with an insulin pump (continuous subcutaneous insulin infusion [CSII]) was introduced almost 40 years ago[24] but it took another 20 years for CSII therapy to become broadly available. The CSII infuses a short-acting, rapid-acting, or ultrarapid-acting insulin analogue to subcutaneous tissue via self-inserted Teflon or steel catheters at slow and variable basal rates to match the individual's needs, and additional bolus doses to cover meals and correct hyperglycemia.[25,26] The pump is a battery-powered programmable device that holds multiple settings that can be tailored to each individual specifically. Health care providers and users can program multiple insulin delivery settings based on the time of day, and in multiple profiles for different circumstances (eg, activity, sick days). Within a user profile, there are variable basal rates for day and night, and typically preprogrammed carbohydrate/insulin ratios, insulin sensitivity factors, and target glucose ranges (bolus calculators) to facilitate the calculation of prandial and correction boluses. Advanced bolus profiles can include immediate and/or extended delivery of a calculated bolus dose to meet postprandial insulin requirements, and temporary basal rates to adapt to physical activity that usually requires less insulin,[27–29] or stress or illness that results in acutely increased insulin needs.[30] In addition, settings may include insulin action time to allow the pump to calculate current insulin activity when giving additional boluses. CSII is considered a safe and effective treatment option for all age groups,[31] and, with the increasing reimbursement, its use is steadily increasing.[32–34] Recent data from a large registry including almost 100,000 individuals with type 1 diabetes reported an increase from 1% to 53% in a 20-year observational period.[35] A similar increase was reported in other large registries, but mostly from affluent societies.[15,32,36,37]

In the decades of CSII use, it was proved that its use is associated with better glycemic control and lower rates of severe hypoglycemia and diabetic ketoacidosis.[38–40] In addition, a recent study showed reduced cardiovascular mortality.[41] This form of therapy has become the insulin treatment modality of choice in many countries, particularly for the pediatric population.[42–44]

GLUCOSE MONITORING

Regular glucose monitoring allows individuals with diabetes to guide their insulin therapy and assess whether their glycemic targets are being safely achieved. Historically, glucose concentration was assessed from the urine using copper (Benedict) reagent and later glucose oxidase–based reagent strip, detecting only glucose levels when the renal threshold for glucose was reached. Nowadays, glucose concentration is measured from capillary blood using a portable handheld glucose meter or from the interstitial fluid using a continuous glucose monitoring (CGM) device.

Self-Monitoring of Blood Glucose

Frequent self-monitoring of blood glucose (SMBG) from capillary blood has considerably improved metabolic control and is considered a fundamental component of effective treatment and daily management of individuals on insulin therapy. The development of smaller and easier-to-use blood glucometers for use at home in the 1980s, and the introduction of electrochemical principle to measure glucose level, substantially changed the approach to the treatment of type 1 diabetes by giving users the ability to self-control and individually intensify insulin treatment. Similar to bolus calculators in CSII, modern smart glucometers can have incorporated bolus advisors to calculate insulin dosages, algorithm-driven message response to each glucose reading, and can transfer data wirelessly to a health care professional or parent/caregiver.[45,46]

Glucometers for personal use must meet regulated minimum requirements for accuracy for the SMBG to be safe and clinically meaningful, and a recent study showed that many cleared devices do not meet the level of accuracy currently required for regulatory clearance.[47]

SMBG has important drawbacks because blood is sampled intermittently, providing only glimpses of glucose concentrations, and it fails to expose ongoing glucose fluctuations even if performed frequently. Episodes of hyperglycemia and hypoglycemia might, therefore, be missed and not factored into treatment decisions.

Continuous Glucose Monitoring

CGM started humbly in 1999, with the first randomized controlled trial (RCT) published in 2006,[48] and subsequently made it all the way to the replacement of SMBG based on a considerable body of evidence. CGM systems currently consist of a disposable sensor that measures glucose concentration in the interstitial fluid (usually at intervals of 1–5 min) and a transmitter that sends or/and stores the sensor values (usually at intervals of 5–15 min) to a dedicated receiver and/or other mobile devices (eg, smartphone, smart-watch, the cloud, shared with family members); intermittently scanned CGM (isCGM) is a variety displaying glucose concentration only on demand,[49,50] but with open alarms it is coming closer to standard CGM systems. The only currently approved implantable CGM system has a sensor that is fully implanted under the skin by a health care provider and functions for 90 to 180 days, with data visualization through an on-body device.[51] The CGM sensor values usually narrowly correlate with blood glucose concentration when it is stable, with a mean time lag of less than 5 minutes; however, during episodes of rapid glucose changes such as after a simple-carbohydrate meal or exercise, the time lag can exceed 10 minutes.[52] The first major CGM RCT was funded by the Juvenile Diabetes Research Foundation (JDRF; www.jdrf.org) and showed the efficacy of CGM in reducing HbA1c levels and hypoglycemia in adults,[53] and in per-protocol analysis also in children and adolescents using CGM for at least 6 d/wk.[54] Additional RCTs using comparable CGM versions with HbA1c or time in hypoglycemia changes as primary outcomes confirmed efficacy and safety.[55–58] These initial results boosted the advancements of sensor technology, which become more user friendly, more accurate, and more readily available. Although CGM sensors are still not as accurate as the most accurate blood glucose meters, modern CGM systems currently exceed the accuracy of many US Food and Drug Administration (FDA)–cleared blood glucose meters.[47]

Recent RCTs using contemporary sensor technology again confirmed the efficacy of CGM (both reducing HbA1c level and hypoglycemia) in individuals with type 1 diabetes treated with MDIs[42,43]; in addition, user satisfaction and consequently mean sensor usage was significantly higher, including significant improvement of QOL measures.[59] Importantly, several QOL measures were also significantly improved in the pediatric population.[60] In addition, several recent RCTs focused on individuals with severe hypoglycemia and/or hypoglycemia unawareness using different treatment modalities, showing a significant reduction in both total and severe hypoglycemia.[61–64] Large international registry studies essentially confirmed results from RCTs: in a European registry, the CGM use was associated with better mean glucose levels and less hypoglycemia,[65] in the T1D Exchange Registry, CGM or CSII usage was associated with lower HbA1c levels,[15] and similarly in the DPV Registry CSII usage was associated with lower HbA1c levels and hypoglycemia rate.[35]

The use of CGM was particularly successful during pregnancy complicated by type 1 diabetes: the CONCEPTT (Continuous Glucose Monitoring in Women with Type 1 Diabetes in Pregnancy Trial) RCT showed that CGM use was associated with a reduction in hyperglycemia, increase in pregnancy-specific time in range (TIR), and improved neonatal outcomes compared with a control group using SMBG.[66] Importantly, these positive outcomes were associated with a projected yearly reduction in cost worth several million US dollars.[67]

The use of CGM is increasing exponentially in all age groups. Most recent data from the T1D Exchange Registry reported that about 30% of participants had been using CGM in the period from 2016 to 2018.[15] The most recent DPV Registry reported CGM use in most children with type 1 diabetes aged less than 10 years, and overall usage in 38% of individuals with type 1 diabetes.[35] This increase is likely related to the approval of isCGM and CGM systems for nonadjunctive use (no SMBG confirmation for insulin-dosing decisions is needed for a CGM, an isCGM, and an implantable CGM), as well as to the coverage of both CGM systems by the US Centers for Medicare and Medicaid Services (CMS) for all individuals with type 1 and type 2 diabetes on intensive insulin treatment, as well as by many European national medical insurance systems (eg, Sweden, Belgium, Germany), some with demonstrated cost reduction.[68]

Further enhancement of CGM technology has involved calibration of sensors: CGM and an isCGM devices are now factory calibrated and do not require SMBG measurements for calibration; however, all other CGM devices still require 2 calibrations per day (**Table 1**).

The use of CGM and isCGM devices by people with type 1 diabetes has been endorsed by the American Diabetes Association (ADA) in its 2019 Standards of Medical Care in Diabetes,[43] the American Association of Clinical Endocrinologists (AACE),[69,70] the International Society for Pediatric and Adolescent Diabetes (ISPAD),[44] and the Endocrine Society.[42] However, the most important endorsement will be the adoption by individuals with diabetes: in order to make CGM and isCGM data meaningful for day-to-day diabetes management, clear guidance on CGM-derived glycemic targets should be provided. Consensus groups have agreed on a core set of 10 CGM metrics for reports.[71] Studies have shown that 10 to 14 days of data from a CGM device generally provide a good approximation of 3 months of glucose data,[72] as well as calculating an estimated HbA1c level, termed glucose management indicator .[73] Recently, the ADA, AACE, American Association of Diabetes Educators (AADE), European Association for the Study of Diabetes (EASD), Foundation of European Nurses in Diabetes, ISPAD, JDRF, and Pediatric Endocrine Society (PES) formally endorsed an international consensus report on clinical targets for CGM data[74]; importantly, the consensus participants also included individuals with diabetes outside the medical profession. The consensus proposed easy-to-understand TIR targets, along with time below range (TBR) and time above range (TAR) targets for routine management of type 1 and type 2 diabetes, as presented in **Table 2**.

The consensus participants solicited the input of professional societies for diabetes in pregnancy and agreed on targets for type 1 diabetes complicated by pregnancy, as presented in **Table 3**.

The reporting, presentation, and visualization of CGM data now greatly facilitate the communication between health care professionals and individuals with diabetes, particularly when a standardized report, such as the ambulatory glucose profile ,[75] shows the core CGM metrics, including proportions of glucose values in different ranges over a specified time period, the recommended target for each CGM data

Table 1
Main characteristics of available continuous glucose monitoring devices

Device	Manufacturer	Type of Monitoring	Insertion	Sensor Lifetime (Days)	MARD (%)	Sensor Calibration	Nonadjunctive Use	Alarms, Trends, Alerts	Data Sharing
G6	Dexcom	CGM	Sensor inserter	10	10	Factory	Yes	Yes	Yes
Guardian Sensor 3	Medtronic	CGM	Sensor inserter	7	10.6, 9.1[b]	Every 12 h	No	Yes	Indirectly
Eversense	Senseonics	CGM	Implantation[a]	90 (United States); 180 (EU)	11.4	Every 12 h	Yes (United States); No (EU)	Yes	Indirectly
FreeStyle Libre/Libre 2	Abbott	isCGM	Sensor inserter	14 d	11.4/NA	Factory	Yes	No	No/yes

Abbreviations: EU, European Union; isCGM, intermittently scanned continuous glucose monitoring; MARD, mean absolute relative difference; NA, not applicable.
[a] Surgically implanted subcutaneously in clinic, with an on-body external transmitter.
[b] MARD for abdomen, arm.

Table 2
Targets for assessment of glycemic control: type 1/type 2 and older/high-risk individuals

	TIR		TBR		TAR	
Diabetes	**% of Readings Time/d**	**Target Range**	**% of Readings Time/d**	**Below Target Level**	**% of Readings Time/d**	**Above Target Level**
Type 1[a]/ type 2	>70	70–180 mg/dL	<4	<70 mg/dL	<25	>180 mg/dL
			<1 h	<3.9 mmol/L	<6 h	>10.0 mmol/L
	>16 h, 48 min	3.9–10.0 mmol/L	<1	<54 mg/dL	<5	>250 mg/dL
			<15 min	<3.0 mmol/L	<1 h, 12 min	>13.9 mmol/L
Older/high risk[b]	>50	70–180 mg/dL	<1	<70 mg/dL	<10	>250 mg/dL
Type 1/ type 2	>12 h	3.9–10 mmol/L	<15 min	<3.9 mmol/L	<2 h, 24 min	>13.9 mmol/L

Each incremental 5% increase in TIR is associated with clinically significant benefits for type 1/ type 2.

[a] For age less than 25 years, if the HbA1c goal is 7.5%, then set TIR target to approximately 60%, and aim at incremental improvements toward the target.

[b] Older and/or high-risk individuals with diabetes: targets should be agreed on in individual context.

Adapted from Battelino T, Danne T, Bergenstal RM, et al. Clinical targets for continuous glucose monitoring data interpretation: recommendations from the international consensus on time in range. Diabetes Care. 2019; 42(8):1593-1603; with permission.

range, and a pictorial demonstration of the CGM values distribution according to the time of day.

This international consensus on TIR targets is being implemented by numerous national diabetes associations and received a welcoming note by many groups of people with diabetes. Presentation and communication CGM data will continue to improve and will be complemented with decision support systems and artificial intelligence, which will integrate behavioral data, identify concerns, and propose solutions for better diabetes management plans.

Table 3
Targets for assessment of glycemic control: pregnancy

	TIR		TBR		TAR	
Diabetes Group	**% of Readings Time/d**	**Target Range**	**% of Readings Time/d**	**Below Target Level**	**% of Readings Time/d**	**Above Target Level**
Pregnancy type 1	>70	63–140 mg/dL[a]	<4	<63 mg/dL[a]	<25	>140 mg/dL
	>16 h, 48 min	3.5–7.8 mmol/L[a]	<1 h	<3.5 mmol/L[a]	<6 h	>7.8 mmol/L
			<1	<54 mg/dL		
			<15 min	<3.0 mmol/L		

Each incremental 5% increase in TIR is associated with clinically significant benefits for pregnancy type 1.

[a] Glucose levels are physiologically lower during pregnancy.

Adapted from Battelino T, Danne T, Bergenstal RM, et al. Clinical targets for continuous glucose monitoring data interpretation: recommendations from the international consensus on time in range. *Diabetes Care*. 2019; 42(8):1593-1603; with permission.

AUTOMATED GLUCOSE-RESPONSIVE INSULIN DELIVERY

The first model of glucose-responsive automated insulin therapy or closed loop was initially introduced around 50 years ago, followed by the first commercial closed-loop system produced in the late 1970s (Biostator, Miles Laboratories, Elkhart, IN, USA).[76–78] However, its broader usage was limited because of algorithm simplicity, the size of the device, the need for intravenous access, and greater wastage of blood. The idea of closed loop was revitalized around 15 years ago when several pediatric and adult diabetologists gathered to formally restart the closed-loop initiative.[79] The JDRF Artificial Pancreas Project (APP) initiative was launched in 2006, with the aim to accelerate progress toward closed-loop systems (the Artificial Pancreas Consortium) with a 6-step modernized roadmap toward closing the loop: (1) low-glucose suspend; (2) predictive low-glucose suspend; (3) hypoglycemia/hyperglycemia minimizer; (4) automated basal/hybrid closed loop; (5) fully automated insulin closed loop; and (6) fully automated multihormone closed loop.[80,81]

Low-Glucose Suspend

Automated glucose-responsive interruption of insulin delivery when preset glucose level is reached to reduce hypoglycemia exposure represents an early example of technology-enabled glucose-responsive regulation of insulin therapy. The first CSII with low-glucose suspend (LGS) feature, Medtronic Paradigm Veo (Medtronic Diabetes, Northridge, CA), was released in 2009. In the United States, this device was marketed as the MiniMed 530G system and was eventually substituted by the updated model MiniMed 630G. The device was able to automatically suspend insulin delivery for up to 2 hours when sensor glucose level reached a preset glucose limit. Several multicenter randomized controlled studies and observational studies including children, adolescents, and adults in unrestricted free-living settings have shown that LGS is safe and effective in decreasing both the frequency and duration of hypoglycemic events,[82,83] even in individuals with hypoglycemia unawareness.[84]

Predictive Low-Glucose Insulin Suspend

In an attempt to prevent hypoglycemic excursions and possibly provide protection to users, predictive low-glucose suspend (PLGS) pumps were developed. CSII devices using PLGS technology cease insulin delivery when the sensor glucose value is predicted within 30 minutes to reach or decrease to less than a preset low glucose limit and automatically restores basal insulin delivery after recovery from hypoglycemia. This feature was introduced in Europe and Australia in 2015 with the MiniMed 640G (Medtronic Diabetes, Northridge, CA). Another commercially available device with PLGS technology is Tandem t:slim X2 Insulin Pump with Basal IQ Technology (Tandem Diabetes care, San Diego, CA) using Dexcom G6 CGM (Dexcom, San Diego, CA). In RCTs including adults, children, and adolescents, the use of predictive low-glucose suspend technology reduces the exposure to nocturnal and overall hypoglycemia, including reduced frequency and length of nocturnal hypoglycemic episodes.[85–89] Moreover, predictive low-glucose suspend reduced the overall risk of moderate and severe hypoglycemia in individuals with the highest risk of hypoglycemia, such as recent severe hypoglycemia event or hypoglycemia unawareness.[64] However, these benefits were achieved at the expense of mildly increased glucose levels or increased time in moderate hyperglycemia without an increased risk for severe rebound hyperglycemia or diabetic ketoacidosis after the PLGS.

Automated Insulin Delivery

Automated insulin delivery or closed loop (artificial pancreas) is characterized by glucose-responsive automated insulin delivery and combines glucose monitoring with computer/tablet/telephone-based algorithm–informed insulin delivery. The core of such systems is a control algorithm that translates, in real time, the data it receives from the CGM and computes the amounts of insulin to be delivered by the CSII. The other components include real-time CGM and an insulin pump to titrate and deliver insulin. Several prototypes of control algorithms have been developed and tested around the world, including model predictive control, proportional-integral-derivative controller, and fuzzy logic–based controller.[90] The first 2 approaches are more commonly used in clinical studies and the development of a closed-loop system to control insulin delivery. They use mathematical models that link insulin delivery with glucose excursions. The third approach to algorithms uses fuzzy logic algorithms (such as the MD-Logic) to modulate insulin delivery based on a set of rules that imitates the line of reasoning of diabetes practitioners.[91,92]

Two recent meta-analyses have summarized most of the clinical trials conducted in an outpatient setting showing that AID use is safe and effective in increasing time spent in target range. Wiesman and colleagues[93] reported an increase of 12.6% (3 h/d) based on 27 comparisons from 24 studies including 585 participants, and Bekiari and colleagues[94] reported an increase of 9.6% (2.3 h/d) based on 44 comparisons from 40 studies including 1027 participants. There are several other reports showing the efficacy of AID during and after physical activity,[95–98] and for missed meals.[99,100]

At present, 1 closed-loop system, the Medtronic MiniMed 670G, is in commercial use in the United States and Europe,[101] whereas there are several other systems (t:slim X2 insulin pump with Control-IQ Technology,[102] Diabeloop,[103] FlorenceM [or X] of the University of Cambridge,[104] Omnipod Horizon[105]) that it is hoped will enter the market soon.

Most systems adopt the hybrid closed-loop approach characterized by manual (user-initiated) administration of prandial boluses to mitigate absorption delay of subcutaneously administered rapid-acting insulin. Previous reports have shown that preprandial insulin bolus might be of benefit to prevent postprandial glycemic excursion,[106–109] even when using an ultrarapid insulin formulation.[110]

In contrast with AID, automated multihormone closed-loop systems deliver subcutaneous additional hormone (eg, glucagon) in conjunction with insulin when there is a threatening or predicted hypoglycemic event in the near future. The multihormone approach may mitigate the risk of hypoglycemia or may be used to increase the aggressiveness of insulin therapy to minimize hyperglycemia without an increased risk for hypoglycemia.[111]

In the past 10 years, there have been several studies with this approach, including a head-to-head comparison with a single-hormone system, showing the safety and efficacy of the dual-hormone approach, and there are ongoing trials with this model.[112–115] An analogue of the hormone amylin (pramlintide), which slows gastric emptying and reduces glucagon secretion, is also being studied in automated insulin delivery systems in an effort to reduce postprandial hyperglycemia.[116]

In addition, there is a do-it-yourself approach by a thriving community of users who have rallied behind a patient-driven ecosystem. In such systems, continuous glucose monitors and insulin pumps are reverse engineered and the data shared via open-source platforms in order to help others with diabetes better use their devices, allowing projects to display data in innovative ways and/or to control automated insulin delivery (do-it-yourself artificial pancreas systems). In conjunction with regulators and legal advisors, JDRF is providing funding and regulatory support with an initiative encouraging manufacturers to give device users greater control by opening their communication protocols to enable uniform, secure connectivity with other devices. Meanwhile, this treatment modality is already used by several users all around the world, showing excellent glycemic control.[117]

Automated Decision Support Systems

With the exponential increase of data generated by novel diabetes technologies, automated decision support systems (DSSs) will play a dominant role in diabetes management. A recent review summarized different DSSs based on closed-loop algorithms.[118] The algorithm of the first FDA-cleared DSS Advisor Pro (DreaMed Diabetes, Petah Tikva, Israel) showed decision results statistically not different from those obtained by endocrinologist from 17 different centers from around the world.[119] Multiple clinical trials with DSSs are ongoing. DSSs will be of particular importance when diabetes technology enters into primary care, where so-called digital diabetes clinics will become inevitable.[120]

SUMMARY

In view of the current accelerating pace of diabetes technology development, ever smaller and more accurate CGM sensors, novel implantable sensors for long-term use (>1 year) with no on-body components, and CGM devices with increased connectivity and improved data visualization both on the device and remotely through the cloud can be anticipated. Automated systems for insulin delivery will become more independent and will likely incorporate other physiologic and behavioral data for providing more accurate predictions, particularly related to food and physical activity. With the increasing technical complexity, DSSs will become an inevitable part of digital diabetes clinics, including their use at the primary care level. In addition, all will depend on the cost-effectiveness that will drive the access and reimbursement of different technologies, and ultimately on the acceptance of any particular technology by individuals with diabetes. TIR is being validated as a new clinical marker,[121] and simple clinical guidance on TIR targets and data visualization[74] were broadly endorsed by professionals, and are being introduced to individuals with diabetes. However, the ultimate goal of diabetes technology development remains clear: improved diabetes outcomes with reduced disease burden and increased QOL for all individuals with diabetes and their families.

DISCLOSURE

T. Battelino served on advisory boards of Novo Nordisk, Sanofi, Eli Lilly, Boehringer, Medtronic, and Bayer HealthCare. T. Battelino's institution received research grant support, with receipt of travel and accommodation expenses in some cases, from Abbott, Medtronic, Novo Nordisk, GluSense, Sanofi, Sandoz, and Diamyd. K. Dovc declares that there is no duality of interest associated with his contribution to this article.

REFERENCES

1. Atkinson MA, Eisenbarth GS, Michels AW. Type 1 diabetes. Lancet 2014; 383(9911):69–82.

2. The DCCT Research Group. Effect of intensive diabetes treatment on the development and progression of long-term complications in adolescents with insulin-dependent diabetes mellitus: diabetes control and complications trial. J Pediatr 1994;125(2):177–88.
3. Lind M, Svensson A-M, Kosiborod M, et al. Glycemic control and excess mortality in type 1 diabetes. N Engl J Med 2014;371(21):1972–82.
4. Schade DS, Lorenzi GM, Braffett BH, et al. Hearing impairment and type 1 diabetes in the diabetes Control and complications trial/epidemiology of diabetes interventions and complications (DCCT/EDIC) cohort. Diabetes Care 2018; 41(12):2495–501.
5. Yau JWY, Rogers SL, Kawasaki R, et al. Global prevalence and major risk factors of diabetic retinopathy. Diabetes Care 2012;35(3):556–64.
6. Gibrin PCD, Melo JJ, Marchiori LL de M. Prevalence of tinnitus complaints and probable association with hearing loss, diabetes mellitus and hypertension in elderly. Codas 2013;25(2):176–80.
7. Albernaz PLM. Hearing loss, dizziness, and carbohydrate metabolism. Int Arch Otorhinolaryngol 2016;20(3):261–70.
8. Kamali B, Hajiabolhassan F, Fatahi J, et al. Effects of diabetes mellitus type ı with or without neuropathy on vestibular evoked myogenic potentials. Acta Med Iran 2013;51(2):107–12.
9. Care D, Suppl SS. 6. Glycemic targets: standards of medical care in diabetes—2019. Diabetes Care 2019;42(Supplement 1):S61–70.
10. Dimeglio LA, Acerini CL, Codner E, et al. Glycemic control targets and glucose monitoring for children, adolescents, and young adults with diabetes 2018 IS-PAD Clinical Practice Consensus Guidelines. Pediatr Diabetes 2018;(19 Suppl 27):105–14.
11. Dovc K, Boughton C, Tauschmann M, et al. Young children have higher variability of insulin requirements: observations during hybrid closed-loop insulin delivery. Diabetes Care 2019;42(7):1344–7.
12. Jabbour G, Henderson M, Mathieu ME. Barriers to active lifestyles in children with type 1 diabetes. Can J Diabetes 2016;40(2):170–2.
13. Van Name MA, Hilliard ME, Boyle CT, et al. Nighttime is the worst time: parental fear of hypoglycemia in young children with type 1 diabetes. Pediatr Diabetes 2018;19(1):114–20.
14. Frier BM. Hypoglycaemia in diabetes mellitus: epidemiology and clinical implications. Nat Rev Endocrinol 2014;10(12):711–22.
15. Foster NC, Beck RW, Miller KM, et al. State of type 1 diabetes management and outcomes from the T1D exchange in 2016-2018. Diabetes Technol Ther 2019; 21(2):66–72.
16. Pettus JH, Zhou FL, Shepherd L, et al. Incidences of severe hypoglycemia and diabetic ketoacidosis and prevalence of microvascular complications stratified by age and glycemic control in U.S. Adult patients with type 1 diabetes: a real-world study. Diabetes Care 2019;42(12):2220–7.
17. Beck RW, Riddlesworth TD, Ruedy K, et al. Continuous glucose monitoring versus usual care in patients with type 2 diabetes receiving multiple daily insulin injections. Ann Intern Med 2017;167(6):365–74.
18. Bally L, Gubler P, Thabit H, et al. Fully closed-loop insulin delivery improves glucose control of inpatients with type 2 diabetes receiving hemodialysis. Kidney Int 2019;96(3):593–6.
19. Dicembrini I, Mannucci E, Monami M, et al. Impact of technology on glycaemic control in type 2 diabetes: a meta-analysis of randomized trials on continuous

glucose monitoring and continuous subcutaneous insulin infusion. Diabetes Obes Metab 2019. https://doi.org/10.1111/dom.13845.
20. Thabit H, Hartnell S, Allen JM, et al. Closed-loop insulin delivery in inpatients with type 2 diabetes: a randomised, parallel-group trial. Lancet Diabetes Endocrinol 2017;5(2):117–24.
21. Bally L, Thabit H, Hartnell S, et al. Closed-loop insulin delivery for glycemic control in noncritical care. N Engl J Med 2018;379(6):547–56.
22. Klonoff DC, Aimbe F, Kerr D. Smart pens will improve insulin therapy. J Diabetes Sci Technol 2018;12(3):551–3.
23. Gomez-Peralta F, Abreu C, Gomez-Rodriguez S, et al. A novel insulin delivery optimization and tracking system. Diabetes Technol Ther 2019;21(4):209–14.
24. Pickup JC, Keen H, Parsons JA, et al. Continuous subcutaneous insulin infusion: an approach to achieving normoglycaemia. Br Med J 1978;1(6107):204–7.
25. Evans M, Ceriello A, Danne T, et al. Use of fast-acting insulin aspart in insulin pump therapy in clinical practice. Diabetes Obes Metab 2019;21(9):1–9.
26. Bode BW, Johnson JA, Hyveled L, et al. Improved postprandial glycemic control with faster-acting insulin aspart in patients with type 1 diabetes using continuous subcutaneous insulin infusion. Diabetes Technol Ther 2017;19(1):25–33.
27. Zaharieva DP, Mcgaugh S, Pooni R, et al. Improved open-loop glucose control with basal insulin reduction 90 minutes before aerobic exercise in patients with type 1 diabetes on continuous subcutaneous insulin infusion. Diabetes Care 2019;1–8. https://doi.org/10.2337/dc18-2204/-/DC1.
28. Adolfsson P, Riddell MC, Taplin CE, et al. ISPAD clinical practice consensus guidelines 2018: exercise in children and adolescents with diabetes. Pediatr Diabetes 2018;19(July):205–26.
29. Riddell MC, Gallen IW, Smart CE, et al. Exercise management in type 1 diabetes: a consensus statement. Lancet Diabetes Endocrinol 2017;5(5):377–90.
30. Laffel LM, Limbert C, Phelan H, et al. ISPAD clinical practice consensus guidelines 2018: Sick day management in children and adolescents with diabetes. Pediatr Diabetes 2018;19(July):193–204.
31. Phillip M, Battelino T, Rodriguez H, et al. Use of insulin pump therapy in the pediatric age-group: consensus statement from the European Society for Paediatric Endocrinology, the Lawson Wilkins Pediatric Endocrine Society, and the International Society for Pediatric and Adolescent Diabetes, endorsed by the American Diabetes Association and the European Association for the Study of Diabetes. Diabetes Care 2007;30(6):1653–62.
32. Dovc K, Telic SS, Lusa L, et al. Improved metabolic control in pediatric patients with type 1 diabetes: a nationwide prospective 12-year time trends analysis. Diabetes Technol Ther 2014;16(1):33–40.
33. Pozzilli P, Battelino T, Danne T, et al. Continuous subcutaneous insulin infusion in diabetes: Patient populations, safety, efficacy, and pharmacoeconomics. Diabetes Metab Res Rev 2016;32(1):21–39.
34. Blackman SM, Raghinaru D, Adi S, et al. Insulin pump use in young children in the T1D Exchange clinic registry is associated with lower hemoglobin A1c levels than injection therapy. Pediatr Diabetes 2014;15(8):564–72.
35. van den Boom L, Karges B, Lilienthal E, et al. Temporal trends and contemporary use of insulin pump therapy and glucose monitoring among children, adolescents , and adults with type 1 diabetes between 1995 and 2017. Diabetes Care 2019;1–7. https://doi.org/10.2337/dc19-0345/-/DC1.L.v.d.B.

36. Szypowska A, Schwandt A, Svensson J, et al. Insulin pump therapy in children with type 1 diabetes: analysis of data from the SWEET registry. Pediatr Diabetes 2016;17:38–45.
37. Eeg-Olofsson K, Cederholm J, Nilsson PM, et al. Glycemic and risk factor control in type 1 diabetes: Results from 13,612 patients in a national diabetes register. Diabetes Care 2007;30(3):496–502.
38. Misso ML, Egberts KJ, Page M, et al. Continuous subcutaneous insulin infusion (CSII) versus multiple insulin injections for type 1 diabetes mellitus. In: Misso ML, editor. Cochrane database of systematic reviews. Chichester (United Kingdom): John Wiley & Sons, Ltd; 2010. p. CD005103. https://doi.org/10.1002/14651858.CD005103.pub2.
39. Karges B, Schwandt A, Heidtmann B, et al. Association of insulin pump therapy vs insulin injection therapy with severe hypoglycemia, ketoacidosis, and glycemic control among children, adolescents, and young adults with type 1 diabetes. JAMA 2017;318(14):1358–66.
40. Sherr JL, Hermann JM, Campbell F, et al. Use of insulin pump therapy in children and adolescents with type 1 diabetes and its impact on metabolic control: comparison of results from three large, transatlantic paediatric registries. Diabetologia 2016;59(1):87–91.
41. Steineck I, Cederholm J, Eliasson B, et al. Insulin pump therapy, multiple daily injections, and cardiovascular mortality in 18 168 people with type 1 diabetes: observational study. BMJ 2015;350(jun22 1):h3234.
42. Peters AL, Ahmann AJ, Battelino T, et al. Diabetes technology—continuous subcutaneous insulin infusion therapy and continuous glucose monitoring in adults: an Endocrine Society Clinical Practice Guideline. J Clin Endocrinol Metab 2016; 101(11):3922–37.
43. American Diabetes Association. 7. Diabetes technology: standards of medical care in diabetes-2019. Diabetes Care 2019;42(January):S71–80.
44. Sherr JL, Tauschman M, Battelino T, et al. ISPAD clinical practice consensus guidelines 2018 diabetes technologies. Pediatr Diabetes 2018. https://doi.org/10.1111/pedi.12731.
45. Bollyky JB, Bravata D, Yang J, et al. Remote lifestyle coaching plus a connected glucose meter with certified diabetes educator support improves glucose and weight loss for people with type 2 diabetes. J Diabetes Res 2018;2018:3961730.
46. Christiansen M, Greene C, Pardo S, et al. A new, wireless-enabled blood glucose monitoring system that links to a smart mobile device: accuracy and user performance evaluation. J Diabetes Sci Technol 2017;11(3):567–73.
47. Klonoff DC, Parkes JL, Kovatchev BP, et al. Investigation of the accuracy of 18 marketed blood glucose monitors. Diabetes Care 2018;41(8):1681–8.
48. Deiss D, Bolinder J, Riveline JP, et al. Improved glycemic control in poorly controlled patients with type 1 diabetes using real-time continuous glucose monitoring. Diabetes Care 2006;29(12):2730–2.
49. Langendam M, Luijf YM, Hooft L, et al. Continuous glucose monitoring systems for type 1 diabetes mellitus. In: Langendam M, editor. Cochrane database of systematic reviews, Vol 1. Chichester (United Kingdom): John Wiley & Sons, Ltd; 2012. p. CD008101. https://doi.org/10.1002/14651858.CD008101.pub2.
50. Piona C, Dovc K, Mutlu GY, et al. Non-adjunctive flash glucose monitoring system use during summer-camp in children with type 1 diabetes: the free-summer study. Pediatr Diabetes 2018;19(7):1285–93.
51. Deiss D, Irace C, Carlson G, et al. Real-world safety of an implantable continuous glucose sensor over multiple cycles of use: a post-market registry

study. Diabetes Technol Ther 2019. https://doi.org/10.1089/dia.2019.0159. dia.2019.0159.

52. Zaharieva DP, Turksoy K, McGaugh SM, et al. Lag time remains with newer real-time continuous glucose monitoring technology during aerobic exercise in adults living with type 1 diabetes. Diabetes Technol Ther 2019;21(6):313–21.
53. The Juvenile Diabetes Research Foundation Continuous Glucose Monitoring Study Group*. Continuous glucose monitoring and intensive treatment of type 1 diabetes. N Engl J Med 2008;359(14):1464–76.
54. Beck RW, Buckingham B, Miller K, et al. Factors predictive of use and of benefit from continuous glucose monitoring in type 1 diabetes. Diabetes Care 2009; 32(11):1947–53.
55. DeSalvo DJ, Miller KM, Hermann JM, et al. Continuous glucose monitoring and glycemic control among youth with type 1 diabetes: International comparison from the T1D Exchange and DPV Initiative. Pediatr Diabetes 2018;19(7):1271–5.
56. Dovc K, Cargnelutti K, Sturm A, et al. Continuous glucose monitoring use and glucose variability in pre-school children with type 1 diabetes. Diabetes Res Clin Pract 2018. https://doi.org/10.1016/j.diabres.2018.10.005.
57. Bergenstal RM. Continuous glucose monitoring: transforming diabetes management step by step. Lancet 2018;391(10128):1334–6.
58. Kropff J, Choudhary P, Neupane S, et al. Accuracy and longevity of an implantable continuous glucose sensor in the PRECISE study: a 180-day, prospective, multicenter, pivotal trial. Diabetes Care 2017;40(1):63–8.
59. Polonsky WH, Hessler D, Ruedy KJ, et al. The impact of continuous glucose monitoring on markers of quality of life in adults with type 1 diabetes: further findings from the DIAMOND randomized clinical trial. Diabetes Care 2017; 40(6):736–41.
60. Hilliard ME, Levy W, Anderson BJ, et al. Benefits and barriers of continuous glucose monitoring in young children with type 1 diabetes. Diabetes Technol Ther 2019;21(9):493–8.
61. van Beers CAJ, DeVries JH, Kleijer SJ, et al. Continuous glucose monitoring for patients with type 1 diabetes and impaired awareness of hypoglycaemia (IN CONTROL): a randomised, open-label, crossover trial. Lancet Diabetes Endocrinol 2016;4(11):893–902.
62. Little SA, Speight J, Leelarathna L, et al. Sustained reduction in severe hypoglycemia in adults with type 1 diabetes complicated by impaired awareness of hypoglycemia: two-year follow-up in the HypoCOMPaSS randomized clinical Trial. Diabetes Care 2018;41(8):1600–7.
63. Heinemann L, Freckmann G, Ehrmann D, et al. Real-time continuous glucose monitoring in adults with type 1 diabetes and impaired hypoglycaemia awareness or severe hypoglycaemia treated with multiple daily insulin injections (HypoDE): a multicentre, randomised controlled trial. Lancet 2018. https://doi.org/10.1016/S0140-6736(18)30297-6.
64. Bosi E, Choudhary P, Valk HW, et al. Efficacy and safety of suspend-before-low insulin pump technology in hypoglycaemia-prone adults with type 1 diabetes (SMILE): an open-label randomised controlled trial. Lancet Diabetes Endocrinol 2019;7(June). https://doi.org/10.1016/S2213-8587(19)30150-0.
65. Battelino T, Liabat S, Veeze HJ, et al. Routine use of continuous glucose monitoring in 10 501 people with diabetes mellitus. Diabet Med 2015;32(12): 1568–74.
66. Murphy HR. Continuous glucose monitoring targets in type 1 diabetes pregnancy: every 5% time in range matters. Diabetologia 2019;62(7):1123–8.

67. Murphy HR, Feig DS, Sanchez JJ, et al. Modelling potential cost savings from use of real-time continuous glucose monitoring in pregnant women with Type 1 diabetes. Diabet Med 2019. https://doi.org/10.1111/dme.14046.
68. Charleer S, Mathieu C, Nobels F, et al. Effect of continuous glucose monitoring on glycemic control, acute admissions, and quality of life: a real-world study. J Clin Endocrinol Metab 2018;103(3):1224–32.
69. Grunberger G, Handelsman Y, Bloomgarden ZT, et al. American Association Of Clinical Endocrinologists and American College of Endocrinology 2018 position statement on integration of insulin pumps and continuous glucose monitoring in patients with diabetes mellitus. Endocr Pract 2018;24(3):302–8.
70. Garber AJ, Abrahamson MJ, Barzilay JI, et al. Consensus statement by the American association of clinical endocrinologists and American college of endocrinology on the comprehensive type 2 diabetes management algorithm – 2019 executive summary. Endocr Pract 2019;25(1):69–100.
71. Danne T, Nimri R, Battelino T, et al. International consensus on use of continuous glucose monitoring. Diabetes Care 2017;40(12):1631–40.
72. Riddlesworth TD, Beck RW, Gal RL, et al. Optimal sampling duration for continuous glucose monitoring to determine long-term glycemic control. Diabetes Technol Ther 2018;20(4):314–6.
73. Bergenstal RM, Beck RW, Close KL, et al. Glucose Management Indicator (GMI): a new term for estimating A1C from continuous glucose monitoring. Diabetes Care 2018;dc181581. https://doi.org/10.2337/dc18-1581.
74. Battelino T, Danne T, Bergenstal RM, et al. Clinical targets for continuous glucose monitoring data interpretation: recommendations from the international consensus on time in range. Diabetes Care 2019;42(8):1593–603.
75. Bergenstal RM, Ahmann AJ, Bailey T, et al. Recommendations for standardizing glucose reporting and analysis to optimize clinical decision making in diabetes: the Ambulatory Glucose Profile (AGP). Diabetes Technol Ther 2013;15(3):198–211.
76. Santiago JV, Clemens AH, Clarke WL, et al. Closed-loop and open-loop devices for blood glucose control in normal and diabetic subjects. Diabetes 1979;28(1):71–84.
77. Clemens AH, Chang PH, Myers RW. The development of biostator, a Glucose Controlled Insulin Infusion System (GCIIS). Horm Metab Res 1977;(Suppl 7):23–33.
78. Kadish A. Automation control of blood sugar, a servomechanism for glucose monitoring and control. Am J Med Electron 1963;3:82–6.
79. Battelino T, Phillip M. The first meeting of the loop club. J Pediatr Endocrinol Metab 2004;17(3). https://doi.org/10.1515/JPEM.2004.17.3.375.
80. Kowalski A. Pathway to artificial pancreas systems revisited: moving downstream. Diabetes Care 2015;38(6):1036–43.
81. Kowalski AJ. Can we really close the loop and how soon? Accelerating the availability of an artificial pancreas: a roadmap to better diabetes outcomes. Diabetes Technol Ther 2009;11(Suppl 1):S113–9.
82. Bergenstal RM, Tamborlane WV, Ahmann A, et al. Effectiveness of sensor-augmented insulin-pump therapy in type 1 diabetes. N Engl J Med 2010;363(4):311–20.
83. Ly TT, Nicholas JA, Retterath A, et al. Effect of sensor-augmented insulin pump therapy and automated insulin suspension vs standard insulin pump therapy on hypoglycemia in patients with type 1 diabetes: a randomized clinical trial. JAMA 2013;310(12):1240–7.

84. Choudhary P, Shin J, Wang Y, et al. Insulin pump therapy with automated insulin suspension in response to hypoglycemia: Reduction in nocturnal hypoglycemia in those at greatest risk. Diabetes Care 2011;34(9):2023–5.
85. Choudhary P, Olsen BS, Conget I, et al. Hypoglycemia prevention and user acceptance of an insulin pump system with predictive low glucose management. Diabetes Technol Ther 2016;18(5):288–91.
86. Battelino T, Nimri R, Dovc K, et al. Prevention of hypoglycemia with predictive low glucose insulin suspension in children with type 1 diabetes: a randomized controlled trial. Diabetes Care 2017;40(6):764–70.
87. Biester T, Kordonouri O, Holder M, et al. "Let the algorithm do the work": reduction of hypoglycemia using sensor-augmented pump therapy with predictive insulin suspension (SmartGuard) in pediatric type 1 diabetes patients. Diabetes Technol Ther 2017;19(3):173–82.
88. Buckingham BA, Cameron F, Calhoun P, et al. Outpatient safety assessment of an in-home predictive low-glucose suspend system with type 1 diabetes subjects at elevated risk of nocturnal hypoglycemia. Diabetes Technol Ther 2013; 15(8):622–7.
89. Forlenza GP, Li Z, Buckingham BA, et al. Predictive low-glucose suspend reduces hypoglycemia in adults, adolescents, and children with type 1 diabetes in an at-home randomized crossover study: results of the PROLOG trial. Diabetes Care 2018;41(10):2155–61.
90. Pinsker JE, Lee JB, Dassau E, et al. Randomized crossover comparison of personalized MPC and PID control algorithms for the artificial pancreas. Diabetes Care 2016;39(7):1135–42.
91. Atlas E, Nimri R, Miller S, et al. MD-logic artificial pancreas system: a pilot study in adults with type 1 diabetes. Diabetes Care 2010;33(5):1072–6.
92. Nimri R, Phillip M. Artificial pancreas: fuzzy logic and control of glycemia. Curr Opin Endocrinol Diabetes Obes 2014;21(4):251–6.
93. Weisman A, Bai J-W, Cardinez M, et al. Effect of artificial pancreas systems on glycaemic control in patients with type 1 diabetes: a systematic review and meta-analysis of outpatient randomised controlled trials. Lancet Diabetes Endocrinol 2017;5(7):501–12.
94. Bekiari E, Kitsios K, Thabit H, et al. Artificial pancreas treatment for outpatients with type 1 diabetes: systematic review and meta-analysis. BMJ 2018;361: k1310.
95. Ekhlaspour L, Forlenza GP, Chernavvsky D, et al. Closed loop control in adolescents and children during winter sports: use of the tandem control-IQ AP system. Pediatr Diabetes 2019;20(6):pedi.12867.
96. Breton MD, Cherñavvsky DR, Forlenza GP, et al. Closed-loop control during intense prolonged outdoor exercise in adolescents with type 1 diabetes: The artificial pancreas ski study. Diabetes Care 2017;40(12):1644–50.
97. Dovc K, Macedoni M, Bratina N, et al. Closed-loop glucose control in young people with type 1 diabetes during and after unannounced physical activity: a randomised controlled crossover trial. Diabetologia 2017;60(11):2157–67.
98. DeBoer MD, Breton MD, Wakeman C, et al. Performance of an artificial pancreas system for young children with type 1 diabetes. Diabetes Technol Ther 2017;19(5):293–8.
99. Cherñavvsky DR, Deboer MD, Keith-Hynes P, et al. Use of an artificial pancreas among adolescents for a missed snack bolus and an underestimated meal bolus. Pediatr Diabetes 2016;17(1):28–35.

100. Lee MH, Vogrin S, Paldus B, et al. Glucose control in adults with type 1 diabetes using a medtronic prototype enhanced-hybrid closed-loop system: a feasibility study. Diabetes Technol Ther 2019;21(9). dia.2019.0120.
101. Garg SK, Weinzimer SA, Tamborlane WV, et al. Glucose outcomes with the in-home use of a hybrid closed-loop insulin delivery system in adolescents and adults with type 1 diabetes. Diabetes Technol Ther 2017;19(3):155–63.
102. Brown SA, Kovatchev BP, Raghinaru D, et al. Six-month randomized, multicenter trial of closed-loop control in type 1 diabetes. N Engl J Med 2019;1–10. https://doi.org/10.1056/NEJMoa1907863.
103. Benhamou P-Y, Franc S, Reznik Y, et al. Closed-loop insulin delivery in adults with type 1 diabetes in real-life conditions: a 12-week multicentre, open-label randomised controlled crossover trial. Lancet Digit Heal 2019;1(1):e17–25.
104. Tauschmann M, Thabit H, Bally L, et al. Closed-loop insulin delivery in suboptimally controlled type 1 diabetes: a multicentre, 12-week randomised trial. Lancet 2018;392(10155):1321–9.
105. Sherr J, Buckingham BA, Forlenza G, et al. Safety and performance of the omnipod hybrid closed-loop system in adults, adolescents, and children with type 1 diabetes over 5 days under free-living conditions. Diabetes Technol Ther 2019. https://doi.org/10.1089/dia.2019.0286. dia.2019.0286.
106. Olinder AL, Kernell A, Smide B. Missed bolus doses: devastating for metabolic control in CSII-treated adolescents with type 1 diabetes. Pediatr Diabetes 2009; 10(2):142–8.
107. Forlenza GP, Cameron FM, Ly TT, et al. Fully closed-loop multiple model probabilistic predictive controller artificial pancreas performance. Diabetes Technol Ther 2018;20(5):1–9.
108. Weinzimer SA, Steil GM, Swan KL, et al. Fully automated closed-loop insulin delivery versus semiautomated hybrid control in pediatric patients with type 1 diabetes using an artificial pancreas. Diabetes Care 2008;31(5):934–9.
109. Cameron FM, Ly TT, Buckingham BA, et al. Closed-loop control without meal announcement in type 1 diabetes. Diabetes Technol Ther 2017;19(9). dia.2017.0078.
110. Dovc K, Piona C, Yeşiltepe Mutlu G, et al. Faster compared to standard insulin aspart during day- and-night fully closed-loop insulin therapy in type 1 diabetes: a double-blind randomized crossover trial article faster compared to standard insulin aspart during day-and-night fully closed-loop ins. Diabetes Care 2019;DC19–0895. https://doi.org/10.2337/dc19-0895/-/DC1. R2.
111. Haidar A, Smaoui MR, Legault L, et al. The role of glucagon in the artificial pancreas. Lancet Diabetes Endocrinol 2016;4(6):476–9.
112. Russell SJ, El-Khatib FH, Sinha M, et al. Outpatient glycemic control with a bionic pancreas in type 1 diabetes. N Engl J Med 2014;371(4):313–25.
113. Russell SJ, Hillard MA, Balliro C, et al. Day and night glycaemic control with a bionic pancreas versus conventional insulin pump therapy in preadolescent children with type 1 diabetes: a randomised crossover trial. Lancet Diabetes Endocrinol 2016;4(3):233–43.
114. Haidar A, Legault L, Matteau-Pelletier L, et al. Outpatient overnight glucose control with dual-hormone artificial pancreas, single-hormone artificial pancreas, or conventional insulin pump therapy in children and adolescents with type 1 diabetes: an open-label, randomised controlled trial. Lancet Diabetes Endocrinol 2015;3(8):595–604.

115. Haidar A, Rabasa-Lhoret R, Legault L, et al. Single- and dual-hormone artificial pancreas for overnight glucose control in type 1 diabetes. J Clin Endocrinol Metab 2016;101(1):214–23.
116. Sherr JL, Patel NS, Michaud CI, et al. Mitigating meal-related glycemic excursions in an insulin-sparing manner during closed-loop insulin delivery: The beneficial effects of adjunctive pramlintide and liraglutide. Diabetes Care 2016;39(7):1127–34.
117. Braune K, O'Donnell S, Cleal B, et al. Real-world use of do-it-yourself artificial pancreas systems in children and adolescents: self-reported clinical outcomes (Preprint). JMIR MHealth UHealth 2019;7:1–9.
118. Nimri R, Ochs AR, Pinsker JE, et al. Decision support systems and closed loop. Diabetes Technol Ther 2019;21(S1):S42–56.
119. Nimri R, Dassau E, Segall T, et al. Adjusting insulin doses in patients with type 1 diabetes that use insulin pump and continuous glucose monitoring - variations among countries and physicians. Diabetes Obes Metab 2018. https://doi.org/10.1111/dom.13408.
120. O'Connor PJ, Sperl-Hillen JAM. Current status and future directions for electronic point-of-care clinical decision support to improve diabetes management in primary care. Diabetes Technol Ther 2019;21(S2):S2–26. S2-34.
121. Beck RW, Bergenstal RM, Riddlesworth TD, et al. Validation of time in range as an outcome measure for diabetes clinical trials. Diabetes Care 2019;42(3): 400 5.

Use of Diabetes Technology in Children

Role of Structured Education for Young People with Diabetes and Families

Hannah R. Desrochers, MSN, RN, CPNP[a],
Alan T. Schultz, MSN, RN, CPNP[b], Lori M. Laffel, MD, MPH[a,*]

KEYWORDS

- Diabetes technology • Continuous glucose monitoring
- Continuous subcutaneous insulin infusion • Closed-loop system • Children • Youth
- Education

KEY POINTS

- Advanced diabetes technologies are rapidly evolving and include continuous glucose monitoring, continuous subcutaneous insulin delivery, and closed-loop insulin delivery systems.
- Education of young people with diabetes and their family members is a critical cornerstone of care for the proper implementation of advanced diabetes technologies and to identify and overcome barriers to continued use in order to derive maximum benefits with respect to biomedical and psychosocial outcomes.
- The improved performance of continuous glucose monitoring (CGM) devices has led to a revolution in their use, often eliminating the need for traditional fingerstick glucose monitoring, yielding CGM as the standard of care for glucose monitoring in youth.
- Closed-loop insulin delivery systems are the newest addition to advanced diabetes technologies in clinical use; safe and effective use of such tools will require substantial education and support for young persons with diabetes and their family members.

INTRODUCTION

The current era is witness to a technological revolution for the management of type 1 diabetes (T1D) in children. Youth with T1D are routinely using advanced diabetes

[a] Section on Clinical, Behavioral, and Outcomes Research, Pediatric, Adolescent, and Young Adult Section, Joslin Diabetes Center, Harvard Medical School, One Joslin Place, Boston, MA 02215, USA; [b] Emergency Department, Montefiore Medical Center, 111 East 210th Street, The Bronx, NY 10467, USA
* Corresponding author.
E-mail address: lori.laffel@joslin.harvard.edu

Endocrinol Metab Clin N Am 49 (2020) 19–35
https://doi.org/10.1016/j.ecl.2019.11.001 endo.theclinics.com

technologies for glucose monitoring and insulin delivery for their day-to-day management, shifting more and more of the meticulous and calculated tasks of T1D self-care from the individual to external systems. The International Society for Pediatric and Adolescent Diabetes and the American Diabetes Association (ADA) recognize the need for initial and ongoing structured education for youth and families living with diabetes in order to keep them informed and to optimize their chances of attaining benefits from technology use.[1,2]

The goal of this review is to provide an overview of diabetes technologies and the role of structured education in empowering youth and families to succeed with safe and effective use of diabetes technology aimed at optimizing glycemic control and reducing the burden of diabetes management. Given deficiencies in achievement of target glycemic control in youth with T1D,[3] the diabetes community should use the available advanced diabetes technologies to help achieve target glycemic outcomes. To do so, it requires the provision of adequate education and support to avoid unrealistic expectations and increased self-care burden. This review highlights educational approaches for youth with T1D along with their family members and other child caregivers, highlighting the pivotal roles played by multidisciplinary members of the diabetes team. The authors also discuss educational approaches regarding continuous glucose monitoring (CGM) devices and advanced insulin delivery systems, mainly insulin pumps with a brief discussion of smart pens and automated insulin delivery systems. Insulin pumps reduce the need for multiple daily injections, and CGM reduce the need for frequent fingersticks; thus, both are welcomed by youth with T1D and their families. According to recently published data from the T1D Exchange Registry, the number of youth using technologies has increased substantially.[3] From 2010 to 12 to 2016 to 18, insulin pump use increased among children and young teens by about 20%, whereas CGM use increased 10-fold over that time, highlighting the timeliness of this review.

Continuous Glucose Monitoring

Many patients and families seek CGM to optimize glycemic control and detect glycemic excursions.[4–7] In the past, CGM use was not always associated with hemoglobin A1c (HbA1c) improvement in pediatric samples; however, newer CGM devices with improved performance have yielded increases in CGM uptake and use along with glycemic benefit in pediatric, adolescent, and young adult patients.[8–16] Recent data from Mulinacci and colleagues[17] (2019) have shown improved glucose control and fewer diabetes-related emergency visits with early CGM initiation during the new-onset period. Several professional organizations support consideration of CGM use for all children and adolescents with T1D, especially since the advent of CGM devices with improved performance and regulatory approval that includes nonadjunctive use.[18–21] Nonadjunctive CGM use allows for insulin dosing and treatment of hypoglycemia based on the CGM values without need for self-monitoring of blood glucose (SMBG) levels. Indeed, it is the nonadjunctive CGM use that reduces substantial burden of diabetes self-care. Recent data from the T1D Exchange and the German/Austrian Diabetes DPV registries show that mean HbA1c is lower among CGM users regardless of insulin delivery method, and CGM users are more likely to achieve the ADA glycemic target of HbA1c less than 7.5% (56% vs 43% for DPV and 30% vs 15% for T1D Exchange, for CGM users vs nonusers, respectively, both $P < .001$).[22] As interest and clinical integration in pediatrics accelerate, it is essential to educate the youth and their families about the fundamentals of CGM device components, insertion, skin care, and data interpretation to assure safe and effective use of the increasingly sophisticated systems.

As an introduction to CGM, the youth and family need to learn realistic expectations about how CGM can be incorporated into diabetes management. Patients and their families must understand the instances in which confirmatory SMBG checks must be performed for safety, such as when there is a device issue (eg, absent number and/or directional arrow) or symptoms are incongruent with displayed value, or rapid confirmation of blood glucose value. Education includes how CGM devices measure interstitial glucose, not blood levels, and that CGM readings may not be identical to an SMBG value. It can be helpful to show the youth and family members a visual graphic of sensor placement that includes location of the sensor tip in the interstitial space (**Fig. 1**). The concepts of sensor lag, generally 5 to 10 minutes behind the blood glucose level, and factors that affect CGM accuracy are vital information for the youth and caregivers to make safe decisions regarding management.[23]

Education needs to be supportive and realistic in order to maximize uptake and continued CGM use, as glycemic benefit can only be realized if the device is worn consistently. Primary barriers to device uptake and continued use in the pediatric population include cost, nuisance alerts/alarms, concerns with accuracy, discomfort, and hassle of wearing devices, among others.[5,24–30] Maximizing adoption and consistent CGM use can be promoted by addressing both youth developmental stage and psychosocial parameters at the time of initiation, as well as identifying individual patient/family needs and potential provider biases (**Table 1**).[5]

Main Teaching Point: Continuous Glucose Monitoring System Components

Topics to review: continuous glucose monitoring type, physical placement, site issues alerts/alarms

Education involving device selection and component parts comprise the initial steps toward successful CGM use. A CGM device includes a sensor, which is inserted under the skin, a transmitter that receives the glucose signal, and a receiver that receives the glucose signal wirelessly and then displays the glucose value. There can be a dedicated receiver or the signal can be sent to a mobile phone by Bluetooth transmission. CGM devices are classified by modality of device insertion and timing of data delivery. The primary approach for device insertion is into the subcutaneous, interstitial space by puncturing the skin with a replaceable sensor. This approach is used for CGM devices such as the Medtronic Guardian, Dexcom, and Abbot Libre Flash. They are self-inserted every 7, 10, or, 14 days, respectively. These devices provide glucose data in

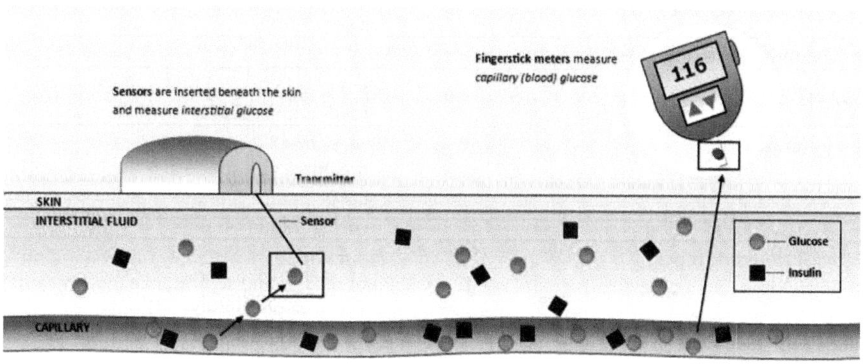

Fig. 1. CGM sensor placement into the interstitial space compared with fingerstick blood glucose monitoring. (*Courtesy of* Lindsay Roethke, BS, Boston, MA.)

Table 1
Challenges and potential strategies for youth and families using continuous glucose monitoring, continuous subcutaneous insulin infusions, and hybrid closed-loop systems

Potential Issue	Educational Opportunity
CGM	
Device Components	
Adhesive issues	Offer adhesive adjunctive options, symptoms of adhesive reaction
Cost/insurance coverage	Advocate for coverage, complete certificate of medical necessity
Supply and reordering	Support consistent supply options
Receiver and/or mobile device	Review features and options of each, mobile device must use up-to-date system
Pump integration	Educate patient about HCL options by device
Device Application	
Sensor site selection	Review symptoms of site problems, rotation to area with sufficient subcutaneous tissue for reading
Safety	MRI incompatible, removal often necessary with radiation exposure or security clearances
Fingerstick requirements	Review parameters for fingerstick confirmation (eg, no number/no arrow, symptoms not matching reading, or glucose rapidly changing or severely low)
Remote treatment and support feasibility	Develop plan for management of severe hypo/hyperglycemia
Data Transmission	
Bluetooth connectivity	Confirm device compatibility, reconnecting Bluetooth if signal lost
WI-FI connectivity for sharing	Data must be received by user in order for share feature; sharing currently only available with Dexcom system
Technological support	Provide access to customer service contact and differentiation between user and device errors
Data Interpretation	
Sensor lag	Discuss interstitial vs blood glucose readings, variability
Trend arrows	Review trend arrow significance, mealtime adjustments
Risk of stacking	Counsel about clinically appropriate correction timeframes
Glucometric report	Assist with patient/family understanding of reports and significance (eg, convert TIR from percentage to hours)
Data overwhelm	Encourage meaningful monitoring of glucose information

(*continued on next page*)

Table 1
(*continued*)

Potential Issue	Educational Opportunity
Data Sharing	
WI-FI connectivity	Dexcom and Share user must be WI-FI connected for data transmission
Privacy rights	Discuss data sharing and glucose reports for age appropriate recipients (minor vs. legal adult status)
Family communication	Support dialogue around youth-family experience including transitions (eg, college), stressors, and successes
CSII	
Glycemic Excursions	Review basal-bolus settings, technical application of device, insulin administration timing, and use of bolus calculator
Risk of DKA	
Hyperglycemia	Review importance of frequent glucose monitoring to detect hyperglycemia and pump failures, administering insulin via injection if pump failure suspected
Ketosis	Discuss need to monitor ketones during hyperglycemia and illness
Running out of insulin	Encourage families to carry back up insulin and set alarms for low insulin reservoir
Missed boluses	Consider bolus reminders, review parent/child responsibility for boluses
Infusion Site Issues	
Site failures	Recommend avoidance of site placement at areas of hypertrophy or scarring, remind family of importance of frequent glucose monitoring
Site disconnections, tubing problem	Offer adjunctive adhesives, recommend frequent visual check of site connection. Confirm appropriate priming technique, cannula and tubing integrity
Adhesive site reactions	Encourage use of adhesive barrier, review site rotation
Body image	Review appropriate application areas, consider untethered pumping
Site infections	Discuss proper skin preparation, changing site every 2–3 d, teaching early signs and symptoms of infection
Hypertrophy	Counsel on importance of site rotation, avoiding overuse of frequent sites

(*continued on next page*)

Table 1
(continued)

Potential Issue	Educational Opportunity
Misc.	
Travel	Offer heath care provider letter, review need to bring extra supplies and keep in carry-on luggage
School	Confirm school has ketone monitoring supplies, back up insulin/syringes in case of pump failure, assist with education of school staff
HCL	
See "CSII" and "CGM" Issues	
Mental burden	
System complexity	Encourage formalized training for initial use to learn system-specific "clinical rules," as well as ongoing education, evaluation, and support with diabetes team, updating pump settings for use in open-loop mode as needed
Terminology	Define brand-specific terms relating to the individual's system
Rapid upgrades and changes to systems	Encourage ongoing education and follow-up for both patient and clinicians
Cost	Review insurance benefits, submit Certificate of Medical Necessity, explore participation in clinical trials
Human vs system conflicts related to automated insulin delivery	Assess user comprehension with system, especially automation vs manual modes; review fundamental concepts of diabetes management routinely; encourage prompt reporting and resolution of device-related issues
Diabetes burnout	Teach benefits of system, reiterate diabetes goals, share and interpret glucometrics
Technology vacation	Assess and review fundamental diabetes management, manual pump use guidelines
Physical activity	Encourage use of system tools (eg, temp target, basal suspension), hypoglycemia and hyperglycemia treatment recommendations by exercise type and duration

Abbreviations: HCL, hybrid closed-loop; TIR, time-in-range.

real-time CGM (for Medtronic and Dexcom) or by intermittent scanning (Abbott Freestyle Libre).[31] The second route for device insertion involves professional placement of an implantable sensor into the subcutaneous space with the Senseonics' Eversense device.[31] This includes a sensor that lasts for 90 days (per Food and Drug Administration [FDA] approval) or 180 days (per European Medicines Agency approval).

However, this device does not currently have FDA approval for use in the pediatric population younger than 18 years.

CGM devices are generally inserted on the arms, abdomen, buttocks/hips, or anterior thighs although different devices have received regulatory approval for only certain sites. Nonetheless, in the clinical arena, educators generally work individually with young persons and their families to identify the easiest sites for sensor insertions. Indeed, site selection and insertion can be challenging for pediatric patients, especially for the very young where available "real estate," or space on the body, can be limited, especially given that the CGM device should be separated from areas of insulin delivery by 3 inches. Unanticipated or accidental sensor removal can be common in children, especially in young children, when the sensor can be knocked off during routine childhood activities. One can often help to ensure durability of the sensor placement with use of additional adhesive products. Occasionally, skin irritations can arise at the sites of sensor insertions. Such skin reactions can generally be handled with topical care or with barrier tapes, which should be managed on an individual basis with the health care team. Continual education and guidance around technique for insertion can help support families overcome challenges with CGM wear.[5,23,28,32]

CGM devices generally have alerts and alarms that can be set for the individual's needs. The alerts and alarms include threshold alarms that are set for high and low glucose levels. There can also be alerts for signal loss and alerts for rapidly changing glucose levels, so-called trend arrow alarms (see later discussion). It is important to avoid too many alerts or alarms, as they can be viewed as a "nuisance" by the youth who may then tend to ignore the signals and the CGM data. Ongoing support and guidance for the youth and family are important.

Main Teaching Point: Glucometrics and Interpretation

Topics to review: data transmission, sensor lag, glucose reports, calibration, sharing data

CGM is a valuable tool for detecting and tracking of glucose levels, trends, and patterns. CGM data generally provide an updated glucose value every 5 minutes, yielding 288 readings daily. CGM data can be nearly 50 times the amount of glucose data provided by SMBG. CGM provides directional information as well as actual glucose levels. CGM data can be taught as offering an understanding of the magnitude (how high or low) as well as the direction (increasing, decreasing, or stable) of the glucose values. Such detailed information allows both the person with diabetes and the provider to better understand cause and effect relationships between glucose values and responsible factors, related to dietary intake or exercise, for example.[23]

CGM data can be viewed in real time to reflect glucose excursions over the past few hours or can be viewed retrospectively via downloaded reports that can be printed out for ease of review and interpretation. Such reports can be helpful visual aids for teaching youth and families about how medication, physical activity, and food affect glucose levels. Retrospective data can be viewed in multiple, adjustable formats to show daily, weekly, and monthly trends, allowing comparisons of glucose levels over time. Real-time CGM data can help families make appropriate and timely management decisions, especially when glucose levels are rapidly changing (see later section on trend arrow).

Several recent publications have highlighted the use of retrospective CGM data to help both clinicians and people with diabetes along with their family members/caregivers to understand glycemic patterns, including the impact of food, exercise, illness, stress, among other things, on glycemic control.[33,34] As noted earlier, retrospective

CGM data can be reviewed over the past few hours to the past few months. A recent publication highlights how 14 days of CGM data provide sufficient information to reflect on the recent 3-month interval.[35] Further, data from a 2-week interval are easier to review for clinicians as well as for the youth and families. A very recent publication highlights the critical importance of assessing glucose time-in-range, generally accepted as 70 to 180 mg/dL (3.9–10 mmol/L),[36] which now appears on apps and downloads of most CGM devices. Youth and families can learn how to review glucose time-in-range as well as time below range, time above range, and glycemic variability in their efforts to optimize glycemic control.

Nonadjunctive CGM devices are rapidly becoming the primary source of glucose data. Thus, it is important to teach youth and their families about the potential limitations of CGM and to confirm their ability to perform SMBG when indicated. There may be a need to calibrate certain CGM devices, depending on the recommendations of the manufacturer. For other devices, there may be opportunities to calibrate at times of suspected inaccuracy or when symptoms do not match the CGM reading. SMBG calibrations should be entered into the CGM system generally when the CGM arrow is steady or indicating only modestly changing glucose levels, again according to the manufacturer's recommendations. At the time of this publication, the Dexcom CGM system is the only CGM currently approved by the FDA for treatment decisions without confirmatory SMBG and without calibration for use in the pediatric population.

Some CGM systems offer "share" features that allow caregivers to receive RT-CGM data. The glucose data are transmitted wirelessly in real time from the child's CGM device if the youth has a cellular or Wi-Fi–enabled device that sends the data to the "cloud," which can then be received by others, such as parents, school nurses, or other care providers. This feature offers parents an opportunity to assist in the care of their child. Some parents elect to help with insulin dosing at lunch time during school, whereas others may provide guidance before physical education by viewing the glucose trends to determine if additional carbohydrate snacking may be needed. Generally, secondary caregivers, such as school nurses, babysitters, daycare providers, and grandparents, among others, may be unfamiliar with CGM interpretation; therefore, it is prudent that they receive training from parents or by attending school nurse or caregiver classes that are often given by diabetes organizations or large pediatric diabetes centers. Such education generally includes the need for ongoing support and guidance to ensure that the continuous and often fluctuating glucose data along with frequent alerts/alarms does not overwhelm the care providers.[29]

Main Teaching Point: Trend Arrows

Topics to review: arrow meaning, trend arrow dose adjustments

As noted, CGM devices display the glucose level along with an arrow that designates the direction and the rate of change of the glucose levels (**Table 2**). There is no standardization of the trend arrows from the different CGM devices regarding glucose rate of change. Therefore, youth and families should work with their diabetes educators and consult the manufacturer's guide. CGM devices may also include alert features that allow for alarms for rapidly changing glucose levels.

The trend arrows allow youth and caregivers to understand where the glucose levels have been and predict which direction the glucose is likely headed over the next 30 minutes or so. At meal times, insulin dosages can be adjusted upward or downward based on the arrow's directionality, adding to the dose for upward arrows and increasing glucose levels or subtracting insulin from the dose for downward or decreasing glucose levels. Recommendations for insulin adjustments based on trend

Table 2
Trend arrow significance by device

Trend Arrow	Glucose Direction	Change in Glucose
Dexcom G5/Dexcom G6		
↑↑	Increasing: Glucose is rapidly increasing	Increasing >3 mg/dL/min or >90 mg/dL in 30 min
↑	Increasing: Glucose is increasing	Increasing 2–3 mg/dL/min or 60–90 mg/dL in 30 min
↗	Increasing: Glucose is slowly increasing	Increasing 1–2 mg/dL/min or 30–60 mg/dL in 30 min
→	Increasing or decreasing: Glucose is steady	Not increasing or decreasing >1 mg/dL/min
↘	Decreasing: Glucose is slowly decreasing	Decreasing 1–2 mg/dL/min or 30–60 mg/dL in 30 min
↓	Decreasing: Glucose is decreasing	Decreasing 2–3 mg/dL/min or 60–90 mg/dL in 30 min
↓↓	Decreasing: Glucose is rapidly decreasing	Decreasing >3 mg/dL/min or >90 mg/dL in 30 min

Trend Arrow	Corresponding SG Rate per Minute
Medtronic MiniMed Guardian 3	
↑	Increasing at a rate of 1 mg/dL but <2 mg/dL
↓	Decreasing at a rate of 1 mg/dL but <2 mg/dL
↑↑	Increasing at a rate of 2 mg/dL but <3 mg/dL
↓↓	Decreasing at a rate of 2 mg/dL but <3 mg/dL
↑↑↑	Increasing at a rate of 3 mg/dL or more
↓↓↓	Falling at a rate of 3 mg/dL or more

Trend Arrow	Glucose Direction	Change in Glucose
Freestyle Libre™		
↑	Increasing quickly	Increasing >2 mg/dL/min or >60 mg/dL in 30 min
↗	Increasing	Increasing 1–2 mg/dL/min or 30–60 mg/dL in 30 min
→	Changing slowly	Not increasing or decreasing >1 mg/dL/min
↘	Decreasing	Decreasing 1–2 mg/dL/min or 30–60 mg/dL in 30 min
↓	Decreasing quickly	Decreasing >2 mg/dL/min or >60 mg/dL in 30 min

Trend Arrow	Glucose Direction and Velocity
Eversense	
→	Gradually increasing or decreasing at a rate between 0.0 mg/dL and 1.0 mg/dL per min
↗	Moderately increasing glucose level, increasing at a rate between 1.0 mg/dL and 2.0 mg/dL per min
↘	Moderately decreasing glucose levels, decreasing at a rate between 1.0 mg/dL and 2.0 mg/dL
↑	Very rapidly increasing glucose levels, increasing at a rate more than 2.0 mg/dL per min
↓	Very rapidly increasing glucose levels, decreasing at a rate more than 2.0 mg/dL per min

arrows from the Dexcom CGM are based on the youth's correction factor and are outlined in the recent publication by Laffel and colleagues (2017) in **Fig. 2**.

Continuous Subcutaneous Insulin Infusion

Insulin pumps, or continuous subcutaneous insulin infusions (CSII), have been an important part of the management of T1D for many years. Recent data indicate that insulin pump use is the most common modality of insulin delivery for youth with T1D.[3] In the T1D Exchange registry, 60%, 74%, and 67% of youth younger than 6, 6 to 12, and 13 to 17 years, respectively, reported using an insulin pump.[3]

There is potential for benefit with insulin pump therapy, including improved glycemic control, reduced hypoglycemia, and improved quality of life. A recent meta-analysis of 25 randomized controlled trials reported a reduction of 0.32% in children and 0.42% in adults using insulin pump therapy compared with those on multiple daily injections.[37] Severe hypoglycemia is also reduced with insulin pump use compared with injection therapy in youth.[38] Furthermore, insulin pumps offer increased flexibility for the delivery of insulin at various times of the day. Families have reported higher rates of satisfaction and a better perception of their health compared with injections users.[39] Higher diabetes-specific quality of life is reported by pump users along with a decrease in the care burden reported by caregivers.[40]

Topics to review: operation, types, placement

It is important to ensure that youth and families understand the fundamentals of insulin delivery with an insulin pump, specifically that basal insulin is provided continuously, whereas prandial insulin is provided when the user programs the pump to deliver a bolus of insulin according to the planned carbohydrate intake. In addition, correction doses of insulin required at times of elevations must also be programmed for delivery by the user. Thus, it is important that youth and parents understand that although pump use may reduce some of the burdens of self-care related to frequent insulin injections, there remains substantial person input for the bolus insulin delivery. Furthermore, it is critical that the user and/or caregiver be aware of any pump dislodgement, as that would prevent basal delivery and could lead to insulin deficiency within a few hours.

Education must include review of the 2 main types of insulin pumps: a pod pump that resides on the body with a small catheter beneath the skin in the subcutaneous tissue and pumps that use an infusion set into the subcutaneous tissue connected via tubing to the actual pump. Both pump types can be placed on the arms, abdomen, buttocks/hips, or anterior thighs.

Structured education can be provided in group classes or one-on-one. It is important that youth and families receive realistic expectations about pump therapy and recognize the ongoing need for substantial self-care behaviors to ensure safe pump use. Understanding insulin action, carbohydrate counting, correction doses, and sick day management is critical for safe pump use.

In particular, deficient understanding of insulin action can result in insulin stacking and severe hypoglycemia.

Topics to review: potential challenges with pump therapy

Table 1 provides a list of common pump challenges and educational opportunities. Pump use requires families to monitor blood glucose and ketone levels frequently in order to detect pump failure in a timely manner. Most failures are the result of a dislodged infusion site. Insulin pump failure can lead to diabetes ketoacidosis (DKA). Fortunately, recent data from children in England, Wales, Germany, Austria, and the United States did not show higher rates of DKA in those on insulin pumps compared

Suggested Approach to Adjusting Insulin Dose Using Trend Arrows in Pediatric Patients: Pre-meal and ≥3 Hours Post-meal

Trend Arrows		Correction Factor[a] (CF)	Insulin Dose Adjustment (U)
Receiver	App		
↑↑	◯	<25	+4.0
		25–<50	+3.0
		50–<75	+2.0
		75–<125	+1.0
		≥125	+0.5
↑	◯	<25	+3.0
		25–<50	+2.0
		50–<75	+1.0
		75–<125	+0.5
		≥125	No adjustment
↗	◯	<25	+2.0
		25–<50	+1.0
		50–<75	+0.5
		75–<125	No adjustment
		≥125	No adjustment
→	◯	<25	No adjustment
		25–<50	No adjustment
		50–<75	No adjustment
		75–<125	No adjustment
		≥125	No adjustment
↘	◯	<25	-2.0
		25–<50	-1.0
		50–<75	-0.5
		75–<125	No adjustment
		≥125	No adjustment
↓	◯	<25	-3.0
		25–<50	-2.0
		50–<75	-1.0
		75–<125	-0.5
		≥125	No adjustment
↓↓	◯	<25	-4.0
		25–<50	-3.0
		50–<75	-2.0
		75–<125	-1.0
		≥125	-0.5

Insulin adjustments using trend arrows do not replace standard calculations using ICR and CF. Adjustments are increases or decreases of rapid-acting insulin in addition to calculations using ICR and CF. Adjustments using trend arrows are an additional step to standard care.

Note on insulin sensitivity with developmental stages in pediatric patients: We provide five insulin sensitivity ranges. Notably, younger patients tend to be more insulin sensitive (higher CF) and older patients tend to be less insulin sensitive (lower CF). Typical decrease in insulin sensitivity is an important consideration in long-term care. Outliers may exist in any group.

Pre-School-Age/Toddlerhood (ages 2–6): often use CF ≥125
School Age/Middle-Childhood (ages 7–12): greatest variability
Adolescence/Young Adulthood (ages 13–22): often use CF 25–50 or <25

Considerations when adjusting for trend arrows:
If sensor glucose is rapidly rising (2 UP arrows; ↑↑) at pre-meal, consider administering insulin 15–30 min before eating.

If sensor glucose is rapidly falling (2 DOWN arrows; ↓↓) at pre-meal, consider administering insulin closer to the meal.

At bedtime, adjustments may be considered; however, use caution when adding insulin at that time. Suggest a bedtime target of 130 mg/dL with FLAT (→) or ANGLE UP (↗) arrow.

Approach does not require insulin on board to be set to 3 h.

[a]Correction factor (CF) is in mg/dL and indicates glucose lowering per unit of rapid-acting insulin.

Fig. 2. Using trend arrows for dosing at meal times. (*From* Laffel LM, Aleppo G, Buckingham BA, et al. A practical approach to using trend arrows on the dexcom G5 CGM system to manage children and adolescents with diabetes. *J Endocr Soc.* 2017;1(12):1461-1476; with permission.)

with injection therapy.[41] The cost of insulin pump therapy is another factor that parents may worry about when considering insulin pump therapy.[42] The cost of the insulin pump, infusion sets, and supplies can be expensive for families.[43]

To best prepare youth and families for success and best manage the challenges with CSII, structured education is needed. Health care providers' approach to educating families varies around the globe. For example, in France, youth may be hospitalized for a few days to start the pump, whereas in New Zealand, there can be substantial within-country variation, including both inpatient and outpatient training.[44] Their approach also varies with timing of the discontinuation of long-acting insulin and the use of CGM to assist with dosage changes.

The timing of when to initiate insulin pump use after diagnosis also varies. A recent study has indicated safe and effective use of insulin pump therapy at or shortly after diagnosis.[45] In another recent study that included a randomized controlled trial, there was no clinical difference between pump therapy and injection regimens during the first year of diagnosis.[46] In the United Kingdom, the Dose Adjustment for Normal Eating (DAFNE) trial showed that structured education for adults was beneficial for glycemic control improvement and benefits to quality of life.[47] Specifically, for pump education, after attending the 5-day pump education DAFNE course also yielded a reduction in severe hypoglycemia and improved psychosocial outcomes after 6 months. The DAFNE course covers the topics noted earlier, including insulin action, dosing, reducing hypoglycemia risk, sick day management, and insulin pump problem solving.[47] Specifically for pump education, a 5-day pump education DAFNE course also yielded a reduction in severe hypoglycemia and improved psychosocial outcomes after 6 months. The DAFNE course covers the topics noted earlier and in the table, including insulin action, dosing, reducing hypoglycemia risk, sick day management, and insulin pump problem-solving.[47] There has been a parallel, structured 5-day education course developed for youth with T1D, called KICk-OFF.[48] This program has been evaluated in a clustered-randomized clinical trial involving teens with T1D.[49] This study demonstrated improved quality of life outcomes in those receiving KICk-OFF compared with usual care 6 and 12 months following the structured education program although there were no differences in glycemic control. Such educational topics are usually covered repeatedly for youth with T1D and their families, as refresher education is generally an ongoing requirement during childhood and adolescence, especially when the youth acquires greater self-care responsibility. These topics are usually covered repeatedly for youth with T1D and their families, as refresher education is generally an ongoing requirement during childhood and adolescence, especially when the youth acquires greater self-care responsibility.

Next-Generation Insulin Pens

Smart pens offer technology integration to youth using pen-based, multiple daily injection therapy. Similar to insulin pumps, smart pens feature dose calculators that incorporate active insulin (insulin on board), record of insulin doses and times of administration, and downloadable report generation. The retrospective reports include calculation of total daily insulin dose, identification of missed doses, and potential to observe glycemic patterns to direct dose changes. Other features include notifications to administer rapid or long-acting insulin doses, low battery alerts, and insulin temperature or insulin expiry warnings. In 2016, the Companion InPen became the first FDA-approved insulin pen delivery device to wirelessly transmit such information by Bluetooth to a dedicated mobile application.[50] To date, there have not been any randomized control studies involving smart pen use in pediatrics. Education to use such devices generally involves one-on-one sessions to set-up the InPen application on a smart phone along with its bolus calculator.

Automated Insulin Delivery Systems

The current era of advanced diabetes devices includes some automation of insulin delivery that requires use of both a CGM device and an insulin pump with an imbedded or Bluetooth-connected algorithm.[31] The algorithm generates insulin dose recommendations based on the CGM glucose level and trends. The initial step of automation included pump basal rate suspension for low glucose levels, which was followed by predictive low glucose suspension, whereby the basal rate is suspended in anticipation of decreasing glucose levels. The current era now includes hybrid closed-loop systems that not only suspend basal rate insulin delivery to prevent hypoglycemia but also modulate basal rates upward for increasing or elevated glucose levels to prevent hyperglycemia. Such devices are called hybrid closed-loop systems, because the user still has to bolus for carbohydrate intake for meals and snacks and may need to provide or confirm insulin correction doses at times of hyperglycemia.

It is important for the education of the youth and family to be explicit regarding these remarkable advances, as there remains an ongoing need for youth and family input to set-up the systems, insert the CGM sensor, and set-up the insulin pump. The first hybrid closed-loop system, the MiniMed Medtronic 670G pump with the Guardian Sensor, was approved in the fall of 2016 for youths aged 14 years and older.[51] It has since been approved for children aged 7 years and older during the summer of 2018. Most recently, the Tandem X2 pump with the *Control IQ* algorithm has been successfully evaluated in a randomized control trial that included pediatric patients aged 14 years and older.[52]

Given the novelty of hybrid closed-loop systems, systematic educational approaches are just being introduced. The CARES paradigm can be used to guide clinicians and educators in practical application and teaching.[53] Another recently published approach suggests use of an in-person group class to review CGM and pump use, followed by a live video conference to teach use of the hybrid closed-loop, which is then followed by 3 phone calls over the next few weeks.[54] Other approaches include in-person, one-on-one, or group classes to implement the closed loop systems. With any of these approaches, close phone follow-up is needed.

SUMMARY: RECOGNIZING AND OVERCOMING POTENTIAL BARRIERS TO TECHNOLOGY UPTAKE AND CONTINUED USE IN YOUTH WITH TYPE 1 DIABETES

There can be multiple barriers to the uptake, use, and accessibility of diabetes technologies for youth with T1D.[26,55–57] There is need to ensure provision of realistic expectations when beginning any new device. It is as important to review what devices cannot do as much as it is important to ensure understanding of what devices can do. Further, education and support must extend beyond the youth and family, as multiple caregivers are generally involved in the care. Caregivers can include daycare providers, school nurses, teachers, babysitters, and after-school programs, among others. Structured education and written health care plans for all involved caregivers can provide practical guidance to support the successful adoption and use of technologies.[6,58]

Ongoing training and education in the use of diabetes technologies for youth and their families are needed, as the technologies are constantly being improved and updated. Such education and support can occur at times of routine follow-up care for youth with T1D, who are expected to maintain frequent contact with the health care team due to their frequent need for insulin dose adjustments, especially during periods of growth and development. The extraordinary advances in diabetes technologies have the potential to improve glycemic control and reduce some of the burdens of diabetes self-care for youth with T1D, especially if implemented and maintained with education and support for the person with diabetes and the family.

DISCLOSURE

Dr L.M. Laffel serves as a consultant for Eli Lilly, Sanofi, Novo Nordisk, AstraZeneca, Roche, Dexcom, Insulet, Boehringer Ingelheim, Janssen, Convatec, Insulogic.

ACKNOWLEDGMENTS

This work was partly supported by the National Institutes of Health under grants P30DK036836 and K12DK094721, the Katherine Adler Astrove Youth Education Fund, the Maria Griffin Drury Pediatric Fund, and the Eleanor Chesterman Beatson Fund. The content is solely the responsibility of the authors and does not necessarily represent the official views of these organizations.

REFERENCES

1. Phelan H, Lange K, Cengiz E, et al. ISPAD clinical practice consensus guidelines 2018: diabetes education in children and adolescents. Pediatr Diabetes 2018; 19(Suppl 27):75–83.
2. American Diabetes Association. 13. Children and adolescents: standards of medical care in diabetes-2019. Diabetes Care 2019;42(Suppl 1):S148–64.
3. Foster NC, Beck RW, Miller KM, et al. State of type 1 diabetes management and outcomes from the T1D exchange in 2016-2018. Diabetes Technol Ther 2019; 21(2):66–72.
4. Scaramuzza AE, Iafusco D, Rabbone I, et al. Use of integrated real-time continuous glucose monitoring/insulin pump system in children and adolescents with type 1 diabetes: a 3-year follow-up study. Diabetes Technol Ther 2011;13(2): 99–103.
5. McGill DE, Volkening LK, Butler DA, et al. Baseline psychosocial characteristics predict frequency of continuous glucose monitoring in youth with type 1 diabetes. Diabetes Technol Ther 2018;20(6):434–9.
6. Van Name MA, Miller KM, Commissariat PV, et al. Greater parental comfort with lower glucose targets in young children with Type 1 diabetes using continuous glucose monitoring. Diabet Med 2019;36(11):1508–10.
7. Hilliard ME, Levy W, Anderson BJ, et al. Benefits and barriers of continuous glucose monitoring in young children with type 1 diabetes. Diabetes Technol Ther 2019;21(9):493–8.
8. Deiss D, Bolinder J, Riveline JP, et al. Improved glycemic control in poorly controlled patients with type 1 diabetes using real-time continuous glucose monitoring. Diabetes Care 2006;29(12):2730–2.
9. Juvenile Diabetes Research Foundation Continuous Glucose Monitoring Study Group. Factors predictive of use and of benefit from continuous glucose monitoring in type 1 diabetes. Diabetes Care 2009;32(11):1947–53.
10. Mauras N, Beck R, Xing D, et al. A randomized clinical trial to assess the efficacy and safety of real-time continuous glucose monitoring in the management of type 1 diabetes in young children aged 4 to <10 years. Diabetes Care 2012;35(2): 204–10.

11. Pickup JC, Freeman SC, Sutton AJ. Glycaemic control in type 1 diabetes during real time continuous glucose monitoring compared with self monitoring of blood glucose: meta-analysis of randomised controlled trials using individual patient data. BMJ 2011;343:d3805.
12. Giani E, Snelgrove R, Volkening LK, et al. Continuous glucose monitoring (CGM) adherence in youth with type 1 diabetes: associations with biomedical and psychosocial variables. J Diabetes Sci Technol 2017;11(3):476–83.
13. Beck RW, Riddlesworth T, Ruedy K, et al. Effect of continuous glucose monitoring on glycemic control in adults with type 1 diabetes using insulin injections: the DIAMOND randomized clinical trial. JAMA 2017;317(4):371–8.
14. Miller KM, Foster NC, Beck RW, et al. Current state of type 1 diabetes treatment in the U.S.: updated data from the T1D exchange clinic registry. Diabetes Care 2015;38(6):971–8.
15. Markowitz JT, Harrington KR, Laffel LM. Technology to optimize pediatric diabetes management and outcomes. Curr Diab Rep 2013;13(6):877–85.
16. Laffel L. Improved accuracy of continuous glucose monitoring systems in pediatric patients with diabetes mellitus: results from two studies. Diabetes Technol Ther 2016;18(Suppl 2):S223–33.
17. Mulinacci G, Alonso GT, Snell-Bergeon JK, et al. Glycemic outcomes with early initiation of continuous glucose monitoring system in recently diagnosed patients with type 1 diabetes. Diabetes Technol Ther 2019;21(1):6–10.
18. Sherr JL, Tauschmann M, Battelino T, et al. ISPAD clinical practice consensus guidelines 2018: diabetes technologies. Pediatr Diabetes 2018;19(Suppl 27): 302–25.
19. Klonoff DC, Buckingham B, Christiansen JS, et al. Continuous glucose monitoring: an endocrine society clinical practice guideline. J Clin Endocrinol Metab 2011;96(10):2968–79.
20. Bailey TS, Grunberger G, Bode BW, et al. American Association of Clinical Endocrinologists and American College of Endocrinology 2016 outpatient glucose monitoring consensus statement. Endocr Pract 2016;22(2):231–61.
21. American Diabetes A. 6. Glycemic targets: standards of medical care in diabetes-2019. Diabetes Care 2019;42(Suppl 1):S61–70.
22. DeSalvo DJ, Miller KM, Hermann JM, et al. Continuous glucose monitoring and glycemic control among youth with type 1 diabetes: international comparison from the T1D exchange and DPV initiative. Pediatr Diabetes 2018;19(7):1271–5.
23. Laffel LM, Aleppo G, Buckingham BA, et al. A practical approach to using trend arrows on the dexcom G5 CGM system to manage children and adolescents with diabetes. J Endocr Soc 2017;1(12):1461–76.
24. Phillip M, Danne T, Shalitin S, et al. Use of continuous glucose monitoring in children and adolescents. Pediatr Diabetes 2012;13(3):215–28.
25. Tansey M, Laffel L, Cheng J, et al. Satisfaction with continuous glucose monitoring in adults and youths with type 1 diabetes. Diabet Med 2011;28(9):1118–22.
26. Naranjo D, Tanenbaum ML, Iturralde E, et al. Diabetes technology: uptake, outcomes, barriers, and the intersection with distress. J Diabetes Sci Technol 2016;10(4):852–8.
27. Barnard KD, Breton MD. Diabetes technological revolution: winners and losers? J Diabetes Sci Technol 2018;12(6):1227–30.
28. Rodbard D. Continuous glucose monitoring: a review of successes, challenges, and opportunities. Diabetes Technol Ther 2016;18(Suppl 2):S3–13.

29. Lawton J, Blackburn M, Allen J, et al. Patients' and caregivers' experiences of using continuous glucose monitoring to support diabetes self-management: qualitative study. BMC Endocr Disord 2018;18(1):12.
30. Forlenza GP, Argento NB, Laffel LM. Practical considerations on the use of continuous glucose monitoring in pediatrics and older adults and nonadjunctive use. Diabetes Technol Ther 2017;19(S3):S13–20.
31. Beck RW, Bergenstal RM, Laffel LM, et al. Advances in technology for management of type 1 diabetes. Lancet 2019;394(10205):1265–73.
32. Laffel LM, Pratt KE, Aggarwal J, et al. Psychosocial impact of real-time continuous glucose monitoring (CGM) in type 1 diabetes (T1D) [abstract]. Diabetes 2009;58(Suppl 1):A485.
33. Danne T, Nimri R, Battelino T, et al. International consensus on use of continuous glucose monitoring. Diabetes Care 2017;40(12):1631–40.
34. Beyond A1C Writing Group. Need for regulatory change to incorporate beyond A1C glycemic metrics. Diabetes Care 2018;41(6):e92–4.
35. Riddlesworth TD, Beck RW, Gal RL, et al. Optimal sampling duration for continuous glucose monitoring to determine long-term glycemic control. Diabetes Technol Ther 2018;20(4):314–6.
36. Battelino T, Danne T, Bergenstal RM, et al. Clinical targets for continuous glucose monitoring data interpretation: recommendations from the international consensus on time in range. Diabetes Care 2019;42(8):1593–603.
37. Benkhadra K, Alahdab F, Tamhane SU, et al. Continuous subcutaneous insulin infusion versus multiple daily injections in individuals with type 1 diabetes: a systematic review and meta-analysis. Endocrine 2017;55(1):77–84.
38. Johansen A, Kanijo B, Fredheim S, et al. Prevalence and predictors of severe hypoglycemia in Danish children and adolescents with diabetes. Pediatr Diabetes 2015;16(5):354–60.
39. Hussain T, Akle M, Nagelkerke N, et al. Comparative study on treatment satisfaction and health perception in children and adolescents with type 1 diabetes mellitus on multiple daily injection of insulin, insulin pump and sensor-augmented pump therapy. SAGE Open Med 2017;5. 2050312117694938.
40. Mueller-Godeffroy E, Vonthein R, Ludwig-Seibold C, et al. Psychosocial benefits of insulin pump therapy in children with diabetes type 1 and their families: the pumpkin multicenter randomized controlled trial. Pediatr Diabetes 2018;19(8):1471–80.
41. Maahs DM, Hermann JM, Holman N, et al. Rates of diabetic ketoacidosis: international comparison with 49,859 pediatric patients with type 1 diabetes from England, Wales, the U.S., Austria, and Germany. Diabetes Care 2015;38(10):1876–82.
42. Commissariat PV, Boyle CT, Miller KM, et al. Insulin pump use in young children with type 1 diabetes: sociodemographic factors and parent-reported barriers. Diabetes Technol Ther 2017;19(6):363–9.
43. Toresson Grip E, Svensson AM, Miftaraj M, et al. Real-world costs of continuous insulin pump therapy and multiple daily injections for type 1 diabetes: a population-based and propensity-matched cohort from the Swedish National Diabetes register. Diabetes Care 2019;42(4):545–52.
44. AbdulAziz YH, Al-Sallami HS, Wiltshire E, et al. Insulin pump initiation and education for children and adolescents - a qualitative study of current practice in New Zealand. J Diabetes Metab Disord 2019;18(1):59–64.

45. Lang EG, King BR, Miller MN, et al. Initiation of insulin pump therapy in children at diagnosis of type 1 diabetes resulted in improved long-term glycemic control. Pediatr Diabetes 2017;18(1):26–32.
46. Blair JC, McKay A, Ridyard C, et al. Continuous subcutaneous insulin infusion versus multiple daily injection regimens in children and young people at diagnosis of type 1 diabetes: pragmatic randomised controlled trial and economic evaluation. BMJ 2019;365:l1226.
47. Heller S, Lawton J, Amiel S, et al. Improving management of type 1 diabetes in the UK: the Dose Adjustment for Normal Eating (DAFNE) programme as a research test-bed. A mixed-method analysis of the barriers to and facilitators of successful diabetes self-management, a health economic analysis, a cluster randomised controlled trial of different models of delivery of an educational intervention and the potential of insulin pumps and additional educator input to improve outcomes. Southampton (United Kingdom): NIHR Journals Library; 2014.
48. Price K. KICk-OFF. Available at: www.dafne.uk.com/uploads/443/documents/KICK-OFF%20-%20Dr%20Kath%20Price.pdf. Accessed November 4, 2019.
49. Price KJ, Knowles JA, Fox M, et al. Effectiveness of the Kids in Control of Food (KICk-OFF) structured education course for 11-16 year olds with Type 1 diabetes. Diabet Med 2016;33(2):192–203.
50. Department of Health and Human Services, Food and Drug Administration. 510(k) summary letter correspondence for Companion Medical InPen System, indications for use approval form. Available at: www.accessdata.fda.gov/cdrh_docs/pdf16/k160629.pdf. Accessed May 20, 2019.
51. Bergenstal RM, Garg S, Weinzimer SA, et al. Safety of a hybrid closed-loop insulin delivery system in patients with type 1 diabetes. JAMA 2016;316(13):1407–8.
52. Brown SA, Kovatchev BP, Raghinaru D, et al. Six-month randomized, multicenter trial of closed-loop control in type 1 diabetes. N Engl J Med 2019;381(18):1707–17.
53. Messer LH, Berget C, Forlenza GP. A clinical guide to advanced diabetes devices and closed-loop systems using the CARES paradigm. Diabetes Technol Ther 2019;21(8):462–9.
54. Garg SK, Weinzimer SA, Tamborlane WV, et al. Glucose outcomes with the in-home use of a hybrid closed-loop insulin delivery system in adolescents and adults with type 1 diabetes. Diabetes Technol Ther 2017;19(3):155–63.
55. Forlenza GP, Messer LH, Berget C, et al. Biopsychosocial factors associated with satisfaction and sustained use of artificial pancreas technology and its components: a call to the technology field. Curr Diab Rep 2018;18(11):114.
56. Wong JC, Foster NC, Maahs DM, et al. Real-time continuous glucose monitoring among participants in the T1D exchange clinic registry. Diabetes Care 2014;37(10):2702–9.
57. Telo GH, Volkening LK, Butler DA, et al. Salient characteristics of youth with type 1 diabetes initiating continuous glucose monitoring. Diabetes Technol Ther 2015;17(6):373–8.
58. Bratina N, Battelino T. Insulin pumps and continuous glucose monitoring (CGM) in preschool and school-age children: how schools can integrate technology. Pediatr Endocrinol Rev 2010;7(Suppl 3):417–21.

Diabetes Technology Use in Adults with Type 1 and Type 2 Diabetes

Jelena Kravarusic, MD, PhD, Grazia Aleppo, MD*

KEYWORDS

- Continuous glucose monitoring (CGM)
- Continuous subcutaneous insulin infusion (CSII) • Sensor-augmented pump (SAP)
- Hybrid closed loop • Patch pump

KEY POINTS

- Continuous glucose monitoring systems have become established tools in diabetes management to provide real-time glucose information that can be used for treatment decisions in patients with type 1 and insulin-treated type 2 diabetes.
- Insulin pumps are useful tools for diabetes management, offering insulin dosing flexibility and reducing hypoglycemia risk; patch pumps are also emerging as useful tools for simplified insulin therapy in patients with type 2 diabetes.
- Sensor-augmented pumps and hybrid closed-loop systems are evolving into sophisticated diabetes management tools to improve glucometrics such as time in range and glycemic variability, as well as decreasing the burden of diabetes disease management.

INTRODUCTION

Management of patients with type 1 diabetes mellitus (T1DM) and type 2 diabetes mellitus (T2DM) on intensive insulin therapy consists of 2 integral parts: glucose measurement and insulin delivery. Both have undergone substantial evolution and enhancement in the past several years. Over time, self-monitoring of blood glucose (SMBG) systems have become easier to use and have achieved improved accuracy[1]; however, they offer only static information about glucose levels without taking into consideration the dynamic nature of glucose changes. By contrast, CGM technology has enabled patients and clinicians to gain a more comprehensive view of glycemic trends and patterns, uncovering a wealth of information not available in the past.[2] With increased sensor duration, improved accuracy, and reduced mean absolute

Funding Sources: None.
Division of Endocrinology, Metabolism and Molecular Medicine, Feinberg School of Medicine, Northwestern University, 645 North Michigan Avenue, Suite 530, Chicago, IL 60611, USA
* Corresponding author.
E-mail address: aleppo@northwestern.edu

Endocrinol Metab Clin N Am 49 (2020) 37–55
https://doi.org/10.1016/j.ecl.2019.10.006 endo.theclinics.com

relative difference (MARD) to 10% or less, most available CGM systems can now be safely used to make therapeutic dose decisions.[3–5]

Continuous subcutaneous insulin infusion (CSII) systems, or insulin pumps, have evolved from rudimentary mechanical syringes with limited dosing flexibility, to "smart" systems with bolus calculators and advanced features that can modulate insulin delivery with greater flexibility and accuracy; in addition, their integration with CGM has enhanced insulin pumps into semiautomated systems able to decrease, suspend, or resume the delivery of basal insulin doses based on feedback from CGM data.[6,7]

CONTINUOUS GLUCOSE MONITORING SYSTEMS

CGM systems have become integral tools for diabetes management in less than 2 decades. Guidelines published by professional societies such as the Endocrine Society, the American Diabetes Association, and the American Association for Clinical Endocrinologists have endorsed CGM as standard of care for use in people with T1DM.[6–9] In November 2018, a supplement to the Endocrine Society Technology Guideline was published with additional reported evidence that CGM benefits are also observed in people with T2DM.[7] Presently, multiple systems are available as stand-alone systems or integrated systems with insulin pumps[10–15] (**Table 1**). Of note, the Dexcom G6 (San Diego, CA) system was recently approved by the US Food and Drug Administration (FDA) as the first interoperable CGM system, compatible with other medical devices (class II special controls).[24] CGM systems measure glucose levels continuously in the interstitial fluid; most systems use an enzymatic reaction with glucose oxidase as a substrate, whereas the implantable Eversense system from Senseonics (Germantown, MA) uses a fluorescence-sensing technology.[25] Data from the sensors are sent to a transmitter and displayed in various devices. Stand-alone CGM systems display the information on either a receiver (Dexcom G4 Platinum/Dexcom G5/G6, FreeStyle Libre 14 day) or via mobile applications on smartphones and smartwatches (Apple/Android for Dexcom G5/G6 Mobile; Apple for Medtronic Guardian Connect Mobile, Apple/Android for FreeStyle Libre 14 days).[10–15,26]

CGM systems can be divided into 2 categories: professional (or diagnostic) and personal. Professional CGM devices can be blinded or unblinded to the patient. In the blinded version, the wearer cannot see any CGM recorded information until the data are uploaded and reviewed with the clinician in a retrospective fashion; at that time, targeted regimen changes can be made based on glucose trends and patterns revealed by the CGM tracings.[27] Professional blinded CGM systems record information for 6, 7, or up to 14 days.[28–30] The unblinded professional CGM systems allow patients to view their glucose levels in real time during the procedure (up to 7 days), receive alerts and alarms, and make therapeutic interventions during the procedure and/or after evaluation of the data with the health care provider.

Personal CGM systems are approved by the FDA for use in T1DM and in general for patients with T2DM treated with intensive insulin regimen; the sensor life ranges from 7 to 90 days.[10–15] In January 2017, CGM coverage was extended for the first time to Centers for Medicare and Medicaid Services (CMS) beneficiaries with diabetes, treated with at least 3 insulin injections per day, measuring glucose levels by fingerstick 4 times per day, and requiring frequent insulin adjustments.[31] At the time of this writing, the CMS-approved systems are Dexcom G5 and G6 systems and Abbott FreeStyle Libre 14 days (Abbott Diabetes Care, Alameda, CA).[32–34] Personal CGM systems are in 2 categories: real-time CGM (rt-CGM) and intermittent scanned CGM (is-CGM) systems. rt-CGM systems[10–15] (see **Table 1**) provide users with current

Table 1
Key features of current personal and professional continuous glucose monitoring systems

	Personal							Professional		
	rt-CGM						is-CGM			
CGM Category	Dexcom G6[13]	Dexcom G5[12]	Dexcom G4 Platinum[16]	Medtronic Guardian 3[10,11]	Medtronic Enlite 2[17]	Senseonic Eversense[18]	Abbott Freestyle Flash Libre[19,20]	Medtronic Enlite iPro2[21]	Dexcom G4 Professional[22]	Abbott Freestyle Libre Pro[23]
Population Age (y)	≥2	≥2	≥2	≥7	≥16	≥18	United States: ≥18 Non–United States: ≥4	≥7	≥2	United States: ≥18
Pregnancy Approval	No	No	No	No	No	No	United States: no Non–United States: yes	No	No	No
Warm-up time (h)	2	2	2	2	2	24	10 d: 12 14-d: 1	2	2	2
Sensor wear (d)	10	7	7	7	6	United States: 90 Non–United States: 180	10–14	6	7	14
Calibrations	None	2/d	2/d	2–4/d	2/d	2/d	None	NA	2/d	NA
Nonadjunctive Use	Yes	Yes	No	No	No	Yes	Yes	NA	NA	NA
Audible Alarms/Alerts	Yes Hypoglycemia predictive alerts	Yes	Yes	Yes Predictive alerts	Yes Predictive alerts	Yes Predictive alerts (vibrates)	No	NA	Blinded: no Unblinded: yes	NA
Trend Arrows	Yes	Yes	Yes	Yes	Yes	Yes	Yes	NA	Blinded: no Unblinded: yes	NA

(*continued on next page*)

Table 1 (continued)

	Personal							Professional		
	rt-CGM						is-CGM			
CGM Category	Dexcom G6[13]	Dexcom G5[12]	Dexcom G4 Platinum[16]	Medtronic Guardian 3[10,11]	Medtronic Enlite 2[17]	Senseonic Everserse[18]	Abbott Freestyle Flash Libre[19,20]	Medtronic Enlite iPro2[21]	Dexcom G4 Professional[22]	Abbott Freestyle Libre Pro[23]
Share features	Yes	Yes	Yes	Guardian Connect Mobile only (Apple)	No	Yes	14-d system only (LibreLink)	NA	NA	NA
Pump integration	Tandem t:slim X2 with Basal IQ	Tandem t:slim X2	Animas Vibe Tandem t:slim G4	Medtronic 670G	Medtronic Revel, 530G, 630G	None	None	NA	NA	NA
Software Compatibility	Dexcom CLARITY Glooko Tidepool	Dexcom CLARITY Glooko Tidepool	Dexcom Studio Glooko Tidepool	Medtronic CareLink Tidepool	Medtronic CareLink	Glooko	LibreView Tidepool (reader only)	iPro CareLink	Dexcom Studio	LibreView
Acetaminophen Interference	No	Yes	Yes	Yes	Yes	No	No	Yes	Yes	No
MARD (%)	9	9	9	Abdominal 10.6[a]-9.6[b] Arm 9.1[a]-8.7[b]	13.6	8.8	10 d: 9.7 14 d: 9.4	13.6	9	12.3
Radiograph/MRI Compatible	No	No	No	No	No	Yes	No	No	No	No

Abbreviations: is-CGM, intermittent scanned CGM; NA, not available; rt-CGM, real-time CGM.

[a] Two calibrations per day.

[b] Four calibrations per day.

Data from Refs.[10–13,16–23]

sensor glucose visualization, its direction with rate-of-change trend arrows, as well as alerts and alarms for current and impending hypoglycemia or hyperglycemia. Some systems also have predictive alerts for urgent low sensor glucose levels,[13] whereas others alert the user with on-body transmitter vibration.[15] is-CGM systems measure glucose levels continuously and record readings every 15 minutes; however, they require that the user actively scan (flash) the sensor/transmitter unit using a reader or through a smartphone application in order to display the glucose information.[26] The only US-approved is-CGM, Abbott FreeStyle Libre, currently does not have audible alerts or alarms; an updated FreeStyle Libre 2 system has recently received Conformité Européene mark in Europe and will have optional alerts or alarms for hypoglycemia or hyperglycemia.[35] Because of these cardinal differences, individual patients' needs must be considered when making a recommendation for therapeutic CGM. In general, rt-CGM systems should be considered in most patients with T1DM, as well as individuals at risk of hypoglycemia, with history of hypoglycemia unawareness and history of frequent nocturnal hypoglycemia. In contrast, is-CGM can be useful in patients with T2DM who are not on intensive insulin therapy, who have intact hypoglycemia awareness, and who are unable to monitor their glucose by finger-stick as frequently as is recommended.[36] Most available CGM systems are approved for nonadjunctive use, and although recent factory-calibrated CGM systems have virtually eliminated the need for confirmatory blood glucose levels by finger-stick (see **Table 1**), it should be emphasized that, when symptoms do not match CGM readings, if the user suspects the reading is inaccurate, or if there are no trend arrows displayed, a finger-stick for insulin dosing decisions may be prudent.

CGM reports can be reviewed by the user through mobile applications and by clinicians on various platforms (Dexcom CLARITY, Diasend-Glooko, Tidepool, LibreView, and Medtronic CareLink). Consensus reports for the standardization of clinically meaningful outcome measures as well as clinical targets for CGM data interpretation have recently been published.[37–39] The ambulatory glucose profile has become the standard CGM report, and it includes a variety of glucometrics, from time in range (70–180 mg/dL or 3.9–10 mmol/L), time below range (<70 mg/dL or <3.9 mmol/L), and time above range (>180 mg/dL or >10 mmol/L), to glycemic variability and glucose management indicator.[39] Review of the CGM tracings provides insights into the duration and frequency of glucose fluctuations and can assist patients and clinicians to identify problematic areas with excess hypoglycemia or hyperglycemia to formulate personalized therapy adjustments.

CGM systems use trend arrows to convey rates of glucose change to the user, who can then anticipate future glucose concentrations and make adjustments in insulin dosing. To date there are several published methods for using trend arrow data to adjust insulin doses.[40–46] Available recommendations on interpretation of trend arrows for insulin adjustments are mostly based on expert opinion[41–46] and have yet to be validated in randomized controlled trials. With this in mind, it is imperative that health care providers take an individualized approach when applying trend arrows to treatment decisions. Of note, available CGM systems have different rate-of-change trend arrows meanings. To avoid confusion and dosing errors, education should be focused on the specific system patients are using.[43–46]

CLINICAL BENEFITS OF CONTINUOUS GLUCOSE MONITORING USE IN TYPE 1 AND TYPE 2 DIABETES

Since the introduction of CGM technology 2 decades ago, more than 30 clinical trials have been completed, with more than 4000 subjects enrolled over time.[47] These data have shown that, even with older CGM systems, patients experienced improved hemoglobin A1c (HbA1c) levels and/or decrease in hypoglycemia. In some studies, CGM use was found to be particularly beneficial for patients with higher risk for hypoglycemia or hypoglycemia unawareness.[48,49] In the seminal JDRF CGM study, 322 adults and children with T1DM were randomly assigned to either CGM or usual glucose monitoring. The results showed age-based and use-related decrease in HbA1c level of 0.53% (*P* = .003) in adults more than 25 years old, but not in children or adolescents.[50] In a subsequent analysis, the JDRF study group evaluated the effect of CGM therapy on time spent in hypoglycemia, HbA1c, and severe hypoglycemia in 129 adults and children using either multiple daily injections of insulin (MDI) or CSII with a baseline HbA1c level less than 7% (53 mmol/mol). CGM use in this group of well-controlled T1DM reduced significantly HbA1c level (≥0.3%, *P*≤.001) and duration of time spent in glucose less than 60 mg/dL (3.3 mmol/L) (*P* = .05).[51] In the COMISAIR study, 65 patients with T1DM, using either sensor-augmented CSII or MDI, versus CSII alone or MDI alone, were followed for up to 1 year. CGM users experienced the greatest HbA1c reduction of 1.2% (*P*≤.0001) regardless of the method of insulin delivery. In addition, CGM users had less hypoglycemia compared with other groups (*P*<.01).[52]

Although earlier studies included mostly patients on insulin pump therapy, more recent studies have focused on patients using MDI. In 2017, the DIAMOND study examined the effectiveness of using CGM in improving glycemic control in participants with T1DM using MDI, and randomized 152 participants to CGM plus SMBG or SMBG alone for 24 weeks. The CGM group participants experienced not only a greater reduction in HbA1c, with an adjusted treatment-group difference of −0.6% (*P*<.001), but also a greater reduction of time in hypoglycemia (<70 mg/dL or 3.9 mmol/L) (*P* = .002) and greater percentage of time spent in the targeted range (70–180 mg/dL or 3.9–10 mmol/L) (*P* = .005).[53] Of note, in the same cohort, significant improvement of diabetes-specific quality of life measures (diabetes distress, hypoglycemia confidence) were noted with CGM use.[54] In the DIAMOND type 2 trial, 158 patients with T2DM were randomly assigned to CGM versus usual care. At the end of the study, the adjusted difference in mean change in HbA1c level from baseline was −0.3% (*P* = .022) in the CGM group.[55] Published the same year, the GOLD trial enrolled 161 participants with T1DM in a crossover design of CGM versus SMBG. HbA1c level was again reduced by 0.43% (*P*<.001) when on CGM. Of note, time spent in hypoglycemia was 2.79% during the CGM period and 4.79% during conventional therapy.[56] In a subsequent study, the GOLD-3 trial, T1DM participants using MDI and CGM experienced less daytime and nocturnal hypoglycemia and improved hypoglycemia-related confidence, especially in social situations, thus contributing to greater well-being and quality of life.[57]

Similar results have been observed when studying the effect of is-CGM FreeStyle Libre in patients with T1DM and T2DM. The IMPACT study enrolled 241 participants with T1DM (MDI and CSII), and, at 6 months, is-CGM users experienced a 38% reduction of time spent in hypoglycemia (*P*<.0001). In the same group, time in range (70–180 mg/dL or 3.9–10 mmol/L) increased by 1 hour (*P* = .0006).[58] Similarly, the REPLACE study on patients with T2DM (n = 224) showed reduction of time spent in hypoglycemia by 43% (*P* = .0006),[59] although neither study showed any change in HbA1c level.

Most recently, the efficacy and safety of CGM initiation within 12 months of T1DM diagnosis was evaluated. In this retrospective study (n = 396; 94% aged <18 years, 6% aged >18 years), early initiation of CGM, irrespective of mode of insulin use, was effective in lowering and maintaining HbA1c level for 2.5 years (MDI + CGM −2.2%, *P*<.001, and CSII + CGM −1.1%, *P*<.001). In addition, reduced emergency department–related visits were noted. The investigators concluded that early initiation of CGM at diagnosis may help to improve long-term glycemic control and may reduce future diabetes-related complications.[60] Taken together, all these studies confirm the benefits of CGM therapy regardless of the type of diabetes or insulin therapy modality.

INSULIN PUMP THERAPY

CSII systems or insulin pumps were initially introduced in the late 1970s[61] and have undergone substantial modifications over the years to provide flexible insulin delivery. Preset variable basal rates or patterns can be programmed, and on-demand changes to basal rates (temporary basal rates) can be implemented for increased or decreased insulin requirements, such as for the management of noncritical illnesses or at the time of physical activity. Similarly, simple and advanced mealtime bolus types can be programmed with the assistance of various types of bolus calculators in all commercially available systems (**Table 2**). Insulin pumps differ from conventional MDI in that they use only rapid-acting insulin delivered via tubing to a subcutaneously placed cannula. Nontubed insulin pump systems, or patch pumps, eliminate the need for tubing because the infusion cannula is connected to the insulin reservoir component that is placed directly on the skin. In the early 2000s, several insulin pump systems became integrated with CGM, initially just showing CGM tracings on the insulin pump screen. Subsequently, these systems were enhanced to enable glucose-responsive automated insulin adjustments, from the threshold-suspend features and suspension of basal insulin for up to 2 hours, to predictive low-glucose suspend features based on predicted hypoglycemia trend on CGM, with suspension of basal infusion and resumed insulin infusion on normalization or up-trending of CGM data.[73–78] In addition, with the approval of the MiniMed 670G system (Medtronic, Northridge, CA) in 2016, the first hybrid closed-loop system appeared on the market.[79] This system, when in auto mode, allows fully automated basal insulin through a proportional-integral derivative control algorithm, which enables variable insulin delivery doses every 5 minutes to a target of 120 mg/dL (6.6 mmol/L). Approved for T1DM and T2DM, insulin pumps are used by more than 1 million people worldwide and about 400,000 in the United States to manage their diabetes.[80] In February 2019, the FDA authorized the marketing of the Tandem t:slim X2 with Basal IQ (Tandem Diabetes, San Diego, CA) pump as the first alternate controller-enabled (ACE) pump or interoperable pump, intended to allow patients to customize treatment through their individual diabetes management devices.[68] Several additional automated insulin delivery systems are under investigation and excitement is building that future systems will reduce the burden of diabetes management.[81]

BENEFITS OF INSULIN PUMP THERAPY IN TYPE 1 AND TYPE 2 DIABETES

Although insulin pumps have been available for almost 3 decades, most clinical trials investigating their benefits have shown generally modest (−0.3% to −0.6%) reduction in HbA1c levels.[6] Challenges in identifying pump therapy benefits include small cohorts and the use of non-analog insulin in earlier studies.[6] Nevertheless, a consistent benefit in severe hypoglycemia risk reduction has been noted in patients using CSII.[82] Early meta-analyses favored CSII for improved glycemic control without concomitant increase in the rate of hypoglycemia in T1DM.[83] In the 2016 Endocrine Society Diabetes Technology Clinical Practice Guidelines, the use of CSII was recommended rather than MDI in patients with T1DM with above-target HbA1c levels or with target HbA1c levels but with persistent severe hypoglycemia or glucose variability. In addition, the use of insulin pump therapy in T1DM was suggested for individuals with

Table 2
Key features of current United States Food and Drug Administration–approved insulin pump systems

	Population (y)	Medicare Coverage	Reservoir Capacity	Bolus Calculator	Advanced Bolus Features	Food Database	Temporary Basal Rates Features and Duration	CGM Integration	Software Compatibility
Medtronic MiniMed 630G[62,63]	≥14	Yes, part B	Up to 300 units	Yes, on pump	Yes	No	Yes. From 0% to 200% or units per hour 30 min to 24 h. Limited by maximum basal rate	Yes, Enlite 2	Medtronic CareLink
Medtronic MiniMed 670G[62,64]	>7	No	Up to 300 units	Yes, on pump	Yes	No	Suspend before low: yes From 0% to 200% or units per hour 30 min to 24 h. Limited by maximum basal rate Auto mode: temperature target Target blood glucose increased to 150 mg/dL up to 12 h	Yes, Guardian 3	Medtronic CareLink Tidepool Glooko
Tandem t:slim[62,65]	>6	Yes, part B	Up to 300 units	Yes, on pump	Yes	No	Yes. From 0% to 250% of current basal 15 min to 72 h. Limited by maximum basal rate	Yes, Dexcom G4	t:Connect Tidepool Glooko
Tandem t:slim X2[62,66]	>6	Yes, part B	Up to 300 units	Yes, on pump	Yes	No	Yes. From 0% to 250% of current basal 15 min to 72 h. Limited by maximum basal rate	Yes, Dexcom G5	t:Connect Tidepool Glooko
Tandem t:slim X2 with Basal IQ[62,67,68]	>6	Yes, part B	Up to 300 units	Yes, on pump	Yes	No	Yes. From 0% to 250% of current basal 15 min to 72 h. Limited by maximum basal rate	Yes, Dexcom G6	t:Connect Tidepool Glooko

Insulet Omnipod[62,69]	All ages	Yes, part D	Up to 200 units	Yes, on PDM	Yes	Yes, 1000 foods database	Yes. From −100% to +95% or units per hour 30 min to 12 h. Limited by maximum basal rate	No	Tidepool Glooko
Insulet Omnipod DASH[62,70]	All ages	Yes, part D	Up to 200 units	Yes, on DASH	Yes	Yes, Calorie King database (>80,000 foods)	Yes. From −100% to +95% or units per hour 30 min to 12 h. Limited by maximum basal rate	No	Tidepool Glooko
Valeritas V-Go[71]	>18	Yes, part B	Basal: 20–30–40 units/d Bolus: up to 36 units/d	No	No	No	No	No	None
PAQ Meal (CeQur)[72]	>18	NA	Up to 200 units Bolus only	No	No	No	No	No	None

Abbreviation: PDM, personal diabetes manager.
Data from Refs.[62–72]

increased insulin delivery flexibility requirements.[6] Similarly, the American Diabetes Association and the American Association of Clinical Endocrinologists have endorsed the use of insulin pump therapy for patients with T1DM who have not achieved their target HbA1c goals and have increased risk for hypoglycemia.[9,73] In 2017, a meta-analysis of 25 randomized controlled trials directly compared MDI and CSII, measuring the absolute and relative change in HbA1c levels during the study period of each clinical trial. Also, it measured the impact of MDI and CSII therapy on severe and nocturnal hypoglycemia, measured as the absolute number of recorded events as well as time spent in hypoglycemia. The results showed an absolute reduction in HbA1c level of 0.42% in adults on CSII (P = .001) compared with MDI. There was no significant difference in severe hypoglycemia between the two groups. However, in adult patients, the use of CSII was associated with fewer nocturnal hypoglycemia episodes compared with MDI (P = .003).[84]

More significant changes in glucometrics have been observed in clinical trials using sensor-augmented insulin pumps (SAPs). In the Sensor-augmented Pump Therapy for A1C Reduction (STAR) 3 trial, 485 patients with inadequately controlled T1DM were followed for 1 year using SAP therapy versus MDI. At 1 year, SAP therapy was superior to MDI, with a between-group difference in HbA1c level in the SAP group of −0.6% (P<.001) without differences in rates of severe hypoglycemia.[75] In the continuation phase study, crossover participants experienced significant decrease in HbA1c level (−0.4%, P = .001), whereas patients who continued on SAP maintained lower HbA1c levels.[85]

Recently, the use of SAP systems in a real-world experience was reported in an anonymized data analysis from CareLink in 920 patients with T1DM. The median time spent with sensor glucose (SG) level less than 54 mg/dL (3 mmol/L) was 0.8% in the SAP group, versus 0.3% in the sensor-integrated pump with low-glucose suspend group, and 0.3% in the sensor-integrated pump with predictive low-glucose management group.[86] In a prospective study assessing the long-term effects of the treatment change to CSII and CGM, patients with T1DM on MDI were followed for almost 7 years. A decrease in HbA1c level from baseline was observed at 12 months in the CSII group (−0.84%, P = .0001); at 24 months, HbA1c level decreased further once CGM was introduced (−0.41%, P = .051). At the end of the study period, no change in rate of newly diagnosed microvascular complications was observed.[87] Additional studies on the use of hybrid closed-loop systems have been published emphasizing the effects on reduction of hypoglycemia and increased time in range.[88]

The use of insulin pumps for patients with T2DM is a more recent practice, but with small numbers of patients until 2014, when the first large-scale trial, OpT2imise, was reported, in which 331 patients with T2DM were randomized to CSII or MDI for 6 months, with between-group improvement in HbA1c level (−0.7%, P<.0001) for CSII and smaller total daily insulin doses (TDDs) (P<.0001) without weight changes.[89] In a recent meta-analysis of insulin pump use in T2DM, CSII users also achieved greater reduction of HbA1c level (−0.4%) than MDI and a 26% reduction in insulin requirements without weight changes.[90] Similarly, a review of CSII studies in patients with T2DM suggested that CSII use can be applicable to T2DM, with caveats of cost, capability, and willingness to manage a technical device.[91] To improve adherence and simplify insulin regimens, insulin delivery options specifically designed for T2DM have been developed to allow simpler basal-bolus therapy and easier incorporation into daily living. The V-Go (Valeritas, Inc, Bridgewater, NJ) is a disposable, mechanical insulin device that delivers a continuous, preset basal rate of insulin (20, 30, or 40 U/24 h) with an additional 36 units of insulin per day for bolus administration. The V-Go is worn like a patch, and, after activation of the needle button perpendicularly to the skin surface, the patient can deliver on-demand bolus doses available in 2-unit increments.[92] The V-Go is replaced daily and filled by the patient using the adapter (EZfill) with rapid-acting insulin.[93,94] In a study comparing V-Go with MDI, V-Go users had lower HbA1c levels with decrease in mean TDD by 26 units.[93] Similar results were observed in a retrospective analysis of V-Go versus MDI in 116 patients with T2DM from a large multicenter diabetes system; the HbA1c difference was −0.64% (P = .0201) at 27 weeks, favoring V-Go.[94] Lower total daily dose and greater decrease in fasting plasma glucose were also observed. In a larger retrospective study, 103 subjects (T1DM = 4, T2DM = 99) were placed on V-Go and followed at 2, 6, 10, and 14 months. Subjects experienced mean reductions in HbA1c level at every follow-up time point compared with baseline.[95] In addition, a new type of insulin delivery system for meals only (PAQ MEAL; CeQur, Marlborough, MA, formerly of Calibra Medical, Wayne, PA) was recently compared with insulin pen for efficacy and safety in type 2 patients with uncontrolled diabetes added to basal insulin over 48 weeks. The patch is a small, wearable mechanical pump worn on the body for up to 3 days for delivery of mealtime insulin. In the United States, the patch is approved for use with rapid-acting insulin and holds up to 200 units with bolus delivery of 2-unit increments via a subcutaneous cannula. HbA1c level improved in both arms from baseline to week 24 and was maintained at 44 weeks. Two-thirds of the subjects reached HbA1c levels less than 7% (53 mmol/mol), and in a subject-preference survey more subjects preferred the patch to pen for all measures. Similarly, 91% of the health care providers preferred the patch to the pen to advance subjects with T2DM from basal to basal-bolus insulin.[96]

CONTINUOUS GLUCOSE MONITORING AND INSULIN PUMP THERAPY IN PREGNANCY

Pregnancy in preexisting diabetes presents a series of specific challenges for diabetes management, because narrow glucose levels targets are needed throughout gestation for optimal outcomes. Although this is not a comprehensive review of diabetes management during pregnancy, it is appropriate to describe in this setting the use of diabetes technology and its benefits during pregnancy with diabetes. MDI and CSII are both effective approaches to control diabetes in pregnancy, but there are insufficient data to recommend one rather than another. If patients are to use insulin pump, they should be trained on MDI also in the event of pump failure and allow ample time preconception to achieve optimal glycemic control and be comfortable with pump use.[97] Both CGM and CSII have been studied for use in pregnancy and have been shown to have beneficial effects related to maternal and offspring outcomes, even though, at the time of this writing, CGM therapy is not yet approved for use during pregnancy.

In 2017, the CONCEPTT trial enrolled 215 women with T1DM either preconception or at less than 14 weeks of gestation. Participants, whether on MDI or CSII, were randomized to wear CGM versus usual home glucose monitoring for the duration of the pregnancy.[98] Although there was no difference between the methods of insulin delivery used, a small but statistically significant reduction in HbA1c level (−0.19%, P = .02) was observed at 34 weeks compared with baseline in subjects using CGM. Women using CGM spent on average 100 min/d more in the targeted range (70–140 mg/dL or 3.9–7.8 mmol/L) and 72 fewer minutes per day in hyperglycemia (>140 mg/dL or >7.8 mmol/L). The most dramatic outcomes were seen in the offspring, with significant reductions in the rate of large-for-gestational-age birthweight, admission to neonatal intensive care units, and episodes of neonatal hypoglycemia requiring intravenous dextrose infusion. Further studies are needed to determine the cost of CGM implementation in the antenatal care; however, the investigators concluded that CGM should be offered to all pregnant women with T1DM during the first trimester.

Although CSII offers more flexibility than MDI during pregnancy, hybrid closed-loop systems (MiniMed 670G) currently available have preset glucose targets that are too high for pregnancy, with an algorithm-driven target of 120 mg/dL (6.7 mmol/L), which is more than the currently recommended fasting goal of less than 95 mg/dL (5.3 mmol/L). Similarly, although predictive low-glucose suspend systems protect against hypoglycemia, they do not account for lower glucose goals in pregnancy. Nevertheless, closed-loop systems may still result in comparable glycemic control with less hypoglycemia in some women.[99–102]

In an open-label, randomized study of 16 pregnant women with T1DM in whom a 4-week overnight closed-loop system was compared with SAP therapy,[102] the percentage of overnight time spent within the target range (63–140 mg/dL or 3.5–7.8 mmol/L) was higher during closed-loop therapy than during control therapy (74.7% vs 59.5%; absolute difference, 15.2% points; 95% confidence interval, 6.1–24.2; $P = .002$) with no significant differences between closed-loop and control therapy for insulin doses or adverse event rates.

This study is in line with recently published consensus for time in range, recommending that pregnant women with T1DM spend more than 70% of the time between 63 and 140 mg/dL (3.5–7.8 mmol/L).[38] Larger studies are needed to draw conclusions regarding routine use of insulin pumps in pregnancy.[103]

SUMMARY

Diabetes technology has rapidly evolved in the last few decades, developing a wide array of tools for daily diabetes management, from simple patch pumps to sophisticated hybrid closed-loop systems. CGM therapy has shown clinical benefits regardless of the type of diabetes and method of insulin therapy. It is hoped that the continued improvement of sensor accuracy and ease of use will make them available to patients on a larger scale and likely replace SMBG in the near future. Insulin pump therapy has been present for the last 3 decades and has improved HbA1c levels and decreased hypoglycemia; in addition, the combination of CGM and pumps has shown enhanced benefits. With this rapidly growing new research and the increasing number of automated insulin delivery system under development, the quest for artificial pancreas is likely to become a reality in the near future.

DISCLOSURE

J. Kravarusic has nothing to disclose. G. Aleppo has received research support to her employer from Novo Nordisk (Denmark), Eli Lilly (United States), and Dexcom. G. Aleppo reports consulting for Dexcom, Insulet, and Medtronic.

REFERENCES

1. Klonoff DC, Parkes JL, Kovatchev BP, et al. Investigation of the accuracy of 18 marketed blood glucose monitors. Diabetes Care 2018;41:1681–8.
2. Rodbard D. Continuous glucose monitoring: a review of recent studies demonstrating improved glycemic outcomes. Diabetes Technol Ther 2017;19:S25–37.
3. Kovatchev BP, Patek SD, Ortiz EA, et al. Assessing sensor accuracy for non-adjunct use of continuous glucose monitoring. Diabetes Technol Ther 2015; 17:177–86.

4. Aleppo G, Ruedy KJ, Riddlesworth TD, et al. REPLACE-BG: a randomized trial comparing continuous glucose monitoring with and without routine blood glucose monitoring in adults with well controlled type 1 diabetes. Diabetes Care 2017;40:538–45.
5. Senseonics, Inc. Available at: https://www.senseonics.com/investor-relations/news-releases/2019/06-06-2019-213456270. Accessed June 10, 2019.
6. Peters AL, Ahmann AJ, Battelino T, et al. Diabetes technology continuous subcutaneous insulin infusion therapy and continuous glucose monitoring in adults: an endocrine society clinical practice guideline. J Clin Endocrinol Metab 2016; 101:3922–37.
7. Peters AL, Ahmann AJ, Hirsch IB, et al. Advances in glucose monitoring and automated insulin delivery: supplement to endocrine society clinical practice guidelines. J Endocr Soc 2018;2(11):1214–25.
8. Fonseca VA, Grunberger G, Anhalt H, et al. Continuous glucose monitoring: a consensus conference of the American Association of Clinical Endocrinologists and American College of Endocrinology. Endocr Pract 2016;22(8):1008–21.
9. American Diabetes Association. Diabetes technology: standards of medical care in diabetes -2019. Diabetes Care 2019;42(Supp 1):S71–80.
10. Medtronic, Inc. Available at: https://professional.medtronicdiabetes.com/guardian-sensor-3. Accessed June 16, 2019.
11. Medtronic, Inc. Available at: https://hcp.medtronic-diabetes.com.au/guardian-connect#collapseOne1. Accessed June 10, 2019.
12. Dexcom G5 continuous glucose monitoring systems user guide. Dexcom, Inc; 2018. Available at: https://s3-us-west-2.amazonaws.com/dexcompdf/G5-Mobile-Users-Guide.pdf. Accessed June 10, 2019.
13. DexcomG6 continuous glucose monitoring systems user guide. Dexcom, Inc; 2018. Available at: https://s3-us-west.amazonaws.com/dexcompdf/Using-Your-G6.pdf. Accessed June 10, 2019.
14. Abbott Diabetes Care, Inc. FreeStyle Libre. Available at: https://www.freestylelibre.us/system-overview/freestyle-14-day.html. Accessed June 16, 2019.
15. Senseonic, Inc. Available at: https://www.eversensediabetes.com/. Accessed June 16, 2019.
16. Dexcom G4 continuous glucose monitoring systems user guide. San Diego (CA): Dexcom, Inc; 2018.
17. Important safety information: indications, contraindications, warnings and precautions (MiniMed 670G system). Northridge (CA): Medtronic, Inc. Available at: https://www.medtronicdiabetes.com/important-safety-information#minimed-670g. Accessed June 10, 2019.
18. Eversense user guide. Germantown (MD): Senseonics, Inc. Available at: https://resources.eversensediabetes.com/resource/patient/eversense-cgm-quick-reference-guide. Accessed June 19, 2019.
19. Abbott Diabetes Care, Alameda, CA. Available at: https://www.freestylelibre.us/#safety-information. Accessed June 10, 2019.
20. Abbot Diabetes Care, Alameda, CA. Available at: https://freestyleserver.com/Payloads/IFU/2018/ART39764-001_rev-A-Web.pdf. Accessed June 10, 2019.
21. Medtronic, Inc. Northridge, CA. Available at: https://www.medtronicdiabetes.com/sites/default/files/library/download-library/user-guides/iPro2-with-Enlite-User-Guide.pdf. Accessed June 17, 2019.
22. Dexcom, Inc. San Diego, CA. Available at: https://s3-us-west-2.amazonaws.com/dexcompdf/HCP_Website/LBL-012206+Rev+05+User's+Guide%2C+G4+PLATINUM+Pro+US+Web.pdf. Accessed June 17, 2019.

23. Abbott Diabetes Care, Alameda, CA. FreeStyle libre pro flash glucose monitoring system operator's manual. Alameda (CA): Abbott; 2017.
24. Dexcom, Inc. Available at: https://www.fda.gov/news-events/press-announcements/fda-authorizes-first-fully-interoperable-continuous-glucose-monitoring-system-streamlines-review. Accessed June 16, 2019.
25. O'Connor CE, Aleppo G. Status of continuous glucose monitoring technology in clinical practice. In: Draznin B, editor. Diabetes technology: science and practice. American Diabetes Association; 2019. p. 43–74.
26. FreeStyle LibreLink. Available at: https://www.freestylelibre.us/system-overview/continous-glucose-monitor-app.html. Accessed June 16, 2019.
27. Aleppo G, Webb K. Continuous glucose monitoring integration in clinical practice: a stepped guide to data review and interpretation. J Diabetes Sci Technol 2019;13(4):664–73.
28. Medtronic, Inc. Available at: https://professional.medtronicdiabetes.com/ipro2-professional-cgm. Accessed June 10, 2019.
29. Dexcom, Inc. Available at: https://provider.dexcom.com/products/professional-cgm. Accessed June 10, 2019.
30. Abbot Diabetes Care, Inc. Available at: https://www.myfreestyle.com/freestyle-libre-pro-cgm-system. Accessed June 10, 2019.
31. Centers for Medicare & Medicaid services. Available at: https://www.cms.gov/Regulations-and-Guidance/Guidance/Rulings/Downloads/CMS1682R.pdf. Accessed June 10, 2019.
32. Dexcom, Inc. Available at: https://provider.dexcom.com/industry-news/medicare-announces-criteria-covering-dexcom-g5-mobile-cgm-all-people-diabetes. Accessed June 10, 2019.
33. Dexcom, Inc. Available at: https://dexcom.gcs-web.com/news-releases/news-release-details/dexcom-g6r-continuous-glucose-monitoring-system-will-be. Accessed June 10, 2019.
34. Abbot Diabetes Care, Inc. Available at: https://abbott.mediaroom.com/2018-01-04-Abbotts-Revolutionary-Continuous-Glucose-Monitoring-System-FreeStyle-R-Libre-Now-Available-To-Medicare-Patients. Accessed June 10, 2019.
35. Abbott Diabetes Care, Inc. Available at: https://abbott.mediaroom.com/2018-10-01-Abbott-s-FreeStyle-R-Libre-2-with-Optional-Real-Time-Alarms-Secures-CE-Mark-for-Use-in-Europe. Accessed June 16, 2019.
36. Edelman SV, Argento NB, Pettus J, et al. Clinical implications of real-time and intermittently scanned continuous glucose monitoring. Diabetes Care 2018;41(11):2265–74.
37. Agiostratidou G, Anhalt H, Ball D, et al. Standardizing clinically meaningful outcome measures beyond HbA1c for type 1 diabetes: a consensus report of the American Association of Clinical Endocrinologists, the American Association of Diabetes Educators, the American Diabetes Association, the Endocrine Society, JDRF International, The Leona M. and Harry B. Helmsley Charitable Trust, the Pediatric Endocrine Society, and the T1D Exchange. Diabetes Care 2017;40:1622–30.
38. Battelino T, Danne T, Bergenstal RM, et al. Clinical targets for continuous glucose monitoring data interpretation: recommendations from the international consensus on time in range. Diabetes Care 2019;42(8):1593–603.
39. Bergenstal RM, Beck RW, Close KL, et al. Glucose management indicator (GMI): a new term for estimating A1C from continuous glucose monitoring. Diabetes Care 2018;41(11):2275–80.

40. Buckingham B, Xing D, Weinzimer S, et al, Diabetes Research in Children Network (DirecNet) Study Group. Use of the DirecNet applied treatment algorithm (DATA) for diabetes management with a real-time continuous glucose monitor (the FreeStyle Navigator). Pediatr Diabetes 2008;9(2):142–7.
41. Scheiner G. Practical CGM: improving patient outcomes through continuous glucose monitoring. 4th edition. Alexandria (VA): American Diabetes Association; 2015.
42. Pettus J, Edelman SV. Recommendations for using real-time continuous glucose monitoring (rtCGM) data for insulin adjustments in type 1 diabetes. J Diabetes Sci Technol 2017;11(1):138–47.
43. Klonoff DC, Kerr D. A simplified approach using rate of change arrows to adjust insulin with real-time continuous glucose monitoring. J Diabetes Sci Technol 2017;11(6):1063–9.
44. Aleppo G, Laffel LM, Ahmann AJ, et al. A practical approach to using trend arrows on the Dexcom G5 CGM system for the management of adults with diabetes. J Endocr Soc 2017;1(12):1445–60.
45. Kudva YC, Ahmann AJ, Bergenstal RM, et al. Approach to using trend arrows in the freestyle libre flash glucose monitoring systems in adults. J Endocr Soc 2018;2(12):1320–37.
46. Aleppo G. Approaches for successful outcomes with continuous glucose monitoring. In: Hirsch IB, Battelino T, Peters AL, et al, editors. Role of continuous glucose monitoring in diabetes treatment. Arlington (VA): American Diabetes Association; 2018. p. 13–8.
47. Peters A. The evidence base for continuous glucose monitoring. In: Hirsch IB, Battelino T, Peters AL, et al, editors. Role of continuous glucose monitoring in diabetes treatment. Arlington (VA): American Diabetes Association; 2018. p. 3–7.
48. Bailey TS, Grunberger G, Bode BW, et al. American Association of Clinical Endocrinologists and American College of Endocrinology 2016 outpatient glucose monitoring consensus statement. Endocr Pract 2016;22(2):231–61.
49. van Beers CA, DeVries JH, Smits MM, et al. Continuous glucose monitoring for patients with type 1 diabetes and impaired awareness of hypoglycaemia (IN CONTROL): a randomised, open-label, crossover trial. Lancet Diabetes Endocrinol 2016;4:893–902.
50. Juvenile Diabetes Research Foundation Continuous Glucose Monitoring Study Group. Continuous glucose monitoring and intensive treatment of type 1 diabetes. N Engl J Med 2008;359:1464–76.
51. Juvenile Diabetes Research Foundation Continuous Glucose Monitoring Study Group. The effect of continuous glucose monitoring in well-controlled type 1 diabetes. Diabetes Care 2009;32:1378–83.
52. Šoupal J, Petruželková L, Flekač M, et al. Comparison of different treatment modalities for type 1 diabetes, including sensor-augmented insulin regimens, in 52 weeks of follow-up: a COMISAIR study. Diabetes Technol Ther 2016;18(9):532–8.
53. Beck RW, Riddlesworth T, Ruedy K, et al, DIAMOND Study Group. Effect of continuous glucose monitoring on glycemic control in adults with type 1 diabetes using insulin injections: the DIAMOND randomized clinical trial. JAMA 2017;317:371–8.
54. Polonsky WH, Hessler D, Ruedy KJ, et al. The impact of continuous glucose monitoring on markers of quality of life in adults with type 1 diabetes: further

findings from the DIAMOND randomized clinical trial. Diabetes Care 2017;40(6): 736–41.
55. Beck RW, Riddlesworth TD, Ruedy K, et al, DIAMOND Study Group. Continuous glucose monitoring versus usual care in patients with type 2 diabetes receiving multiple daily insulin injections: a randomized trial. Ann Intern Med 2017;167: 365–74.
56. Lind M, Polonsky W, Hirsch IB, et al. Continuous glucose monitoring vs conventional therapy for glycemic control in adults with type 1 diabetes treated with multiple daily insulin injections: the GOLD randomized clinical trial. JAMA 2017;317:379–87.
57. Ólafsdóttir AF, Polonsky W, Bolinder J, et al. A randomized clinical trial of the effect of continuous glucose monitoring on nocturnal hypoglycemia, daytime hypoglycemia, glycemic variability, and hypoglycemia confidence in persons with type 1 diabetes treated with multiple daily insulin injections (GOLD-3). Diabetes Technol Ther 2018;20(4):274–84.
58. Bolinder J, Antuna R, Geelhoed-Duijvestijn P, et al. Novel glucose-sensing technology and hypoglycaemia in type 1 diabetes: a multicentre, non-masked, randomised controlled trial. Lancet 2016;388:2254–63.
59. Haak T, Hanaire H, Ajjan R, et al. Flash glucose-sensing technology as a replacement for blood glucose monitoring for the management of insulin-treated type 2 diabetes: a multicenter, open-label randomized controlled trial. Diabetes Ther 2017;8:55–73.
60. Mulinacci G, Alonso GT, Snell-Bergeon JK, et al. Glycemic outcomes with early initiation of continuous glucose monitoring system in recently diagnosed patients with type 1 diabetes. Diabetes Technol Ther 2019;21(1):6–10.
61. Skyler JS. Continuous subcutaneous insulin infusion—a historical perspective. Diabetes Technol Ther 2010;12(Suppl 1):S5–9.
62. Available at: https://www.diabeteshealth.com/wp-content/uploads/2019/pdf/2019/InsulinPumps.pdf. Accessed June 17, 2019.
63. MiniMed 630G system user guide. Medtronic MiniMed, Inc; 2018. Available at: https://www.medtronicdiabetes.com/sites/default/files/library/download-library/user-guides/MiniMed%20630G%20System%20User%20Guide%20-%2020-Mar-2018.pdf. Accessed June 18, 2019.
64. MiniMed 670G system user guide. Medtronic MiniMed, Inc; 2017. Available at: https://www.medtronicdiabetes.com/sites/default/files/library/download-library/user-guides/MiniMed-670G-System-User-Guide.pdf. Accessed June 18, 2019.
65. T:slim G4 insulin pump user guide. San Diego (CA): Tandem Diabetes; 2015. Available at: https://www.tandemdiabetes.com/docs/default-source/product-documents/t-slim-g4-insulin-pump/tslim-g4-insulin-pump-user-guide-b005630_c.pdf?sfvrsn=3bb93ad7_4. Accessed June 18, 2019.
66. T:slim X2 insulin pump user guide. Tandem Diabetes; 2019. Available at: https://www.tandemdiabetes.com/docs/default-source/product-documents/t-slim-x2-insulin-pump/user-guide_tslim_x2_g5b989599775426a79a519ff0500a9fd39.pdf?sfvrsn=dfec3cd7_81. Accessed June 18, 2019.
67. Tandem diabetes t:slim X2 with basal IQ user guide, 2019. Available at: https://www.tandemdiabetes.com/docs/default-source/product-documents/t-slim-x2-insulin-pump/patient_pack_tslimx2_g5_can_eng359d599775426a79a519ff0500a9fd39.pdf?sfvrsn=41a83ed7_28. Accessed June 18, 2019.
68. Tandem ACE PUMP. Available at: https://www.fda.gov/news-events/press-announcements/fda-authorizes-first-interoperable-insulin-pump-intended-allow-patients-customize-treatment-through. Accessed June 18, 2019.

69. Omnipod user guide. Insulet Corporation; 2017. Available at: https://www.myomnipod.com/sites/default/files/inline-files/17845-5A%20Guide%2C%20Eros%20US%20User%20Guide%20Rev%20B.pdf. Accessed June 18, 2019.
70. Omnipod DASH user guide. Insulet Corporation; 2018. Available at: https://www.myomnipod.com/sites/default/files/media/documents/18296-ENG-AW%20Rev%20B_USA%20DASH%20User%20Guide.pdf. Accessed June 18, 2019.
71. Valeritas, Inc. V-Go instructions for patient use. ART-037 Rev: H 09/2011. Available at: http://www.go-vgo.com/wp-content/uploads/2018/06/instructions-for-patient-use.pdf. Accessed June 18, 2019.
72. CeQur PAQ Meal. Available at: https://www.cequrcorp.com/hcp-info. Accessed June 19, 2019.
73. Grunberger G, Handelsman Y, Bloomgarden ZT, et al. American association of clinical endocrinologists and American college of endocrinology 2018 position statement on integration of insulin pumps and continuous glucose monitoring in patients with diabetes mellitus. Endocr Pract 2018;24(3):302–8.
74. Slover RH, Welsh JB, Criego A, et al. Effectiveness of sensor augmented pump therapy in children and adolescents with type 1 diabetes in the STAR 3 study. Pediatr Diabetes 2012;13:6–11.
75. Bergenstal RM, Tamborlane WV, Ahmann A, et al, STAR 3 Study Group. Effectiveness of sensor-augmented insulin-pump therapy in type 1 diabetes. N Engl J Med 2010;363(4):311–20.
76. Bergenstal RM, Klonoff DC, Garg SK, et al. Threshold based insulin-pump interruption for reduction of hypoglycemia. N Engl J Med 2013;369:224–32.
77. Buckingham BA, Raghinaru D, Cameron F, et al. Predictive low-glucose insulin suspension reduces duration of nocturnal hypoglycemia in children without increasing ketosis. Diabetes Care 2015;38:1197–204.
78. Buckingham BA, Bailey TS, Christiansen M, et al. evaluation of a predictive low-glucose management system in-clinic. Diabetes Technol Ther 2017;19:288–92.
79. Food and Drug Administration, Center for Devices and Radiological Health: MiniMed 670G system approval letter. 2016. Available at: https://www.fda.gov/NewsEvents/Newsroom/PressAnnouncements/ucm522974.htm. Accessed June 19, 2019.
80. Heinemann L, Fleming GA, Petrie JR, et al. Insulin pump risks and benefits: a clinical appraisal of pump safety standards, adverse event reporting, and research needs: a joint statement of the European Association for the Study of Diabetes and the American Diabetes Association Diabetes Technology Working Group. Diabetes Care 2015;38(4):716–22.
81. Kovatchev B. A century of diabetes technology: signals, models, and artificial pancreas control. Trends Endocrinol Metab 2019;30(7):432–44.
82. Pickup JC, Sutton AJ. Severe hypoglycaemia and glycaemic control in Type 1 diabetes: meta-analysis of multiple daily insulin injections compared with continuous subcutaneous insulin infusion. Diabet Med 2008;25:765–74.
83. Fatourechi MM, Kudva YC, Murad MH, et al. Clinical review: hypoglycemia with intensive insulin therapy: a systematic review and meta-analyses of randomized trials of continuous subcutaneous insulin infusion versus multiple daily injections. J Clin Endocrinol Metab 2009;94(3):729–40.
84. Benkhadra K, Alahdab F, Tamhane SU, et al. Continuous subcutaneous insulin infusion versus multiple daily injections in individuals with type 1 diabetes: a systematic review and meta-analysis. Endocrine 2017;55(1):77–84.

85. Bergenstal RM, Tamborlane WV, Ahmann A, et al. Sensor-augmented pump therapy for A1C reduction (STAR 3) study: results from the 6-month continuation phase. Diabetes Care 2011;34(11):2403–5.
86. Choudhary P, De Portu S, Arrieta A, et al. Use of sensor-integrated pump therapy to reduce hypoglycaemia in people with type 1 diabetes: a real-world study in the UK. Diabet Med 2019;36(9):1100–8.
87. Senn JD, Fischli S, Slahor L, et al. Long-term effects of initiating continuous subcutaneous insulin infusion (CSII) and continuous glucose monitoring (CGM) in people with type 1 diabetes and unsatisfactory diabetes control. J Clin Med 2019;8(3):394.
88. Forlenza GP, Li Z, Buckingham BA, et al. Predictive low-glucose suspend reduces hypoglycemia in adults, adolescents, and children with type 1 diabetes in an at-home randomized crossover study: results of the PROLOG trial. Diabetes Care 2018;41(10):2155–61.
89. Reznik Y, Cohen O, Aronson R, et al. Insulin pump treatment compared with multiple daily injections for treatment of type 2 diabetes (OpT2mise): a randomised open-label controlled trial. Lancet 2014;384(9950):1265–72.
90. Pickup JC, Reznik Y, Sutton AJ. Glycemic control during continuous subcutaneous insulin infusion versus multiple daily insulin injections in type 2 diabetes: individual patient data meta-analysis and meta-regression of randomized controlled trials. Diabetes Care 2017;40:715–22.
91. Landau Z, Raz I, Wainstein J, et al. The role of insulin pump therapy for type 2 diabetes mellitus. Diabetes Metab Res Rev 2017;33(1):e2822.
92. Winter A, Lintner M, Knezevich E. V-Go insulin delivery system versus multiple daily insulin injections for patients with uncontrolled type 2 diabetes mellitus. J Diabetes Sci Technol 2015;9(5):1111–6.
93. Gilbert M, Pratley RE. V-Go™—a novel device for delivering basal–bolus insulin therapy to patients with type 2 diabetes mellitus. US Endocrinol 2007;(2):30–2.
94. Lajara R, Davidson JA, Nikkel CC, et al. Clinical and cost-effectiveness of insulin delivery with V-Go (®) disposable insulin delivery device versus multiple daily injections in patients with type 2 diabetes inadequately controlled on basal insulin. Endocr Pract 2016;22(6):726–35.
95. Sutton D, Higdon CD, Nikkel C, et al. Clinical benefits over time associated with use of V-go wearable insulin delivery device in adult patients with diabetes: a retrospective analysis. Adv Ther 2018;35(5):631–43.
96. Bergenstal RM, Peyrot M, Dreon DM, et al. Implementation of basal–bolus therapy in type 2 diabetes: a randomized controlled trial comparing bolus insulin delivery using an insulin patch with an insulin pen. Diabetes Technol Ther 2019;21:273–85.
97. Farrar D, Tuffnell DJ, West J. Continuous subcutaneous insulin infusion versus multiple daily injections of insulin for pregnant women with diabetes. Cochrane Database Syst Rev 2007;(3):CD005542.
98. Feig DS, Donovan LE, Corcoy R, et al. Continuous glucose monitoring in pregnant women with type 1 diabetes (CONCEPTT): a multicenter international randomized controlled trial. Lancet 2017;390(10110):2347–59.
99. Stewart ZA, Wilinska ME, Hartnell S, et al. Day-and-night closed-loop insulin delivery in a broad population of pregnant women with type 1 diabetes: a randomized controlled crossover trial. Diabetes Care 2018;41(7):1391–9.
100. Murphy HR, Kumareswaran K, Elleri D, et al. Safety and efficacy of 24-h closed-loop insulin delivery in well-controlled pregnant women with type 1 diabetes: a randomized crossover case series. Diabetes Care 2011;34(12):2527–9.

101. Murphy HR, Elleri D, Allen JM, et al. Closed-loop insulin delivery during pregnancy complicated by type 1 diabetes. Diabetes Care 2011;34(2):406–11.
102. Stewart ZA, Wilinska ME, Hartnell S, et al. Closed-loop insulin delivery during pregnancy in women with type 1 diabetes. N Engl J Med 2016;375(7):644–54.
103. Alexopoulos AS, Blair R, Peters AL. Management of preexisting diabetes in pregnancy: a review. JAMA 2019;321(18):1811–9.

Benefits and Challenges of Diabetes Technology Use in Older Adults

Elena Toschi, MD[a,b,*], Medha N. Munshi, MD[a,b,c]

KEYWORDS

- Older adults • Technology • Type 1 diabetes mellitus • Type 2 diabetes mellitus
- Subcutaneous continuous insulin infusion • Continuous glucose monitoring

KEY POINTS

- Recent studies have shown that the use of the technology for insulin administration and glucose monitoring can be used in older adults with type 1 and type 2 diabetes.
- Some medical conditions more commonly seen in older adults can act as barriers to the successful use of technology, including cognitive and physical decline.
- Periodic assessment of cognitive and physical function, as well as overall health, is important in older adults using diabetes-related technologies.
- Guidelines on the use of technology in older adults, impact of medical comorbidities, screening tests for these conditions, and educational materials are needed.

INTRODUCTION

Over the past few decades, there has been an increase in the use of technology for the management of diabetes, primarily in young and middle-aged patients with type 1 diabetes (T1D). However, as technology has become more common, less expensive, and easier to use, its use has expanded to those with type 2 diabetes (T2D). In addition, in recent years, a growing number of older adults have started using technology to improve their diabetes. This phenomenon provides opportunities and challenges to understand the benefits and barriers in the use of technology in the aging population (**Table 1**).

Currently, major advances in diabetes technology include (1) insulin delivery systems, such as smart insulin pens and insulin pumps, (2) blood glucose monitoring, such as continuous glucose monitoring systems (CGM), and (3) hybrid devices that combined glucose monitoring systems and insulin delivery systems.[1] The overall goal in the use

[a] Joslin Diabetes Center, United States, One Joslin Place, Boston, MA 02215, USA; [b] Harvard Medical School, 330 Brookline Avenue, Boston, MA, USA; [c] Beth Israel Deaconess Medical Center, Boston, MA, USA
* Corresponding author. Joslin Diabetes Center, One Joslin Place, Boston, MA 02215.
E-mail address: Elena.toschi@joslin.harvard.edu

Endocrinol Metab Clin N Am 49 (2020) 57–67
https://doi.org/10.1016/j.ecl.2019.10.001

Table 1
Diabetes technology systems: benefits and challenges in aging population

Technology System	Benefits in Older Adults	Challenges in Older Adults
Insulin administration systems		
Pump or CSII	Reduce hypoglycemia Improve hemoglobin A1c Availability of bolus calculators Smaller accurate doses Keep track of active insulin Downloadable reports	Maintenance in context of getting and changing various parts Need for intact dexterity High cost Visual impairment Burden/negative impact on quality of life
Bluetooth-enabled insulin pen	Bolus calculator Keep track of active insulin Downloadable reports Useful to assess adherence	Maintenance in context of changing cartridges Need for dexterity High cost Visual impairment
Monitoring systems		
CGM	Reduce hypoglycemia Reduce glucose variability Improve glucose control Reduce need for fingersticks measurement Downloadable reports Alarm/alerts are available in most SHARE feature can help involve caregivers	Maintenance in context of changing sensor Need for dexterity High cost Visual impairment Hearing impairment Perception of data overload causing anxiety Alarm/alert fatigue
Hybrid systems	Reduce hypoglycemia Reduce glucose variability Improve glucose control Downloadable reports Alarm/alert	Maintenance in context of many parts need replacement Need for dexterity Very high cost Visual impairment Hearing impairment Perception of data overload causing anxiety Alarm/alert fatigue

of these technologies is to improve glycemic control, lower the risk of hypoglycemia, decrease the burden of living with diabetes, and improve quality of life.[2–7]

In this article we review the evidence supporting the use of diabetes technologies in the older population and discuss recommendations based on current data and the authors' clinical knowledge and experience.

INSULIN DELIVERY SYSTEMS

Insulin Pens and Bluetooth-Enabled Insulin Pens

Insulin pens have been a major advance in technology and have improved accuracy of insulin doses and ease of administration for patients who were using vial and syringe methods. Insulin pens are available as prefilled syringes, disposable or reusable with replaceable insulin cartridges that allow push-button injections. Some of these insulin pens have the ability to administer insulin by 0.5-U increments, improving the accuracy of dosing.

Recently, Bluetooth-enabled insulin pens (smart pens) have further improved this technology with their ability to record the dose and the time of the insulin delivery. In addition, some of these smart pens have built-in bolus calculators to help with insulin dosing calculations. They also provide downloadable data reports to the clinicians and/or patients.[1] Until now, clinicians were adjusting insulin dosing based on blood glucose monitoring records, along with the assumption that the patient is taking their insulin as prescribed (both timing and dose). However, for patients with diabetes taking multiple insulin injection, omissions or errors in doses and timing of insulin are fairly common.[8,9] The use of Bluetooth-enabled insulin pens in participants with T1D or T2D on insulin injection was shown to capture deviation from insulin prescriptions in a recent study.[10] Twenty-two percent of the older subgroup in this study showed nonadherence with bolus insulin dosing, and 27% showed nonadherence with basal insulin administration. The study results also showed that the nonadherence measured by these methods was associated with poor glycemic control.

Benefits for older population

Insulin pens are easier to use for older adults with vision impairment or dexterity problems compared with a vial and syringes. Bluetooth-enabled pens can be used to assess missed or extra doses in patients with cognitive impairment. This information can be used by formal (aids or nurses) or informal (family members) caregivers to remind patients to take their insulin or eat meals on time. As mentioned elsewhere in this article, some of the Bluetooth-enabled insulin pen systems have a built-in bolus calculator that can help with dosing calculation for those people who have difficulty with problem solving (see **Table 1**).

Challenges in older adults

Some older adults with cognitive decline have difficulty operating insulin pens, especially changing cartridges. There is also a problem with identifying missed or incorrect doses, because most pens do not have memory for given doses. The numbers on the pen are sometimes hard to read for visually impaired patients. Although Bluetooth pens are better for some of these issues, they are much more expensive and some of the pens require the need for daily charging to keep system functioning. These additional steps add an extra level of complexity (see **Table 1**; **Table 2**).

Insulin Pump or Continuous Subcutaneous Insulin Infusion

Insulin pumps administer insulin continuously throughout the day. Most insulin pumps use tubing to deliver insulin through a cannula; a few attach directly to the skin, without tubing (patch pump). This insulin delivery system is more accurate and precise than insulin administration via injections, and the amount of basal dose can be as small as 0.1 U/h. Insulin pumps have a bolus calculator that can determine bolus doses based on preprogrammed insulin to carbohydrate ratio, sensitivity factor, and set glucose target. Infusion sets are required to be changed every 2 to 3 days, requiring cannula insertion in the subcutaneous tissues and cartridge refill. Data can be downloaded from the pump; these reports can be reviewed by clinicians and can help to identify problems such as missed doses or too many boluses causing stacking of insulin, often leading to hypoglycemia.[1]

Until recently, the use of insulin pump was mostly seen in younger adults and in those with T1D. Large registry cohorts in this population have shown benefits of pump use by improvement in glucose control (hemoglobin A1c), decrease in hypoglycemia, and improvement in quality of life.[11,12] Several studies have evaluated the use of insulin pumps in the older population with T1D and T2D. A retrospective chart

Table 2
Barriers to technology use in older adults

Barriers	Glucose Monitoring Systems	Insulin Delivery Systems
Cognitive dysfunction	Unable to troubleshoot CGM data readings May under bolus or over bolus owing to information overload of glucose readings Challenge to remember multiple steps to change sensor Overreacting to CGM alarms Frustration when device seems too complicated Unable to problem solve when issues arise (failed sensors, problems with connectivity)	Unable to remember multiple steps to change tubing and cannula May administer repeated boluses owing to forgetfulness, leading to insulin stacking Unable to problem solve when issues arise (kinked tubes, bent cannulas, pump failure)
Dexterity problems	Difficulty calibrating CGM Difficulty inserting CGM sensor Difficulty dealing with CGM adhesion tape Difficulty manipulating CGM transmitter to change sensor Difficulties tapping on button on CMG receiver	Difficulty changing cartridges in the insulin pen Difficulty working with pump tubing and insertions Difficulty pressing buttons on insulin pump required to administer insulin Difficulty reaching insertion sites for pump
Visual impairment	Unable to read CGM readings Unable to read calibration prompts	Unable to see numbers on insulin pen Unable to see pump display Unable to notice pump damage that can lead to malfunction
Hearing impairment	Unable to hear CGM alarms and alerts	Unable to hear alarm from insulin pump malfunction
Social isolation/lack of support	No one to help during times of confusion Unable to find assistance changing sensors	Unable to administer insulin injections alone Unable to find assistance changing pump sites

review to compare pump therapy in older and younger adults with T1D has shown similar benefits in both age groups in the risk of severe hypoglycemia and hospitalization.[13] Another retrospective study evaluating electronic medical records showed that the pump therapy can be used effectively and safely in carefully selected older adults with T1D.[14] A prospective, randomized study of older adults with T2D on either insulin pump or multiple daily injections (MDI) showed equal improvement in glucose variability over time with both modalities.[15] However, it did not show any difference between people using pump versus MDI with regard to glucose control, episodes of severe hypoglycemia, glucose variability, or treatment satisfaction.

Benefits in older adults

Many older adults enjoy the convenience of insulin pumps, because they do not need to carry multiple insulin pens with them. Although cost can be a problem, currently, all insulin pump systems are covered by Medicare, which is beneficial to the older population (see **Table 1**).

Challenges in older adults

Obtaining and keeping up with various pump parts and supplies can be challenging at any age, but can be especially burdensome in older adults (see **Tables 1** and **2**). Although the Centers for Medicare & Medicaid Services cover the expenses for insulin pump use in older adults with T1D, there is a caveat that the patients using the pump technology have a face-to-face encounter with a clinician every 3 months to receive disposable supplies needed for insulin pump use. A survey of older adults with T1D showed that obtaining supplies in a timely fashion remains a challenge.[16] More than 50% of the people interviewed in this study reported that, because of these challenges, they changed pump-related behaviors such as leaving the infusion site in place longer than prescribed, reusing pump supplies, using injections to supplement pump use, or temporarily stopping the insulin pump use. As a consequence, there was an increased risk for adverse outcomes, including more erratic blood glucose, irritation at insertion sites, and a greater number of episodes of hypoglycemia and hospitalizations.

Another major concern is the risk of diabetic ketoacidosis associated with insulin pump use. This risk is thought to be a result of issues with infusion sets (dislodgement, occlusion). Although there are no studies specifically looking at the older population, the risk of malfunction of pump and diabetic ketoacidosis needs careful consideration (see **Tables 1** and **2**).

Aging is also associated with a higher prevalence of a number of conditions that interfere with diabetes self-care. Cognitive decline with aging is not uncommon and can impact mental flexibility and mental speed.[17] Patients with diminished mental flexibility and processing speed may do well with a simple regimen or technology, but may fail if the regimen is too complex or the technology requires multiple steps. In general, when patients develop cognitive dysfunction, they are less likely to be involved in diabetes self-care and glucose monitoring.[18] It is important to reassess patient's ability to use inulin pumps periodically when cognitive decline is noted (**Fig. 1**, **Table 3**). Aging is associated with an increased incidence of conditions such as osteoarthritis and tremors that can impact dexterity. A study conducted in people with T1D and T2D evaluating hand function and motoric performances showed that reduced skills are common in those people with diabetes, compared with the general population.[19] Assessment of dexterity in clinical practice is not part of diabetes-related clinical visit and may result in a failure of insulin pump use if not considered beforehand (see **Tables 1** and **2**). Vision and hearing impairment can also be barriers for many aspects of insulin pump use. Insulin pump screens may be difficult to see owing to their small size and lack of magnification abilities. Alarms and alerts regarding malfunctions and reminders may be missed by those people with hearing difficulties.

GLUCOSE MONITORING SYSTEMS

Self-monitoring of blood glucose (SMBG) is a key component of diabetes management. Older people with diabetes have been using SMBG values for several decades, however, this measure is a static value compared with the dynamic data obtained from the CGM, with information not only on the absolute value, but also trends. Over the last decade, CGM has dramatically improved in technology, ease of use, and accuracy. Real-time CGM (rtCGM), which continuously reports glucose levels and includes alarms for hypoglycemic and hyperglycemic excursions, is primarily used in the management of T1D. Professional CGM is used for pattern management and for the assessment of glucose excursions in the management of both T1D and T2D. Two CGM devices are now approved by the US Food and Drug Administration for making treatment decisions without SMBG confirmation, sometimes called nonadjunctive use.[1]

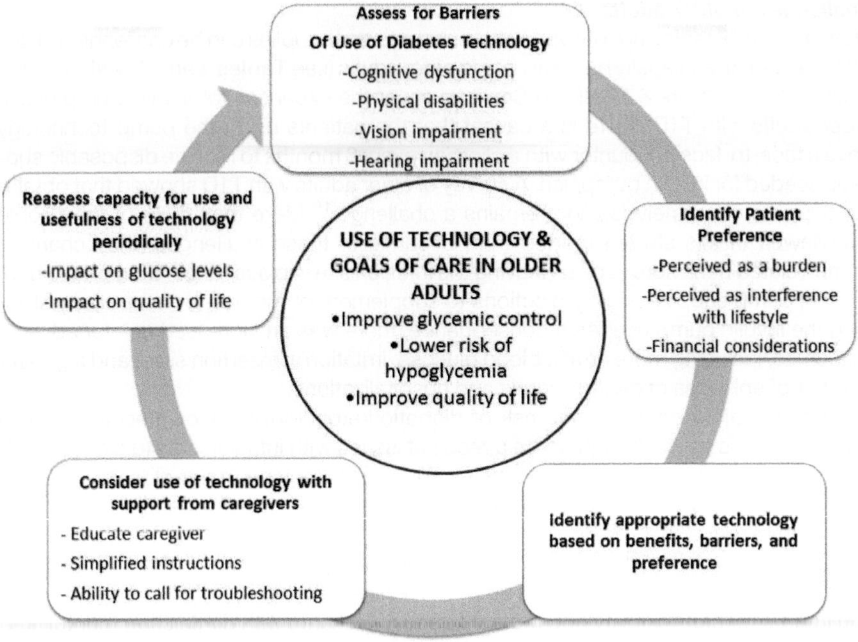

Fig. 1. Steps to consider in the use of diabetes technology and goals of care in older adults to improve diabetes and quality-of-life outcomes.

A pivotal study conducted in 2008 showed that the use of CGM was associated with improved glycemic control and a lower risk of hypoglycemia in adults and children with T1D.[5] Similar results with improved glycemic control were also shown in 2 randomized controlled trials using CGM in adults with T1D and T2D using MDI.[7,20] A subanalysis of this study evaluated the use of CGM versus usual self-monitoring in older adults (>60 years age) with T1D and T2D using MDI, and showed that 97% of the older participants used the CGM ≥6 d/wk at 6 months, and the use of CGM was associated with improved glycemic control and glycemic variability.[21] A few small retrospective studies have evaluated use of CGM in older population in community setting. In 2014, a community endocrine practice looked at retrospective data on a small number of older adults (≥65 years of age) using CGM at that time, when CGM was not covered by the Medicare, and found that the older patients using rtCGM had a lower hemoglobin A1c and fewer episode of severe hypoglycemia compared with non-CGM users.[22]

Recently, the Wireless Innovation for Seniors With Diabetes Mellitus (WISDM trial) prospectively assessed the potential benefits and risks of CGM use in older adults (>60 years) with T1D. The study showed a high retention rate up to 98% along with improvement in hemoglobin A1c, hypoglycemia (time spent at <70 mg/dL or 3.9 mmol/L) and severe hypoglycemia.[23]

A few studies have also evaluated the impact of CGM on quality of life by surveying patients using CGM. They have shown that in older adults with either T1D or T2D using CGM, rtCGM users had fewer moderate and severe hypoglycemic episodes and greater reductions in severe hypoglycemia compared with non-CGM users. The rtCGM users also reported significantly better well-being, less hypoglycemic fear, and less diabetes distress than non-CGM users.[24,25]

Table 3
Consideration for use of diabetes technology systems based on patient characteristics, health status, and glycemic goals

Patient Characteristics and Health Status	Glycemic Goal	Potential Benefits on Use of Diabetes Technology	Potential Limitations of Use of Diabetes Technology
Healthy (few coexisting chronic illnesses, intact cognitive and functional status)	Hemoglobin A1c goal of 7.5% (58 mmol/L)	Bluetooth pen Can be used to keep track of adherence and educate patients regarding impact of missed or inaccurate dosing Pump Capacity for small dose of insulin Assistance with insulin calculator and active insulin on board Provide flexibility CGM Reduced need for finger sticks Alarm and alert can help with hypoglycemia fear and unawareness Share feature can be used to involve caregivers as needed	Need to evaluate cognitive function periodically Caregivers need to be trained to help, especially with Share feature Alarms and alert fatigue can cause anxiety
Community-dwelling patients receiving care in a skilled nursing facility for short-term rehabilitation	Hemoglobin A1c is not a reliable measure, glycemic goal between 100 and 200 mg/dL (5.5 and 11.0 mmol/L)	Pump May maintain tighter control needed during rehabilitation CGM Can help to lower risk of hypoglycemia, especially if on an insulin regimen	Need to train staff at the facility
Very complex/poor health (long-term care or end-stage chronic illnesses or moderate-to-severe cognitive impairment or 21 activity of daily living dependencies)	Hemoglobin A1c of <8.5% (69 mmol/L)	Pump: Consider continuing pump in older adult with T1D if staff is able to support CGM Continue CGM therapy to prevent unrecognized hypoglycemia episodes in those on multiple insulin injections or those who are not tolerating fingersticks	Need to train nursing home staff
Patients at end of life	Avoid extreme of glucose level as hypoglycemia or hyperglycemia	Not much role in person with T2D CGM can help those with T1D to reduce burden of multiple fingersticks	

Benefits in Older Adults

The use of rtCGM in older adults has shown effectiveness in decreasing the risk of hypoglycemia. This finding is of particular importance, because hypoglycemia leads to poorer outcomes in older adults, owing to its association with increased risks of falls and potential injury, myocardial infarcts, arrhythmias, temporary or permanent cognitive impairment, and death.[26–28] Older adults have a high risk of hypoglycemia unawareness and do not recognize many episodes of mild to moderate hypoglycemia, because they are asymptomatic.[29,30] Thus, alarms and alerts built in the CGM can help older patients to manage their hypoglycemia episodes in time and improve safety.

In addition, now there is an availability to use a smart device in conjunction with the CGM, which allows patients to enable mobile applications and use the SHARE feature. The SHARE application allows the user to share CGM data with up to 5 designated individuals who can monitor glucose levels remotely on compatible smart devices. This data-sharing capability can be helpful to caregivers of elderly and frail patients, especially if they have cognitive decline (see **Tables 1** and **2**). In January 2017, the Centers for Medicare & Medicaid Services started providing coverage for rtCGM as durable medical equipment, which has helped to make this technology more affordable for older adults.

Challenges in Older Adults

rtCGM provides an abundance of data, which sometimes creates challenges in troubleshooting and diabetes self-management decisions, especially in older adults. In addition, the constant problem solving that is needed in interpreting and reacting to CGM readings can become a burden when other competing medical conditions or socioeconomic problems arise.

In older adults with diabetes, Medicare covers the CGM, however, it requires limitation on the use of glucometer to only 3 fingerstick checks per day. This limitation can be challenging in some, because SMBG has been used so diligently for many decades as a point of reference. Moreover, SMBG by glucometer are needed in certain situations, for example, CGM can have a warm-up period of a few hours where the patient does not have real-time information regarding their glucose level or when sensor glucose reads less than 80 mg/dL or greater than 250 mg/dL (<4.4 or >13.9 mmol/L) because CGM accuracy is decreased in these ranges.

As mentioned in the insulin delivery system discussion, cognitive decline and physical decline along with dexterity and visual impairment can be a challenge also in using CGM for older adults. In addition, hearing impairment, which is common in older subjects with diabetes, may interfere with hearing alarm and alert causing distress and impact appropriate use of the CGM system[31] (see **Tables 1** and **2**). Some medications and comorbidities occurring frequently in older adults can also create problems. Older adults are more likely to use medications that contain acetaminophen. The use of acetaminophen interferes with some of the sensors, making reading inaccurate (false hyperglycemic readings).[32] Older adults with diabetes may also have altered renal function. However, thus far, CGM accuracy has not been tested for chronic kidney disease and an estimated glomerular filtration rate of less than 30 mg/mL/min.

GLUCOSE-RESPONSIVE INSULIN DELIVERY SYSTEM OR HYBRID SYSTEM

Two major class of glucose responsive insulin delivery system are currently on the market. The first is a sensor-augmented insulin pump that can automatically suspend insulin to prevent hypoglycemia.[33] The hybrid closed-loop systems (also called the artificial pancreas or automated insulin delivery systems) is the other one, that can modulate insulin delivery less than and greater than the preset rate based on sensor glucose levels to mitigate both hyperglycemia and hypoglycemia.[34] In the United States, a system with predictive low glucose suspend (Tandem t:slim ×2 with Basal IQ) is approved by the US Food and Drug Administration. Once covered by Medicare, this system will be available for use in older adults. The goal of the hybrid closed loop systems is to decrease the daily engagement by the person who wears it and provide help with the daily burden of diabetes decision making, based on food intake (or lack thereof), exercise, and acute illnesses. There are no studies to assess the use of this technology in the older age group; however, a case report highlights the potential power of this system in the older and frail population.[35] In this report, the use of closed loop insulin delivery systems was continued in a hospitalized individual during a period of terminal illness. Glucose control was kept within good range with minimal hypoglycemia while using a factory-calibrated CGM, which decreased the burden of SMBG measurements, and an insulin pump, which is less intrusive than insulin injections.

SUMMARY

Newer diabetes-related technologies, such as insulin pump and CGM, are being more commonly used in older adults with both T1D and T2D. Study data have shown that healthy older adults can use these technologies successfully and derive benefits through improvement of glycemic control and glucose variability, reduced hypoglycemia, and improvement of overall quality of life. However, aging brings challenges associated with competing medical conditions, comorbidities, polypharmacy, and cognitive and functional decline (see **Table 3**). Careful evaluation and thoughtful discussion between clinicians, patients, and their caregivers should be performed to continually reevaluate the use of technology and its benefits and burdens. If an older patient chooses to use technology, it is important to assess their support system and offer training and education to the caregivers. **Fig. 1** show the steps needed for successful use of technology with the overall goal of improved diabetes and quality of life outcomes.

ACKNOWLEDGMENTS

The authors thank Christine Slyne for editorial assistance. Drs E. Toshi and Dr M.N. Munshi are supported by NIH DP3 Grant "Technological Advances in Glucose Management in Older Adults (The Tango Study)"– Clinicaltrials.gov: NCT03078491?

DISCLOSURE

Dr M.N. Munshi is a consultant for Lilly and Sanofi. No disclosure for Dr E. Toschi.

REFERENCES

1. American Diabetes Association. 7. Diabetes technology: standards of medical care in diabetes-2019. Diabetes Care 2019;42:S71–80.
2. Jeitler K, Horvath K, Berghold A, et al. Continuous subcutaneous insulin infusion versus multiple daily insulin injections in patients with diabetes mellitus: systematic review and meta-analysis. Diabetologia 2008;51:941–51.
3. Pickup JC, Sutton AJ. Severe hypoglycaemia and glycaemic control in type 1 diabetes: meta-analysis of multiple daily insulin injections compared with continuous subcutaneous insulin infusion. Diabet Med 2008;25:765–74.

4. Karges B, Schwandt A, Heidtmann B, et al. Association of insulin pump therapy vs insulin injection therapy with severe hypoglycemia, ketoacidosis, and glycemic control among children, adolescents, and young adults with type 1 diabetes. JAMA 2017;318:1358–66.
5. Tamborlane WV, Beck RW, Bode BW, et al. Continuous glucose monitoring and intensive treatment of type 1 diabetes. N Engl J Med 2008;359:1464–76.
6. Lind M, Polonsky W, Hirsch IB, et al. Continuous glucose monitoring vs conventional therapy for glycemic control in adults with type 1 diabetes treated with multiple daily insulin injections: the GOLD randomized clinical trial. JAMA 2017;317:379–87.
7. Beck RW, Riddlesworth T, Ruedy K, et al. Effect of continuous glucose monitoring on glycemic control in adults with type 1 diabetes using insulin injections: the DIAMOND randomized clinical trial. JAMA 2017;317:371–8.
8. Peyrot M, Barnett AH, Meneghini LF, et al. Insulin adherence behaviours and barriers in the multinational Global Attitudes of Patients and Physicians in Insulin Therapy study. Diabet Med 2012;29:682–9.
9. Brod M, Rana A, Barnett AH. Adherence patterns in patients with type 2 diabetes on basal insulin analogues: missed, mistimed and reduced doses. Curr Med Res Opin 2012;28:1933–46.
10. Munshi MN, Slyne C, Greenberg JM, et al. Nonadherence to insulin therapy detected by bluetooth-enabled pen cap is associated with poor glycemic control. Diabetes Care 2019;42:1129–31.
11. Fazeli Farsani S, Brodovicz K, Soleymanlou N, et al. Incidence and prevalence of diabetic ketoacidosis (DKA) among adults with type 1 diabetes mellitus (T1D): a systematic literature review. BMJ Open 2017;7:e016587.
12. Sherr JL, Hermann JM, Campbell F, et al. Use of insulin pump therapy in children and adolescents with type 1 diabetes and its impact on metabolic control: comparison of results from three large, transatlantic paediatric registries. Diabetologia 2016;59:87–91.
13. Matejko B, Cyganek K, Katra B, et al. Insulin pump therapy is equally effective and safe in elderly and young type 1 diabetes patients. Rev Diabet Stud 2011;8:254–8.
14. Briganti EM, Summers JC, Fitzgerald ZA, et al. Continuous subcutaneous insulin infusion can be used effectively and safely in older patients with type 1 diabetes: long-term follow-up. Diabetes Technol Ther 2018;20:783–6.
15. Johnson SL, McEwen LN, Newton CA, et al. The impact of continuous subcutaneous insulin infusion and multiple daily injections of insulin on glucose variability in older adults with type 2 diabetes. J Diabetes Complications 2011;25:211–5.
16. Argento NB, Liu J, Hughes AS, et al. Impact of Medicare continuous subcutaneous insulin infusion policies in patients with type 1 diabetes. J Diabetes Sci Technol 2019. [Epub ahead of print].
17. Munshi MN. Cognitive dysfunction in older adults with diabetes: what a clinician needs to know. Diabetes Care 2017;40:461–7.
18. Sinclair AJ, Girling AJ, Bayer AJ. Cognitive dysfunction in older subjects with diabetes mellitus: impact on diabetes self-management and use of care services. All Wales Research into Elderly (AWARE) Study. Diabetes Res Clin Pract 2000;50:203–12.
19. Pfutzner J, Hellhammer J, Musholt P, et al. Evaluation of dexterity in insulin-treated patients with type 1 and type 2 diabetes mellitus. J Diabetes Sci Technol 2011;5:158–65.

20. Beck RW, Riddlesworth TD, Ruedy K, et al. Continuous glucose monitoring versus usual care in patients with type 2 diabetes receiving multiple daily insulin injections: a randomized trial. Ann Intern Med 2017;167:365–74.
21. Ruedy KJ, Parkin CG, Riddlesworth TD, et al. Continuous glucose monitoring in older adults with type 1 and type 2 diabetes using multiple daily injections of insulin: results from the DIAMOND trial. J Diabetes Sci Technol 2017;11:1138–46.
22. Argento NB, Nakamura K. Personal real-time continuous glucose monitoring in patients 65 years and older. Endocr Pract 2014;20:1297–302.
23. Wireless Innovations for Seniors with Diabetes Mellitus—Primary Results of the WISDM Study. The 79th scientific sessions of the American Diabetes Association. San Francisco, CA, June 7-11, 2019.
24. Polonsky WH, Peters AL, Hessler D. The impact of real-time continuous glucose monitoring in patients 65 years and older. J Diabetes Sci Technol 2016;10:892–7.
25. Litchman ML, Allen NA. Real-time continuous glucose monitoring facilitates feelings of safety in older adults with type 1 diabetes: a qualitative study. J Diabetes Sci Technol 2017;11:988–95.
26. Shah VN, Wu M, Foster N, et al. Severe hypoglycemia is associated with high risk for falls in adults with type 1 diabetes. Arch Osteoporos 2018;13:66.
27. Thorpe CT, Gellad WF, Good CB, et al. Tight glycemic control and use of hypoglycemic medications in older veterans with type 2 diabetes and comorbid dementia. Diabetes Care 2015;38:588–95.
28. Lipska KJ, Ross JS, Miao Y, et al. Potential overtreatment of diabetes mellitus in older adults with tight glycemic control. JAMA Intern Med 2015;175:356–62.
29. Martin-Timon I, Del Canlzo-Gomez FJ. Mechanisms of hypoglycemia unawareness and implications in diabetic patients. World J Diabetes 2015;6:912–26.
30. Bremer JP, Jauch-Chara K, Hallschmid M, et al. Hypoglycemia unawareness in older compared with middle-aged patients with type 2 diabetes. Diabetes Care 2009;32:1513–7.
31. Bainbridge KE, Cowie CC, Gonzalez F 2nd, et al. Risk factors for hearing impairment among adults with diabetes: the Hispanic community health study/study of Latinos (HCHS/SOL). J Clin Transl Endocrinol 2016;6:15–22.
32. Maahs DM, DeSalvo D, Pyle L, et al. Effect of acetaminophen on CGM glucose in an outpatient setting. Diabetes Care 2015;38:e158–9.
33. Bergenstal RM, Garg S, Weinzimer SA, et al. Safety of a hybrid closed-loop insulin delivery system in patients with type 1 diabetes. JAMA 2016;316:1407–8.
34. Forlenza GP, Li Z, Buckingham BA, et al. Predictive low-glucose suspend reduces hypoglycemia in adults, adolescents, and children with type 1 diabetes in an at-home randomized crossover study: results of the PROLOG trial. Diabetes Care 2018;41:2155–61.
35. Boughton CK, Bally L, Hartnell S, et al. Closed-loop insulin delivery in end-of-life care: a case report. Diabet Med 2019. [Epub ahead of print].

Integration of Diabetes Technology in Clinical Practice

Anne L. Peters, MD*

KEYWORDS

• Outpatient clinic • Continuous glucose monitoring • Insulin pump therapy

KEY POINTS

- For the use of technology to be effective, appropriate systems must be implemented for individualization, education, and follow-up.
- Office flow must be structured to allow for downloading of devices so data can be easily accessed for interpretation by the provider.
- If specific requirements for documentation are met, the use and interpretation of continuous glucose monitoring can be a billable procedure.

INTRODUCTION

Integrating technology into a clinic setting means developing the tools to download data and interpret data to help with diabetes management. The first step is helping the patient decide which devices are best for him or her. Providers must stay up to date on technology and match devices to patients based on their unique characteristics such as age, lifestyle, education, health literacy and numeracy, access to health care, and insurance status. It also means having the support and resources to perform device initiation, troubleshooting when devices break or fail to work effectively, and teach data uploading and self-interpretation. New data streams need to be created for data interpretation, decision making, and documentation. Finally, it means navigating systems of reimbursement so that patients can obtain the devices initially and use them over time.

TYPES OF TECHNOLOGY

In clinical practice there are several basic approaches to using technology

One approach is the use of professional or blinded continuous glucose monitoring (CGM) in which a device is placed on a patient in a clinic and started. The data are not

Keck School of Medicine of the University of Southern California, Los Angeles, CA, USA
* USC Westside Center for Diabetes, 9033 Wilshire Boulevard, Suite 406, Beverly Hills, CA 90211.
E-mail address: annepete@med.usc.edu

Endocrinol Metab Clin N Am 49 (2020) 69–77
https://doi.org/10.1016/j.ecl.2019.10.002 endo.theclinics.com
0889-8529/20/

viewable by the patient. Data are uploaded in clinic after up to 14 days for interpretation. The blinded CGM process requires in-office systems for starting the device and then removing it, uploading the data, and giving it to the provider.

Another approach is the use of personal or unblinded devices, such as CGM, self-monitoring of blood glucose (SMBG), insulin pumps (continuous subcutaneous insulin infusion or CSII), and smart pens. These devices are generally started at a training/education session or by a patient watching or reviewing the instructions at home. The devices must be downloaded at every visit for evaluation by the practitioner.

A third approach is clinic-based data interpretation that involves data downloading from devices in the clinic and/or viewing data in the clinic from cloud-based systems. These cloud-based or computer-based systems are either provided by the specific device company or through a site that integrates data from a variety of different devices (eg, Tidepool or Glooko).

DEVICE SELECTION

Which device(s) to use is generally a decision made by the health care provider and the patient. It should be done in the context of what the patient is interested in trying and what is covered by insurance.[1] Patients should be given information on what is available to them and then the opportunity to review it either on-line, through demonstrations in clinic, and/or through feedback of others with diabetes. All patients should have the opportunity to review devices that might be helpful to them. Some people are more interested in technology than others; some are not ready to change, and others become more receptive once they have seen the device and had it explained to them. It is helpful to have an example of each tool available in the office and a handout with Web sites and local contacts for the device companies so a patient knows where to turn for more information.

Table 1 presents the CGM devices available at the time of publication of this article, and **Table 2** show the insulin pumps that are available. This is to provide a framework for the key points of comparison of the devices. Given the rate of change of the field, many will have different specifications and indications on an on-going basis. Additional devices will be added. An important designation for devices has been created by the US Food and Drug Administration (FDA) to signify that a device meets a specific standard that allows it to be integrated with other devices. This designation for continuous glucose monitors is known as interoperable CGM (iCGM)[2] and for pumps as alternate controller enabled pumps (ACE pumps).[3] This should lead to greater integration of device components for the development of automated insulin delivery systems.

Blinded Continuous Glucose Monitoring

Professional CGM (blinded CGM) is used as a blinded snapshot for some duration of time (up to 14 days) that provides retrospective data for the clinician and patient to review.

Table 1
Features of commonly available continuous glucose monitoring systems

	Calibration	Warm up	Duration of Wear	Alerts	Other Features
Dexcom G6	No	2 h	10 d	Yes	iCGM
Abbott Libre	No	1 h	14 d	No	Must be scanned by user for result
Guardian G3	Yes	2 h	7 d	Yes	Works with Sugar IQ Diabetes Assistant
Eversense	Yes	24 h	3 mo	Yes	Implanted through small incision

Table 2
Features of commonly available insulin pumps

	Tethered?	ACE-Pump?	Compatible Sensor	Automated Insulin Delivery?
Omnipod Dash System	No–tubeless	No	None	No
Tandem t:slim X2 pump	Yes	Yes	Dexcom G6	Yes
Minimed 670G	Yes	No	Medtronic Guardian Sensor 3	Yes

Although some advocate only for use of unblinded CGM,[4] this can be helpful in getting a baseline snapshot of how the patient is doing and identifying periods of high and low glucose levels. Moreover it can be used in patients on every type of therapy, from lifestyle alone through insulin.[5] For some it helps motivate changes in diet and exercise; in others it may encourage progression to unblinded CGM. It is useful if patients are taught to keep a log of food, medication, and exercise to correlate with the data.

If blinded CGM is to be used there should be a system for starting the device on the patient at a clinic visit and options for its return. Generally at least 1 or 2 staff members should be trained to start the device and provide brief patient education as to wearing it. Patients need to be instructed as to how to return the device, either in person (which can be coupled with a clinic appointment/education session or appointment with a registered dietitian) or sent back through the mail for analysis. **Fig. 1** shows data from a blinded CGM device worn by a patient on basal insulin who has previously undetected, asymptomatic nocturnal hypoglycemia.

Unblinded Systems

All other systems are used by the patient in real time. This includes CGM devices, insulin pumps, automated insulin delivery systems, smart pens, and glucose meters. Each of these is used by the patient to either monitor glucose levels or deliver insulin. Depending on the patient's circumstances and interest in these tools, as well as their insurance benefits determines which is best for any given individual. This is a patient's choice, with education and input from the provider. Often there is more than 1 type to choose from. Regardless of the device selected, education is always required,[6] from on-line to in-person training. Device prescribers can either have educators available in their own office or have a list of resources a patient can contact for assistance. It is helpful for the patient to have the option of meeting with a diabetes educator should device issues occur or more training is needed. Older patients and those with lower health numeracy/literacy skills may need more education. It is also necessary for patients to have back-up plans in cases of device failure and access to health care for instructions on what to do in an emergency.

DATA FLOW

Technology is allowing provider and patients to have access to more data than ever before. However, data alone change nothing. Data must be integrated into the health care providers' clinical practice and used on a day-to-day basis by the person using the technology. Historically, many providers did not download basic data from glucose meters; now the range of devices that require downloading has expanded including pumps, sensors, insulin dose calculators, and smart pens. Learning how to download data and evaluate and provide recommendations is vital to the education of patients and the treatment of their diabetes.

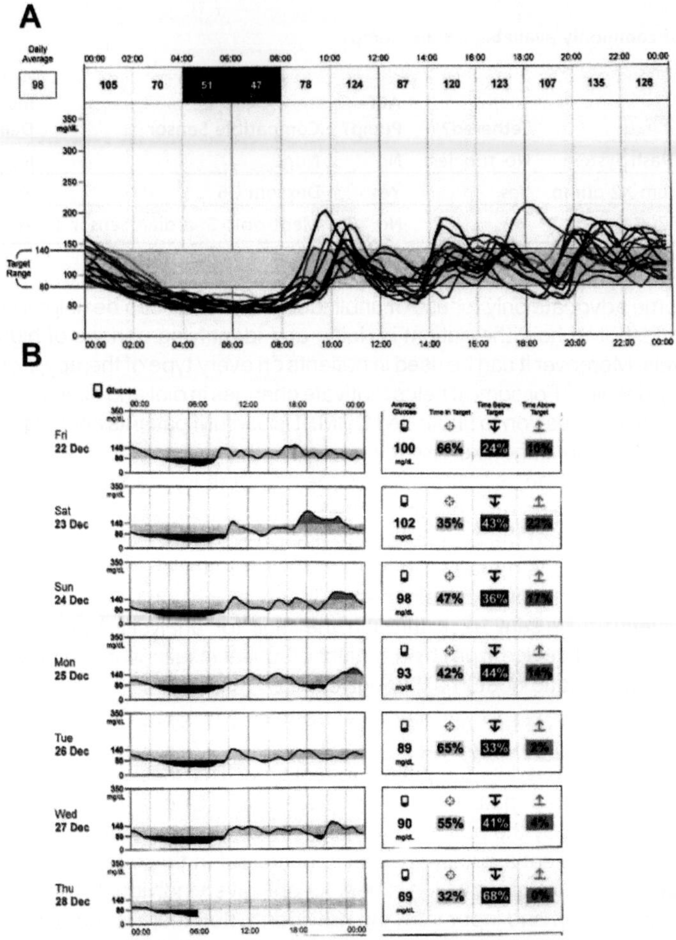

Fig. 1. Professional CGM Printout. (*A*) Data are presented as a modal day, with all the dates from the 14 days of device wear included. The x-axis is time of day—starting at midnight and ending at midnight. (*B*) These are individual day tracings showing the daily nocturnal episodes of hypoglycemia.

Systems must be developed for downloading/viewing data within the clinic setting. The specifics of how this works will be clinic dependent, but general principles apply. First, a place needs to be identified as to where device information assessment/downloading will occur. Second, systems need to be set up, and the staff members who will do this need to be trained; third, how the data will be presented for the provider/patient should be determined.

In general it is helpful for a staff member who does the initial intake to ask patients if they use any diabetes devices (from glucose meters and beyond) and whether they have uploaded to the cloud (**Fig. 2**). If they have, then the patient's account should be accessed and the data prepared for the visit (in some cases this is a printout for the provider, in others the provider will view the data in the actual program on the Internet.) In other cases the devices will need to be downloaded in clinic and the data provided to the health care providers. In all cases there must be a commitment

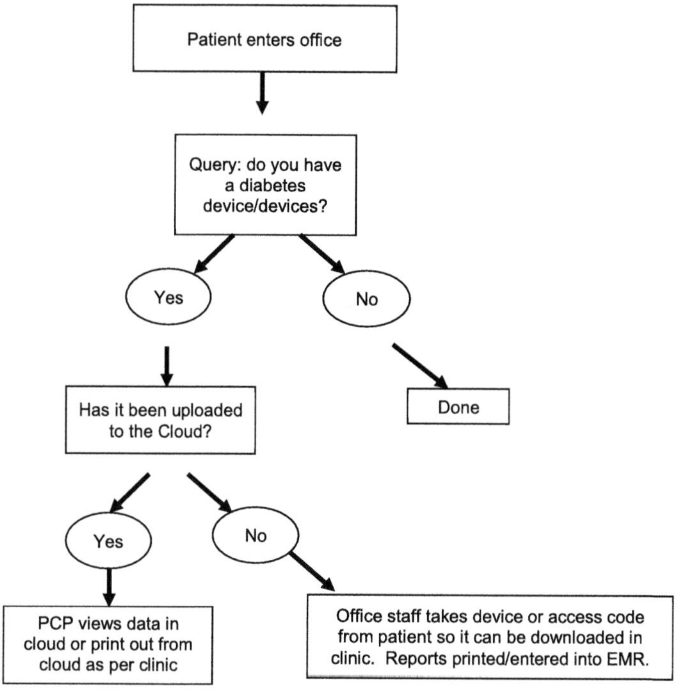

Fig. 2. Suggested office flow. Basic office flow for obtaining data from patient devices. Offices will modify based on their own circumstances.

to making this process work. Often a staff member should be identified as the champion for diabetes devices to ensure that the systems work. This is in part because these systems can be fraught with issues, including updates to programs that may require institutional information technology (IT) intervention to change, forgotten passwords, and lack of device connectivity.

The data flow must go from patient to device to office and then to the health care providers for interpretation and review with the patient. As much as possible providers should predetermine the format for data review. In general reviewing the past 2 weeks' worth of data is the most useful for assessment and improving outcomes over the next 3 months.[7] Most devices come with their own array of printouts, and some can be uploaded into programs that integrate data and allow for a uniform display of information (eg, Tidepool, Glooko). The Ambulatory Glucose Profile (AGP), is an excellent tool for standard data interpretation and can save time during clinic visits.[8] Patients can engage with the information and learn to track such metrics as time in range (TIR), glucose management indicator (GMI), and coefficient of variation (CV).

PROVIDER ROLE

Providers must work with their team to set expectations and define which information is necessary for each office visit. Providers need to understand the different devices that are available and keep updated as technology advances, as well as possess a willingness to work with technology and help patients succeed.[9] As prescribers of the devices, providers must offer on-going support and education, with emphasis on reinforcing troubleshooting information at each office visit. Pump failures, site occlusions and infections, and CGMs that fall off or stop working after only a day or two can be disruptive for patients who are depending on them. Having a backup plan for each patient, with emergency-injected insulin dosing (if a patient is on a pump), is imperative, as well as providing patients with on-call support 24/7. Patients also need to be aware of whom to call from the device companies if technical assistance is required.

The health care professional should be able to analyze the data from each device and provide succinct feedback to the patient during the course of each visit. Patients should be encouraged to express their frustrations with technology as well as review what is helpful. Plans for going forward should be formulated with motivational interviewing and goal setting.[10] Issues with regards to diabetes distress and burnout should be addressed, as needed, with considered attention to other physical and mental health issues the patient is experiencing.

PATIENT ROLE

In using all devices, from SMBG through automated insulin delivery systems, the patient is the driver of how well these tools are used. Nearly all device reports give some indication of the frequency of use. It is clear that unblinded CGM is most effective when used nearly daily.[6] If a patient is not reaching his or her targets and is not using his or her device(s) regularly, it is important to discuss barriers to the use of technology. If a device is not working or cannot be refilled patients should be encouraged to contact the provider and/or device company to be sure he or she has a functional system. Shared decision making and goal setting are important, to ensure that the patient has a sense of what he or she is aiming for and is in agreement with the plan. If a patient needs more education then sessions with a CDE should be arranged. If meal planning and carbohydrate counting is an issue, then referral to a registered dietitian knowledgeable about diabetes management may be beneficial. For some individuals, referral to a mental health provider can help them deal with issues such as anxiety, fear, depression, eating disorders, and other concerns.

Patients should be encouraged to download and interpret their own data as much as is helpful. Education around data interpretation can lead to a person with diabetes identifying patterns and trends that can result in medication adjustments in between visits with a provider. For some self-titration of medication can be taught; for others communication with the health care team is needed for dose adjustments. Regardless of how the data are used, changes made more often than at every 3 months clinic visits can lead to more rapid improvements in glycemic control.

INSURANCE COVERAGE AND BILLING

Understanding the insurance coverage for devices can be tricky, and some patients may have copays that are unaffordable. It is important to learn the requirements for prescribing any given device and consider creating automatic text phrases to facilitate adequate documentation (**Table 3**). For Medicare to receive approval for a CGM device for a patient it must be stated that[11]

1. The patient requires a therapeutic CGM and has diabetes mellitus.
2. The patient is performing SMBG at least 4 times daily (although Medicare only provides 3 test strips daily).
3. The patient is insulin treated and is injecting insulin at least 3 times daily or is on an insulin pump.

Table 3
Billing codes for continuous glucose monitoring

Code	Description	Who Can Place and Initiate Sensor?	Who Can Bill for Service?
95,249	Ambulatory initiation of CGM of interstitial tissue fluid via a subcutaneous sensor for a minimum of 72 h Patient-owned equipment, sensor placement, hook-up, calibration of monitor, patient training, and printout of recording The code requires the patient to bring the data receiver into the clinician office where the entire process is performed	RN, PharmD/RPh, RD, CDE or MA within their scope of practice	Only MD/DO, NP, and CNS can bill for services associated with this code
95,250	Ambulatory CGM of interstitial tissue fluid via a subcutaneous sensor for a minimum of 72 h Clinician-owned equipment, sensor placement, hook-up, calibration of monitor, patient training, removal of sensor, and printout of recording	RN, PharmD/RPh, RD, CDE or MA within their scope of practice	Only MD/DO, NP, and CNS can bill for services associated with this code
95,251	This code is used and reported to insurers when clinicians perform an analysis, interpretation, and report on a minimum of 72 h of CGM data The analysis, interpretation, and report may be done with data from patient-owned or clinician-owned CGM device It requires the patient to bring the data receiver into the physician or other qualified health care professional's office, where the entire initial data collection process is performed Importantly, the analysis, interpretation, and report are distinct from an E/M service and do not include an assessment of the patient or indicate a plan of care for the patient	N/A	Only MD/DO, NP, and CNS can bill for services associated with this code

Modified from Kruger DF, Edelman SV, Hinene DA, Parkin CG. A reference guide for integrating continuous glucose monitoring into clinical practice. Diabetes Educ 2019;45(suppl 1):3S-20S; with permission.

4. The patient's insulin treatment regimen requires frequent dose adjusting based on SMBG/CGM results.
5. Within 6 months prior to ordering the CGM the patient had an in-person visit with the treating practitioner to evaluate his or her diabetes control and determine that criteria 1 to 4 are met. Every 6 months following the initial prescription the patient must have an in-person visit to assess adherence to CGM and diabetes treatment plan.

There are billing codes for inserting/analyzing data from CGM devices (both professional and personal) that can help with reimbursement. **Table 2** lists these codes and their descriptions.[12] It is important that the patient visit include certain key elements and that these are clearly documented in the chart.

Documentation for billing includes[13]

1. A brief statement or narrative that glucose sensor data were evaluated
2. Treatment or therapy changes noted
3. Action steps, plan, or after visit summary provided to the patient
4. Electronic or print of data report attached to the patient chart

SUMMARY

Device use has changed the management of diabetes. However, devices alone are not useful unless integrated into the practice of medicine. Patients need education, follow-up, and evaluation on an on-going basis. In-office downloading and assessment of devices make office visits useful and help encourage effective device use. Patients can also use tools for data assessment on their own, which helps them with near real-time feedback as to their progress. Each office must assess resources and determine the best flow for uploading and evaluating device data. If a system is in place, it allows for effective education and communication with the patient and can increase the likelihood of patients reaching their goals.

DISCLOSURE

The author has research that is funded by Dexcom and have been provided devices for use in research by Abbott Diabetes Care. The author has served on an advisory panel for Abbott Diabetes Care.

REFERENCES

1. Aleppo G, Webb K. Continuous glucose monitoring integration in clinical practice: a stepped guide to data review and interpretation. J Diabetes Sci Technol 2018. https://doi.org/10.1177/1932296818813581.
2. Available at: https://www.fda.gov/news-events/press-announcements/fda-authorizes-first-fully-interoperable-continuous-glucose-monitoring-system-streamlines-review. Accessed June 17, 2019.
3. Available at: https://www.fda.gov/news-events/press-announcements/fda-authorizes-first-interoperable-insulin-pump-intended-allow-patients-customize-treatment-through. Accessed June 17, 2019.
4. Ahn D, Pettus J, Edelman S. Unblinded CGM should replace blinded CGM in the clinical management of diabetes. J Diabetes Sci Technol 2016;10:793–8.
5. Sierra JA, Shah M, Gill MS, et al. Clinical and economic benefits of professional CGM among people with type 2 diabetes in the United States: analysis of claims and lab data. J Med Econ 2018;21:225–30.

6. Peters AL, Ahmann AJ, Battelino T, et al. Diabetes technology-continuous subcutaneous insulin infusion therapy and continuous glucose monitoring in adults: an Endocrine Society clinical practice guideline. J Clin Endocrinol Metab 2016;101: 3922–37.
7. Riddlesworth TD, Beck RW, Gal RL, et al. Optimal sampling duration for continuous glucose monitoring to determine long-term glycemic control. Diabetes Technol Ther 2018;20:314–6.
8. Mullen DM, Bergenstal R, Criego A, et al. Time saving using a standardized glucose reporting system and ambulatory glucose profile. J Diabetes Sci Technol 2018;12:614–21.
9. Tanenbaum ML, Adam RN, Lanning MS, et al. Using cluster analysis to understand clinician readiness to promote continuous glucose monitoring adoption. J Diabetes Sci Technol 2018;12:1108–15.
10. Beverly EA, Worley MF, Court AB, et al. Patient-physician communication and diabetes self-care. J Clin Outcomes Management 2016;23(11).
11. Centers for Medicare and Medicaid Services. Medicare coverage of diabetes supplies and devices. Available at: https://www.medicare.gov/Pubs/pdf/11022-Medicare-Diabetes-Coverage.pdf. Accessed June 17, 2019.
12. Kruger DF, Edelman SV, Hinene DA, et al. A reference guide for integrating continuous glucose monitoring into clinical practice. Diabetes Educ 2019; 45(suppl 1):3S–20S.
13. AACE report. CPT codes 95249, 95250, and 95251. Available at: https://www.aace.com/practice-management/cpt-codes-95249-95250-and-95251. And https://www.aace.com/files/socioeconomics/new_revised_codes_2018.pdf. Accessed June 17, 2019.

Diabetes Technology in the Inpatient Setting for Management of Hyperglycemia

Georgia M. Davis, MD, Rodolfo J. Galindo, MD,
Alexandra L. Migdal, MD, Guillermo E. Umpierrez, MD, CDE*

KEYWORDS

• Diabetes • Technology • Inpatient • Hospital • Glycemic control

KEY POINTS

- Ambulatory use of diabetes technology, including continuous glucose monitoring (CGM), continuous subcutaneous insulin infusion (CSII), and closed-loop systems, has rapidly expanded during the past decades, with more recent studies evaluating its translation to the hospital setting.
- Preliminary data show improvement in detection of both hyperglycemia and hypoglycemia with use of CGM in the hospital.
- Recent studies have tested the use of closed-loop systems in diverse populations of hospitalized patients.
- Further investigation is needed regarding the inpatient use of diabetes technology and how it pertains to glycemic control and patient-centered outcomes.

INTRODUCTION

Advances in diabetes technology over the past decades have revolutionized patient care and diabetes management. The use of this technology, including continuous glucose monitoring (CGM) and continuous subcutaneous insulin infusion (CSII), in patients with type 1 (T1) and type 2 (T2) diabetes mellitus (DM) continues to grow in the ambulatory setting. Although substantial data support outpatient use of this technology for improvement in glycemic control and diabetes outcomes, there are limited data regarding its use in the inpatient setting.[1] There is consensus among experts and medical societies that, compared with intermittent capillary blood glucose testing, CGM technology offers benefits in the prevention of severe hyperglycemia and hypoglycemia by identifying glucose trends and allowing insulin doses to be adjusted more accurately.[2–4] In addition, several diabetes clinical guidelines support the continued use of outpatient CSII in patients who are physically able to continue using their insulin

Department of Medicine, Emory University, 69 Jesse Hill Jr Drive Southeast, Glenn Memorial Building, Suite 200, Atlanta, GA 30303, USA
* Corresponding author.
E-mail address: geumpie@emory.edu

Endocrinol Metab Clin N Am 49 (2020) 79–93
https://doi.org/10.1016/j.ecl.2019.11.002 endo.theclinics.com

pump during hospitalization.[3,5] However, randomized controlled trials are needed to determine whether use of CGM and CSII systems in the hospital can improve clinical outcomes compared with intermittent capillary blood glucose monitoring and conventional insulin treatment. As CGM and CSII technologies continue to advance, the use of artificial pancreas technology is being evaluated in the inpatient setting. Use of computerized decision support systems for glycemic control in the hospital is also expanding. Here we review current available diabetes technology as it relates to the management of hospitalized patients.

CONTINUOUS GLUCOSE MONITORING IN THE HOSPITAL

The use of capillary point-of-care (POC) glucose testing has been the mainstay for monitoring and treatment of hospitalized patients with diabetes. POC blood glucose (BG) testing is commonly performed 3 to 4 times daily in hospitalized patients for monitoring of glycemic control and adjustment of diabetes treatment regimens. However, the need for frequent BG testing in certain inpatient populations, the intermittent nature of testing, and the associated time burden for nursing and ancillary hospital staff are significant limitations of POC BG testing. The desire for closer monitoring of glucose values led to the development of CGM beginning in the late 1970s, with approval of the first CGM by the Food and Drug Administration occurring in 1999.[6] The ability of CGM to provide estimated glucose values every 5 to 15 minutes with information regarding glucose trends allows for a more comprehensive assessment of glycemic control, an attractive feature in both inpatient and outpatient settings. Rapid improvements in accuracy and increased commercial availability of CGM technology has led to its widespread use in ambulatory diabetes management. However, use of CGM in the hospital remains investigational, with ongoing studies evaluating its use in diverse inpatient populations.

In the hospital setting, several studies have shown improvement in the detection of both hyperglycemia and hypoglycemia in critically ill and non–critically ill patients.[2,7–9] In contrast to the exclusive use of subcutaneous CGM sensors in the outpatient realm, CGM use in the hospital can also include invasive (intravascular) or noninvasive (transdermal) CGM in intensive care unit (ICU) settings.

Most studies in ICU populations using CGM have focused on accuracy and reliability, and have in general been small and underpowered to detect changes in patient-centered outcomes (ie, incidence of hypoglycemia or complications) (**Table 1**). Of the studies assessing glycemic control, most did not show significant differences in average glycemic control with CGM versus POC glucose testing. Kopecky and colleagues[12] investigated the use of CGM combined with an enhanced model predictive control (eMPC) insulin titration algorithm in postoperative cardiac ICU patients. The use of the eMPC algorithm combined with CGM was compared with standard use of the algorithm with interval POC glucose testing (control group). Overall, there were no significant differences in glycemic control between the eMPC-CGM system with more frequent input of glucose values compared with the eMPC algorithm with intermittent BG values alone.[12] In a larger study, Holzinger and colleagues[11] observed a significant reduction in hypoglycemia (defined as glucose <40 mg/dL or 2.2 mmol/L) with real-time CGM (RT-CGM) use versus POC testing (1.6 vs 11.5%; P = .031) in ICU patients requiring mechanical ventilation. A subgroup analysis in this population revealed improved glycemic control and time in target glucose range (defined as glucose <110 mg/dL or 6.1 mmol/L) in patients with higher illness severity indices. Despite these findings, there were no differences in hospital length of stay (LOS) or mortality between CGM and POC BG testing groups.[11] A recent expert

Table 1
ICU CGM outcomes studies

Authors	CGM Type	Patient Population	Study Design	Outcomes	Results
Logtenberg et al,[10] 2009	Paradigm (Medtronic MiniMed)	Cardiac ICU; non-DM patients undergoing elective cardiothoracic surgery (n = 30)	Prospective RCT: RT-CGM with alerts at 72 mg/dL and 180 mg/dL vs RT-CGM without alerts	Accuracy and glycemic control between alert groups	No significant difference in glycemic control with use of CGM alerts.
Holzinger et al,[11] 2010	Guardian (Medtronic MiniMed)	DM and non-DM ICU patients requiring mechanical ventilation (n = 124)	Prospective RCT: RT-CGM (no alerts) vs standard of care (with blinded CGM)	Glycemic control, LOS, mortality	No significant difference in mean glucose or time with glucose <150 or <110 mg/dL; marked reduction in hypoglycemia with RT-CGM (1.6 vs 11.5%; *P* = .031). No differences in LOS or hospital mortality.
Kopecky et al,[12] 2013	Guardian (Medtronic MiniMed)	Cardiac ICU; patients with DM and non-DM undergoing elective major cardiac surgery (n = 24)	Prospective RCT: eMCP algorithm for BG management alone vs eMPC combined with CGM values every 15 min	Glycemic control	No significant differences in glycemic control between groups; 2 hypoglycemic events in control eMPC vs no events in eMPC-CGM group.
Umbrello et al,[13] 2014	OptiScanner 5000 (OptiScan Biomedical Corporation)	DM and non-DM ICU patients with sepsis (n = 6)	Pilot prospective observational study: use of CGM to evaluate glycemic control protocol	Glycemic control	Adequate glycemic control ([93% of cohort with median time in target range [BG 80–150 mg/dL]). No episodes of severe hypoglycemia (<40 mg/dL).
De Block et al,[14] 2015	GlucoDay S (A. Menarini Diagnostics)	ICU patients (n = 35)	Prospective RCT: RT-CGM vs standard of care and blinded CGM	Accuracy and glycemic control	No significant difference in glycemic control, variability, or hypoglycemic events. No significant difference in LOS or hospital mortality.

Conversion: mg/dL × 0.0555 = mmol/L.

Abbreviations: CGM, continuous glucose monitoring; DM, diabetes mellitus; eMPC, enhanced model predictive control; ICU, intensive care unit; LOS, length of stay; RCT, randomized-controlled trial; RT-CGM, real-time continuous glucose monitoring.

Data from Refs.[10–14]

consensus meeting acknowledged that use of CGM in critical care populations appears to be accurate and reliable, but there continues to be a need for larger studies powered to determine efficacy in improving glycemic control, detection and reduction of hypoglycemic events, and impact on hospital stay and clinical outcomes.[2]

In non–critically ill hospitalized patients, studies with the use of CGM have been mostly observational (**Table 2**). Observational data have provided important insight into glycemic control patterns in hospitalized patients, emphasizing improved detection of hypoglycemia using CGM. Gomez and Umpierrez[7] compared the use of blinded/professional CGM versus POC glucose testing in non–critically ill hospitalized patients with T2DM treated with basal bolus insulin regimens. Even though there was no significant difference in mean daily blood glucose concentration between groups, CGM detected a higher number of hypoglycemic events (52 vs 12, $P = .0001$). More than 50% of the hypoglycemic events occurred between dinner and breakfast, highlighting the utility of CGM use for detection of nocturnal hypoglycemia in this population.[7] A recent pilot study by Spanakis and colleagues[19] in a population of non-ICU hospitalized older adult patients (mean age 70.8 ± 6.2 years) demonstrated feasibility of using CGM data transmitted to nursing personnel in a telemetry-type method, with an alert for hypoglycemia set at a sensor glucose value of 85 mg/dL (4.7 mmol/L). In this group of 5 patients on insulin therapy, there were no episodes of severe hypoglycemia (<54 mg/dL or 3 mmol/L) and potential hypoglycemic episodes were prevented in 2 patients using the CGM alert system during the hospital stay.[19]

CGM technology continues to evolve, with investigations expanding to more diverse inpatient populations with diabetes. More accuracy data are needed in specific hospital patient populations, including those with severe dehydration and volume depletion, anasarca, and end-stage renal disease on hemodialysis or peritoneal dialysis. Although CGM metrics (including time in target glucose range, time in hyperglycemia, time in hypoglycemia, and glycemic variability) continue to be updated and defined for targeting improved glycemic control and outcomes in ambulatory patients,[20] no current consensus exists regarding CGM metrics in hospitalized patients. Further information is needed in this setting on standardization of glycemic control metrics, appropriate target glucose ranges, and impact of CGM use on hospital outcomes and costs to understand how to safely and effectively implement this technology. In addition to targeting improved glycemic control, emerging CGMs that no longer require calibration with POC glucose testing (factory-calibrated) have the potential to decrease both nursing and patient burden associated with frequent POC glucose testing in the hospital. Ongoing studies (NCT03832907) with factory-calibrated CGM are testing its accuracy in diverse inpatient populations, and the use of CGM data by nursing and ancillary staff to detect and prevent glycemic excursions (NCT03877068).

CONTINUOUS SUBCUTANEOUS INSULIN INFUSION IN THE HOSPITAL

With the use of CSII increasing in the ambulatory setting, the importance of guidelines for its continued use in the inpatient setting for health care providers has been addressed by several professional societies, including the American Diabetes Association, the American Association of Clinical Endocrinologists, and The Endocrine Society. These societies advocate for continuation of CSII therapy in appropriate hospitalized patients, with the support of (1) implemented hospital policies on CSII, (2) inpatient endocrinology or diabetes management teams, and (3) a signed agreement from the patient acknowledging responsibilities of CSII therapy.[3,5,21] Continuation of CSII is not recommended in critically ill and hemodynamically unstable

Table 2
Non-ICU CGM studies

Authors	CGM Type	Patient Population	Study Design	Outcomes	Results
Burt et al,[15] 2013	CGMS Gold (Medtronic MiniMed)	T1DM and T2DM admitted to general wards on basal bolus insulin (n = 26)	Observational Prospective Cohort: blinded CGM vs POC glucose testing	Accuracy and glycemic control	No significant difference in glycemic control; most hyperglycemic episodes were postprandial and hypoglycemic episodes more likely to occur between midnight and 7 AM
Schaupp et al,[16] 2015	iPro2 system (Medtronic MiniMed)	T2DM admitted to general wards on basal bolus insulin (n = 84)	Observational Prospective Cohort: blinded CGM vs POC glucose testing	Accuracy	Good agreement between CGM and POC glucose values; Clarke Error Grid analysis with 98.7% of values in Zone A or Zone B (88.2% within Zone A); 15-fold increase in detection of nocturnal hypoglycemia with CGM.
Gómez et al,[17] 2015	iPro2 system (Medtronic MiniMed)	T2DM or hyperglycemia admitted to general wards on basal bolus insulin (n = 38)	Prospective Pilot RCT: blinded CGM vs POC glucose testing	Accuracy	Good agreement between CGM and POC glucose values; Clarke Error Grid analysis with 91.9% of values in Zone A or Zone B. Increased detection of hypoglycemic episodes with CGM (55 vs 12, $P<.01$).
Gu et al,[18] 2017	Paradigm 722 or CGMS Gold (Medtronic MiniMed)	T2DM admitted to general wards for glycemic control (n = 81)	Prospective RCT: SAP vs MDI with blinded CGM	Glycemic control, time to target glucose	21 SAP vs 6 MDI patients achieved glycemic targets within 3 d. SAP vs MDI had less hypoglycemia (sensor glucose <50 mg/dL: 0.04% vs 0.32%; $P<.05$) and hyperglycemia (sensor glucose >180 mg/dL: 21.56% vs 35.03%; $P<.05$).
Spanakis et al,[19] 2018	DEXCOM G4 CGM with Share2 application (DEXCOM)	T2DM admitted to general wards on insulin therapy (n = 5)	Single-arm pilot trial of consecutive patients using glucose telemetry system (CGM alert at 85 mg/dL)	Glucose telemetry system feasibility	Prevention of potential hypoglycemia (CGM BG <70 mg/dL for >20 min) captured by alarm occurred in 2 patients (3 events). No patients had CGM glucose value <54 mg/dL.

Conversion: mg/dL x 0.0555 = mmol/L.

Abbreviations: BG, blood glucose; CGM, continuous glucose monitoring; CGMS, continuous glucose monitoring system; ICU, intensive care unit; MDI, multiple daily injections; POC, point of care; SAP, sensor-augmented pump; T1DM, type 1 diabetes mellitus; T2DM, type 2 diabetes mellitus;

Data from Refs.[15–19]

patients, as well as in those who are not able to demonstrate appropriate use of their insulin pump.[1,3,5] For instance, a retrospective analysis of 50 patients by Kannan and colleagues[22] demonstrated that 24% of patients admitted to the hospital using CSII in the outpatient setting were unable to correctly demonstrate use of critical pump skills during hospitalization. A recent review by Umpierrez and Klonoff[1] illustrates a proposed algorithm for decision-making regarding hospital continuation of CSII therapy (**Fig. 1**), as well as contraindications to its use (**Box 1**).

Most of the data regarding hospital use of CSII have been retrospective and focused on the continuation of outpatient CSII during admission. These studies have suggested that with appropriate patient selection and hospital guidelines, patients on preexisting CSII (with or without concurrent CGM) can safely maintain glycemic control during hospitalization. Review of 125 hospitalizations of 65 patients on insulin pump therapy by Nassar and colleagues[23] showed an increase in prevalence of insulin pump use during hospitalization over a 3-year period. During this time, there were no significant differences in mean hospital glucose levels between patients who continued CSII versus those transitioned to multiple daily insulin injections (MDI).[23] An additional review by Cook and colleagues[24] of 253 hospitalizations of 136 patients on outpatient CSII over a 6-year period showed similar results regarding glycemic control between CSII use and subcutaneous insulin therapy during hospitalization, but there were fewer severe hyperglycemic (BG >300 mg/dL or 16.7 mmol/L) and hypoglycemic (BG <50 mg/dL or 2.8 mmol/L) events in patients remaining on CSII in the hospital. In addition, a recent prospective pilot trial by Levitt and colleagues[25] investigated the feasibility of CSII, both with and without CGM technology, in hospitalized patients with T2DM. Patients were randomized to 3 groups: (1) basal bolus insulin therapy with blinded CGM, (2) CSII with blinded CGM, or (3) CSII with RT-CGM. Although there were no significant differences in time in target glucose range or time in

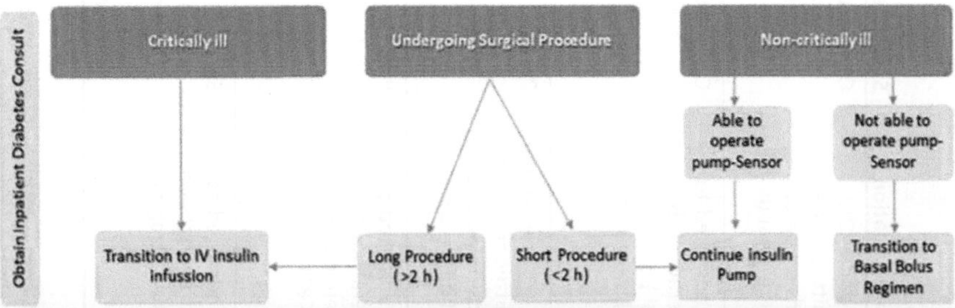

Changes to pump therapy with Imaging Studies	
X-Ray/CT	Pump should be covered by lead apron
MRI	Pump and metal infusion set should be removed
Ultrasound	No need to remove pump but transducer should not be pointed directly at the pump
Cardiac Catheterization	Pump should be covered by lead apron
Pacemaker/Automatic Implantable Cardioverter Defibrillator (AICD)	Pump should be covered by lead apron
Colonoscopy/EGD	Pump can remain in place
Laser Surgery	Pump can remain in place

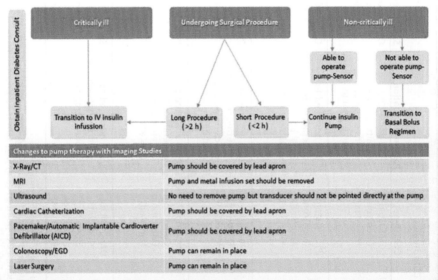

Fig. 1. Algorithm for inpatient continuation of CSII-CGM therapy hospitalization. EGD, upper endoscopy; IV, intravenous. (*From* Umpierrez GE, Klonoff DC. Diabetes Technology Update: Use of Insulin Pumps and Continuous Glucose Monitoring in the Hospital. *Diabetes Care*. 2018;41(8):1579-1589; with permission.)

Box 1
Contraindications to insulin pump therapy in the hospital

Impaired level of consciousness (except during short-term anesthesia)

Patient's inability to correctly demonstrate appropriate pump settings

Critical illness requiring intensive care

Psychiatric illness that interferes with a patient's ability to self-manage diabetes

Diabetic ketoacidosis and hyperosmolar hyperglycemic state

Refusal or unwillingness to participate in self-care

Lack of pump supplies

Lack of trained health care providers, diabetes educators, or diabetes specialist

Patient at risk for suicide

Health care decision

From Umpierrez GE, Klonoff DC. Diabetes Technology Update: Use of Insulin Pumps and Continuous Glucose Monitoring in the Hospital. *Diabetes Care.* 2018;41(8):1579-1589; with permission.

hypoglycemia between groups, this study showed the feasibility of combined CSII-CGM therapy in the inpatient setting. In addition, they reported that CGM detected more episodes of hypoglycemia than POC glucose testing alone (19 vs 12 episodes).[25] A study by Gu and colleagues[18] in China evaluated CSII with CGM versus MDI in non–acutely ill patients with T2DM hospitalized for glycemic optimization over a 2-week period. In 81 patients (40 on CSII-CGM vs 41 on MDI), more patients using CSII-CGM were able to achieve target glucose values between 70 and 180 mg/dL (3.9–10.0 mmol/L) within a 3-day period compared with those on MDI (53% vs 15%, respectively). Overall, those on CSII-CGM also had significantly less hypoglycemia (glucose <50 mg/dL [2.8 mmol/L]; 0.02 vs 0.31%, $P<.05$), and less severe hyperglycemia (glucose >250 mg/dL [13.9 mmol/L]; 3.9 vs 8.3%, $P<.05$).[18]

Although CSII does continue to be used in the inpatient setting, current investigations are moving toward the use of combined CSII-CGM technology with the ability to provide automated modulation of subcutaneous insulin infusion rates (ie, closed-loop or hybrid closed-loop technology).

ARTIFICIAL PANCREAS TECHNOLOGY IN THE HOSPITAL

The artificial pancreas system, also referred to as a "closed-loop" system, "automated insulin delivery" system, or "autonomous system for glycemic control," is composed of a CGM and insulin infusion pump for CSII. Insulin delivery is regulated by a computer algorithm that determines the amount of insulin to administer in response to a given sensor glucose concentration, thereby more closely approximating physiologic insulin action. Initial studies evaluating the use of a closed-loop system in the hospital setting focused on critically ill patients. These small, randomized trials demonstrated good efficacy data with improvement in time in target glucose range, and lower mean glucose levels without an increased risk of hypoglycemia.[26–28]

More recent studies by Hovorka and colleagues[29–32] evaluating the use of a closed-loop system in the non–critically ill hospital setting have shown promising safety and efficacy data. In one study, patients with T2DM were randomized to receive conventional insulin treatment or insulin delivery based on a closed-loop system with ad lib meal intake and activity. Findings from the initial pilot study of 40 patients demonstrated a greater percentage of time spent with sensor glucose in target range (100–180 mg/dL or 5.6–10.0 mmol/L) in the closed-loop intervention compared with control, 59.8% versus 38.1%, and less time in hyperglycemia (difference of 19%).[31] There was no significant difference in mean BG between groups or hypoglycemia rates, and no significant differences in insulin doses. Glucose variability was decreased in the closed-loop group. Patients were overwhelmingly satisfied with the use of the closed-loop system.[31] Similar findings were seen in a larger multicenter study implementing the same protocol with improvement in time in target glucose range in the closed-loop group compared with controls (65.8% ± 16.8% vs 41.5% ± 16.9%, 95% confidence interval [CI], 18.6 to 30.0; $P<.0013$).[29] A post hoc analysis in patients with T2DM admitted to the hospital on hemodialysis found that patients randomized to the closed-loop system spent 37.6% more time with sensor glucose in target range compared with standard-of-care POC glucose monitoring without an increased risk of hypoglycemia.[32]

Nutritional support, either through parenteral or enteral routes, frequently results in hyperglycemia in patients with and without a prior diagnosis of diabetes.[33] Unique challenges exist in this population in that unplanned interruptions in feedings can place patients at risk for hypoglycemia. Use of a closed-loop system in the setting of nutritional support resulted in improved glycemic control with a higher proportion of time with glucose in target range (68.4% [standard deviation (SD) 15.5] vs 36.4% [SD 26.6], $P<.0001$), lower mean glucose (153 mg/dL [SD 1.2] vs 205 mg/dL [SD 3.4], 8.5 vs 11.4 mmol/L, $P = .001$), lower rates of hyperglycemia (32.6% less time with glucose >180 mg/dL or 10.0 mmol/L [95% CI 17.8–47.3], $P<.0001$), although no difference in hypoglycemia when compared with conventional insulin treatment.[30]

A recent observational study reported glycemic control of patients with T1DM (N = 27) who participated in randomized crossover trials during pregnancy using closed-loop during labor, delivery, and postpartum.[34] Use of closed-loop was associated with 82.0% (interquartile range [IQR] 49.3, 93.0) time in target glucose range during labor and delivery and a mean glucose of 124 ± 25 mg/dL (6.9 ± 1.4 mmol/L). Closed-loop resulted in good glycemic control throughout vaginal, elective, and emergency cesarean deliveries. After delivery, women spent 83.3% of time in target glucose range (70–180 mg/dL or 3.9–10.0 mmol/L).[34]

Potential advantages to using a closed-loop system in the hospital setting include the ability to continually adapt insulin administration to changing glucose levels with minimal input from nursing or support staff. Use of a closed-loop system means less active management for nursing staff and therefore less risk of dosing errors compared with MDI or intravenous insulin administration, with improved glycemic control outcomes and a lower risk of iatrogenic hypoglycemia. Previous randomized controlled trials have been limited to patients with T2DM, and have mostly excluded patients with T1DM, which may be a more vulnerable population. There is concern with regard to pump or sensor failure and the need for device removal given the associated potential for diabetic ketoacidosis. Among closed-loop studies, up to 27% of patients had devices removed at least once during hospitalization.[29] It is also important to note that limited data exist evaluating the impact of a closed-loop system on clinical outcomes and hospital costs. These data will be essential to justify widespread adoption of such technology, given high implementation costs and need for specialized training for health care staff.

Table 3
Computerized glycemic management systems

Authors	Glucose Management System	Design	Glycemic Outcome (mg/dL)[a]	Results
Commercially available computerized glycemic management systems				
Juneja et al,[40] 2009	Glucostabilizer (ICU)	Retrospective, descriptive	%Time in target range (80–110) %BG <70 %BG <40	73.4% 0.31% 0.1%
Newton et al,[41] 2010	Glucommander (ICU)	Multicenter, randomized controlled trial, paper-based vs computerized	Mean BG %BG in target Range (80–120) Patients with BG <60	117 vs 103[c] 51% vs 71%[c] 31.9 vs 42.9
Tanenberg et al,[42] 2017	EndoTool (ICU)	Retrospective, descriptive	%BG <70 %BG <40 CV%	0.93% 0.03% 26.5%
John et al,[43] 2018	EndoTool (ICU)	Retrospective, comparative analysis of paper-based vs computerized	Time in target[b] %BG <70 Hours on IV insulin infusion	47.3% vs 45.2% 0.36 vs 0.007 2.39 vs 20.9

(*continued on next page*)

Table 3
(*continued*)

Authors	Glucose Management System	Design	Glycemic Outcome (mg/dL)[a]	Results
Ullal et al,[44] 2018	Glucommander (DKA)	Retrospective, comparative analysis of paper-based vs computerized	%Patients with BG <60 %Patients with BG <40	11%–14% vs 33%–39% 0.2%–0.4% vs 6%–7.5%
Institution-specific computerized glycemic management systems				
Hermayer et al,[37] 2007	Medical University of South Carolina	Retrospective, comparative analysis of paper-based vs computerized	Mean BG %BG in target range (80–120) %BG <70	163 vs 154[c] 82% vs 54%[c] 1.42 vs 1.14
Dortch et al,[45] 2008	Vanderbilt University Hospital, TN	Retrospective, comparative analysis of paper-based vs computerized	%BG 80–110 %BG >150 %BG ≤40	41.8% vs 34%[c] 12.8% vs 15.1%[c] 0.2% vs 0.5%[c]
Pachler et al,[46] 2008	Medical University Graz, Austria	Randomized controlled trial, paper-based vs computerized	Mean BG Hyperglycemic index	106 vs 133[c] 0.4 vs 1.6[c]
Lee et al,[47] 2012	University of California San Diego – Burn Unit	Retrospective, descriptive	%BG in target range (90–150) %BG <50	75.8% 0.07%
Saur et al,[38] 2013	Tufts Medical Center, MA	Retrospective, comparative analysis of paper-based vs computerized	Mean BG %Time in target range (95–135) %Time BG <70	117 vs 135[c] 68% vs 52%[c] 0.51% vs 1.44%[c]

Abbreviations: BG, blood glucose; CV, coefficient of variation; DKA, diabetic ketoacidosis; ICU, intensive care unit; IV, intravenous; SQ, subcutaneous.

[a] BG presented in mg/dL (conversion: mg/dL × 0.0555 = mmol/L).

[b] Range not described.

[c] (*P*<.05).

Data from Refs.[37,38,40–47]

COMPUTERIZED DECISION SUPPORT SYSTEMS FOR GLYCEMIC CONTROL IN THE HOSPITAL

The need for frequent hospital glucose monitoring and insulin titration to maintain glycemic control while avoiding hypoglycemia with the use of intravenous insulin infusion has triggered the emergence of computerized insulin dosing systems, also known as computerized decision support systems for glycemic control.[35]

Several systems have become commercially available to assist with glycemic management in critically ill patients with hyperglycemia, such as Glucommander (Glytec, Greenville, SC), EndoTool System (MD Scientific LLC, Charlotte, NC), and GlucoStabilizer (Medical Decision Network, Charlottesville, VA). In addition, several institutions have developed their own computerized insulin protocols and have integrated these systems into their electronic medical record (EMR), including, among others Vanderbilt University Hospital,[36] Medical University of South Carolina,[37] Tuft Medical Center,[38] and Kaiser Sunnyside Medical Center[39] (**Table 3**).

These systems aim to direct the nursing staff on adjusting insulin infusion rates and frequency of glucose testing to optimize inpatient glycemic control and alleviate some of the increased burden of nursing care associated with titrating insulin infusions in medical or surgical critical care units. The software considers previous glucose values and recommends changes in insulin infusion based on a dynamic insulin sensitivity multiplier derived from glucose changes after insulin dose adjustments.[48] Most of the software is based on proportional-integral-derivative algorithms.

Several prospective and observational studies in critically ill patients,[40–43,49] burn unit patients,[47] and patients with diabetic ketoacidosis[44] have reported that use of these systems resulted in improved glycemic control with low rates of hypoglycemia, and also less glycemic variability, when compared with standard paper-based algorithms.

Some systems also include algorithms for the management of hyperglycemia in non–critically ill patients treated with basal bolus insulin regimens, such as the GlucoTab (Joanneum Research GmbH [Graz, Austria] and Medical University of Graz) and Glucommander.[50–52] As shown in the critically ill population, these computerized decision support systems can improve protocol adherence and glycemic control without increased rates of hypoglycemia.[52]

Still, most institutions use standard paper-based, nursing-driven protocols, likely due to the added licensing and implementation costs associated with these systems. There are also considerations regarding compatibility requirements for integration with the electronic medical records system at each individual institution. These devices may be useful in hospitals without diabetes management teams or diabetes experts on staff; however, considerations need to be given to the potential added costs and implementation needs.

SUMMARY

The rapid evolution of diabetes technology during the past decades has led to increased use of CGM and CSII in the ambulatory setting for management of both T1DM and T2DM. In this volume of the *Endocrine Clinics*, experts have extensively reviewed benefits of outpatient diabetes technology use and the development of new CGM-derived glycemic control metrics. Expanding use of CGM and CSII technology has emphasized the need for more evidence regarding the continuation of these therapies during hospitalization. Recent data in hospitalized patients have shown remarkable progress in the use of diabetes technology in the hospital, including (1) improved accuracy and reliability of CGM, (2) safety of CSII in appropriate hospital populations, (3) improvement of glycemic control with computerized glycemic management systems in ICU and non-ICU settings, and (4) feasibility of inpatient CGM-CSII closed-loop systems for inpatient glycemic control. Ongoing studies are focusing on continued translation of this technology to improve glycemic control and outcomes in hospitalized patients.

DISCLOSURE

G.M. Davis and A.L. Migdal have no disclosures. R.J. Galindo is partly supported by a grant from the National Institute of Diabetes and Digestive and Kidney Diseases of the National Institutes of Health under Award Number P30DK11102. R.J. Galindo has received research grant support to Emory University for investigator-initiated studies from Novo Nordisk, and consulting fees from Abbott Diabetes Care, Sanofi, Valeritas, and Novo Nordisk. G.E. Umpierrez is partly supported by research grants from the National Center for Advancing Translational Sciences of the National Institutes of Health under Award Number UL1TR002378 from the Clinical and Translational Science Award program and a National Institutes of Health (NIH) grant U30, P30DK11102, and has received research grant support to Emory University for investigator-initiated studies from Sanofi, Novo Nordisk, and Dexcom.

REFERENCES

1. Umpierrez GE, Klonoff DC. Diabetes technology update: use of insulin pumps and continuous glucose monitoring in the hospital. Diabetes Care 2018;41(8):1579–89.
2. Wallia A, Umpierrez GE, Rushakoff RJ, et al. Consensus statement on inpatient use of continuous glucose monitoring. J Diabetes Sci Technol 2017;11(5):1036–44.
3. Peters AL, Ahmann AJ, Battelino T, et al. Diabetes technology-continuous subcutaneous insulin infusion therapy and continuous glucose monitoring in adults: an Endocrine Society clinical practice guideline. J Clin Endocrinol Metab 2016;101(11):3922–37.
4. Fonseca VA, Grunberger G, Anhalt H, et al. Continuous glucose monitoring: a consensus Conference of the American Association of Clinical Endocrinologists and American College of Endocrinology. Endocr Pract 2016;22(8):1008–21.
5. Grunberger G, Abelseth JM, Bailey TS, et al. Consensus statement by the American Association of Clinical Endocrinologists/American College of Endocrinology insulin pump management task force. Endocr Pract 2014;20(5):463–89.
6. Clarke SF, Foster JR. A history of blood glucose meters and their role in self-monitoring of diabetes mellitus. Br J Biomed Sci 2012;69(2):83–93.
7. Gomez AM, Umpierrez GE. Continuous glucose monitoring in insulin-treated patients in non-ICU settings. J Diabetes Sci Technol 2014;8(5):930–6.
8. Torimoto K, Okada Y, Sugino S, et al. Determinants of hemoglobin A1c level in patients with type 2 diabetes after in-hospital diabetes education: a study based on continuous glucose monitoring. J Diabetes Investig 2017;8(3):314–20.
9. Levitt DL, Silver KD, Spanakis EK. Mitigating severe hypoglycemia by initiating inpatient continuous glucose monitoring for type 1 diabetes mellitus. J Diabetes Sci Technol 2017;11(2):440–1.
10. Logtenberg SJ, Kleefstra N, Snellen FT, et al. Pre- and postoperative accuracy and safety of a real-time continuous glucose monitoring system in cardiac surgical patients: a randomized pilot study. Diabetes Technol Ther 2009;11(1):31–7.

11. Holzinger U, Warszawska J, Kitzberger R, et al. Real-time continuous glucose monitoring in critically ill patients: a prospective randomized trial. Diabetes Care 2010;33(3):467–72.
12. Kopecky P, Mraz M, Blaha J, et al. The use of continuous glucose monitoring combined with computer-based eMPC algorithm for tight glucose control in cardiosurgical ICU. Biomed Res Int 2013;2013:186439.
13. Umbrello M, Salice V, Spanu P, et al. Performance assessment of a glucose control protocol in septic patients with an automated intermittent plasma glucose monitoring device. Clin Nutr 2014;33(5):867–71.
14. De Block CE, Gios J, Verheyen N, et al. Randomized evaluation of glycemic control in the medical intensive care unit using real-time continuous glucose monitoring (REGIMEN Trial). Diabetes Technol Ther 2015;17(12):889–98.
15. Burt MG, Roberts GW, Aguilar-Loza NR, et al. Brief report: comparison of continuous glucose monitoring and finger-prick blood glucose levels in hospitalized patients administered basal-bolus insulin. Diabetes Technol Ther 2013;15(3):241–5.
16. Schaupp L, Donsa K, Neubauer KM, et al. Taking a closer look–Continuous glucose monitoring in non-critically ill hospitalized patients with type 2 diabetes mellitus under basal-bolus insulin therapy. Diabetes Technol Ther 2015;17(9): 611–8.
17. Gómez AM, Umpierrez GE, Munoz OM, et al. Continuous glucose monitoring versus capillary point-of-care testing for inpatient glycemic control in type 2 diabetes patients hospitalized in the general ward and treated with a basal bolus insulin regimen. J Diabetes Sci Technol 2015;10(2):325–9.
18. Gu W, Liu Y, Chen Y, et al. Multicentre randomized controlled trial with sensor-augmented pump vs multiple daily injections in hospitalized patients with type 2 diabetes in China: Time to reach target glucose. Diabetes Metab 2017;43(4): 359–63.
19. Spanakis EK, Levitt DL, Siddiqui T, et al. The effect of continuous glucose monitoring in preventing inpatient hypoglycemia in general wards: the glucose telemetry system. J Diabetes Sci Technol 2018;12(1):20–5.
20. Battelino T, Danne T, Bergenstal RM, et al. Clinical targets for continuous glucose monitoring data interpretation: recommendations from the international consensus on time in range. Diabetes Care 2019;42(8):1593–603.
21. Association AD. 15. Diabetes care in the hospital: standards of medical care in diabetes—2019. Diabetes Care 2019;42(Supplement 1):S173–81.
22. Kannan S, Satra A, Calogeras E, et al. Insulin pump patient characteristics and glucose control in the hospitalized setting. J Diabetes Sci Technol 2014;8(3): 473–8.
23. Nassar AA, Partlow BJ, Boyle ME, et al. Outpatient-to-inpatient transition of insulin pump therapy: successes and continuing challenges. J Diabetes Sci Technol 2010;4(4):863–72.
24. Cook CB, Beer KA, Seifert KM, et al. Transitioning insulin pump therapy from the outpatient to the inpatient setting: a review of 6 years' experience with 253 cases. J Diabetes Sci Technol 2012;6(5):995–1002.
25. Levitt DL, Spanakis EK, Ryan KA, et al. Insulin pump and continuous glucose monitor initiation in hospitalized patients with type 2 diabetes mellitus. Diabetes Technol Ther 2018;20(1):32–8.
26. Leelarathna L, English SW, Thabit H, et al. Feasibility of fully automated closed-loop glucose control using continuous subcutaneous glucose measurements in critical illness: a randomized controlled trial. Crit Care 2013;17(4):R159.

27. Chee F, Fernando T, van Heerden PV. Closed-loop glucose control in critically ill patients using continuous glucose monitoring system (CGMS) in real time. IEEE Trans Inf Technol Biomed 2003;7(1):43–53.
28. Yatabe T, Yamazaki R, Kitagawa H, et al. The evaluation of the ability of closed-loop glycemic control device to maintain the blood glucose concentration in intensive care unit patients. Crit Care Med 2011;39(3):575–8.
29. Bally L, Thabit H, Hartnell S, et al. Closed-loop insulin delivery for glycemic control in noncritical care. N Engl J Med 2018;379(6):547–56.
30. Boughton CK, Bally L, Martignoni F, et al. Fully closed-loop insulin delivery in inpatients receiving nutritional support: a two-centre, open-label, randomised controlled trial. Lancet Diabetes Endocrinol 2019;7(5):368–77.
31. Thabit H, Hartnell S, Allen JM, et al. Closed-loop insulin delivery in inpatients with type 2 diabetes: a randomised, parallel-group trial. Lancet Diabetes Endocrinol 2017;5(2):117–24.
32. Bally L, Gubler P, Thabit H, et al. Fully closed-loop insulin delivery improves glucose control of inpatients with type 2 diabetes receiving hemodialysis. Kidney Int 2019;96(3):593–6.
33. Pasquel FJ, Spiegelman R, McCauley M, et al. Hyperglycemia during total parenteral nutrition: an important marker of poor outcome and mortality in hospitalized patients. Diabetes Care 2010;33(4):739–41.
34. Stewart ZA, Yamamoto JM, Wilinska ME, et al. Adaptability of closed loop during labor, delivery, and postpartum: a secondary analysis of data from two randomized crossover trials in type 1 diabetes pregnancy. Diabetes Technol Ther 2018;20(7):501–5.
35. Eslami S, Abu-Hanna A, de Jonge E, et al. Tight glycemic control and computerized decision-support systems: a systematic review. Intensive Care Med 2009;35(9):1505–17.
36. Boord JB, Sharifi M, Greevy RA, et al. Computer-based insulin infusion protocol improves glycemia control over manual protocol. J Am Med Inform Assoc 2007;14(3):278–87.
37. Hermayer KL, Neal DE, Hushion TV, et al. Outcomes of a cardiothoracic intensive care Web-based online intravenous insulin infusion calculator study at a medical university hospital. Diabetes Technol Ther 2007;9(6):523–34.
38. Saur NM, Kongable GL, Holewinski S, et al. Software-guided insulin dosing: tight glycemic control and decreased glycemic derangements in critically ill patients. Mayo Clin Proc 2013;88(9):920–9.
39. Olinghouse C. Development of a computerized intravenous insulin application (AutoCal) at Kaiser Permanente Northwest, integrated into Kaiser Permanente HealthConnect: impact on safety and nursing workload. Perm J 2012;16(3):67–70.
40. Juneja R, Roudebush CP, Nasraway SA, et al. Computerized intensive insulin dosing can mitigate hypoglycemia and achieve tight glycemic control when glucose measurement is performed frequently and on time. Crit Care 2009;13(5):R163.
41. Newton CA, Smiley D, Bode BW, et al. A comparison study of continuous insulin infusion protocols in the medical intensive care unit: computer-guided vs. standard column-based algorithms. J Hosp Med 2010;5(8):432–7.
42. Tanenberg RJ, Hardee S, Rothermel C, et al. Use of a computer-guided glucose management system to improve glycemic control and address national quality measures: a 7-year, retrospective observational study at a tertiary care teaching hospital. Endocr Pract 2017;23(3):331–41.

43. John SM, Waters KL, Jivani K. Evaluating the implementation of the EndoTool Glycemic Control Software System. Diabetes Spectr 2018;31(1):26–30.
44. Ullal J, Aloi JA, Reyes-Umpierrez D, et al. Comparison of computer-guided versus standard insulin infusion regimens in patients with diabetic ketoacidosis. J Diabetes Sci Technol 2018;12(1):39–46.
45. Dortch MJ, Mowery NT, Ozdas A, et al. A computerized insulin infusion titration protocol improves glucose control with less hypoglycemia compared to a manual titration protocol in a trauma intensive care unit. JPEN J Parenter Enteral Nutr 2008;32(1):18–27.
46. Pachler C, Plank J, Weinhandl H, et al. Tight glycaemic control by an automated algorithm with time-variant sampling in medical ICU patients. Intensive Care Med 2008;34(7):1224–30.
47. Lee J, Fortlage D, Box K, et al. Computerized insulin infusion programs are safe and effective in the burn intensive care unit. J Burn Care Res 2012;33(3):e114–9.
48. Rattan R, Nasraway SA. The future is now: software-guided intensive insulin therapy in the critically ill. J Diabetes Sci Technol 2013;7(2):548–54.
49. Umpierrez G, Cardona S, Pasquel F, et al. Randomized controlled trial of intensive versus conservative glucose control in patients undergoing coronary artery bypass graft surgery: GLUCO-CABG trial. Diabetes Care 2015;38(9):1665–72.
50. Mader JK, Neubauer KM, Schaupp L, et al. Efficacy, usability and sequence of operations of a workflow-integrated algorithm for basal-bolus insulin therapy in hospitalized type 2 diabetes patients. Diabetes Obes Metab 2014;16(2):137–46.
51. Neubauer KM, Mader JK, Holl B, et al. Standardized glycemic management with a computerized workflow and decision support system for hospitalized patients with type 2 diabetes on different wards. Diabetes Technol Ther 2015;17(10):685–92.
52. Aloi J, Bode BW, Ullal J, et al. Comparison of an electronic glycemic management system versus provider-managed subcutaneous basal bolus insulin therapy in the hospital setting. J Diabetes Sci Technol 2017;11(1):12–6.

HbA_{1c}

The Glucose Management Indicator, Time in Range, and Standardization of Continuous Glucose Monitoring Reports in Clinical Practice

Anders L. Carlson, MD[a,*], Amy B. Criego, MD, MS[b],
Thomas W. Martens, MD[c], Richard M. Bergenstal, MD[c]

KEYWORDS

- Continuous glucose monitoring • Ambulatory glucose profile • Time in range
- Glucose management indicator

KEY POINTS

- Continuous glucose monitoring (CGM) is a rapidly expanding technology used by people with diabetes and their care teams to make treatment decisions and therapeutic adjustments and to monitor for overall safety and efficacy of their treatment plans.
- For CGM data to be as effective a tool as possible, both for patients and for clinicians/researchers, it is important to standardize CGM-based metrics and definitions, and large consensus groups have been working to establish such standards.
- Time in range and the Glucose Management Indicator are emerging as clinically useful tools to assess overall diabetes management and help guide treatment decisions beyond hemoglobin A_{1c} measurements.
- Using the ambulatory glucose profile to review CGM data can help personalize diabetes management by demonstrating not only how much hypoglycemia or time in target range an individual has but also when it is occurring.

INTRODUCTION

The potential for debilitating complications related to diabetes mellitus has been established for decades if not centuries.[1] With the ushering in of contemporary medicine, and the widespread use of insulin and other pharmacotherapies, significant progress has been made in reducing the burden posed by these complications, which have prevented many patients with diabetes from living full and healthy lives. More

[a] International Diabetes Center & Health Partners, 3800 Park Nicollet Boulevard, Minneapolis, MN 55416, USA; [b] International Diabetes Center, Park Nicollet Clinic Pediatric Endocrinology, 3800 Park Nicollet Boulevard, Minneapolis, MN 55416, USA; [c] International Diabetes Center, 3800 Park Nicollet Boulevard, Minneapolis, MN 55416, USA
* Corresponding author.
E-mail address: Anders.L.Carlson@Healthpartners.com

Endocrinol Metab Clin N Am 49 (2020) 95–107
https://doi.org/10.1016/j.ecl.2019.10.010
endo.theclinics.com

recently, clinicians caring for people with diabetes have strived to find a biomarker of some kind to help identify those with the highest glucose levels and therefore most likely at risk for complications. Glycosylated hemoglobin A_{1c} (HbA_{1c}) emerged in the twentieth century as the most widely adopted and well understood of such markers, and its use in diabetes care has remained the gold standard ever since.

To be sure, the reliance on HbA_{1c} is well deserved. In the United Kingdom Prospective Diabetes Study, using intensive therapy to treat newly diagnosed type 2 diabetes mellitus (T2D), HbA_{1c} was lowered to a mean of 7.0% (intensive) compared with 7.9% (control) over a median of 10 years.[2] This intensive therapy reduced the risk of any diabetes-related endpoint by 12% and microvascular disease by 25%, with a 16% trend to a reduced risk of myocardial infarction (P = .052). For patients with type 1 diabetes mellitus (T1D), the Diabetes Control and Complications Trial (DCCT) showed decisively that intensive versus control insulin interventions substantially reduce retinopathy, neuropathy, and nephropathy after a mean of 6.5 years, noting the final achieved HbA_{1c} associated with these improvements was 7.4% (intensive group) compared with 9.1% in the control group.[3] Recently, it was shown that an HbA_{1c} of 6.5% had the lowest risk for all-cause mortality in people with diabetes, with the optimal HbA_{1c} range of 5.6% to 7.4%.[4] It is therefore not surprising that the major organizations charged with setting diabetes targets and standards of care have relied heavily on HbA_{1c}. The American Diabetes Association, for instance, suggests an HbA_{1c} of less than 7% as a target for most individuals with diabetes,[5] whereas the American Association of Clinical Endocrinologists sets the target at less than or equal to 6.5%.[6] Whether they agree or disagree on the value, no society yet has endorsed 1 particular biomarker or metric more valuable for treatment decision making than the HbA_{1c}. Achieving these HbA_{1c} goals while minimizing the risk for severe hypoglycemia has been challenging.

Furthermore, HbA_{1c} is an easy test to take (nonfasting, can take at any time of day, and so forth) and is widely available, making it an ideal tool for busy primary care and endocrine practices. Point-of-care technology has made it even more accessible. In 2010, successful efforts led to the standardization of HbA_{1c} chemistry assays across the world, further facilitating the use of HbA_{1c} in cross-sectional and population analyses.[7] HbA_{1c} is now understood by clinicians and patients alike as their treatment goal and that HbA_{1c} corresponds to the risk for diabetes-related complications.

Despite the robust associations between HbA_{1c} and complications and patient outcomes, it is worth acknowledging the limits of the HbA_{1c} biomarker. HbA_{1c} is impacted by numerous factors, such as race, disorders of red blood cell lifespan (such as hemolytic anemia, cirrhosis, and end-stage renal disease), and hemoglobinopathies.[8] HbA_{1c} also corresponds to a wide range of mean glucoses, making it difficult in isolation to know how accurately HbA_{1c} is estimating the average glucose. Furthermore, for an individual living with diabetes, and for their care team helping make treatment recommendations, a HbA_{1c} reflecting the average glucose over the past 3 months to 4 months does not fully inform such treatment decisions, because HbA_{1c} cannot directly assess for details, such as day/night patterns, risks for hypoglycemia, and glucose variability related to circumstances, such as exercise or illness.

Now with the increasing adoption of continuous glucose monitoring (CGM) technology, there is a new set of metrics to better understand each patient's unique glycemic profile. In 2017, 2 large consensus groups convened to put forward common metrics regarding CGM data.[9,10] One of these international consensus groups published their key metrics for CGM analysis and reporting (**Table 1**).[10]

Table 1
Core continuous glucose monitoring metrics, adapted from the international consensus on continuous glucose monitoring

Measures	Values
Mean glucose	Calculated from all CGM values
GMI (previously eA_{1c})[a]	Derived from CGM mean glucose
Percentage of time in hypoglycemia ranges (mg/dL/mmol/L)	
Very high	>250/>13.9
High	181–250/10.1–13.9
Percentage of TIR (mg/dL/mmol/L)	70–180/3.9–10.0
Percentage of time in hypoglycemic ranges, mg/dL (mmol/L)	
Low	54–69/3.0–3.8
Very low	<54/<3.0
Glucose variability	
%CV	
Stable	%CV ≤36
Unstable	%CV >36
Three time periods for evaluation	
Sleep	12:00 AM–6:00 AM
Wake	6:00 AM–12:00 AM
24 h	12:00 AM–12:00 AM
Recommended data sufficiency	
Collection period	14 d
Percentage of expected CGM readings (minimum percentage)	70% (10 of 14 d)
Standardized CGM report	AGP

[a] GMI (%) = 3.31 + 0.02392 × [mean glucose in mg/dL][14] Jaeb Center for Health Research. HbA_{1c} estimator [Internet]. Available from https://www.jaeb.org/gmi/.

Adapted from Danne T, Nimri R, Battelino T, et al. International consensus on use of continuous glucose monitoring. Diabetes Care. 2017;40(12):1631-40; with permission.

Contemporaneously, another group composed of many of the key stakeholder diabetes organizations internationally published a consensus around definitions of outcomes to be used beyond HbA_{1c}, such as hypoglycemia, hyperglycemia, and time in ranges.[9] Working toward a standardized idea of what is, for instance, time in target range (TIR), will possibly lead to similar conclusions connecting CGM data to clinical outcomes similar to those established with HbA_{1c}. These data are just starting to emerge. A recent study of 3262 patients with T2D showed that more advanced diabetes-related retinopathy is associated with lower CGM-based TIR (70–180 mg/dL [3.9–10.0 mmol/L]), with TIR inversely associated with all stages of retinopathy.[11] Another analysis looking at the DCCT trial 7-point self-monitored blood glucose profiles and the TIR (70–180 mg/dL [3.9–10.0 mmol/L]) for those measurements further validates that TIR may be a reliable metric for predicting complication risk.[12] With these findings, there may be a shift away from reliance solely on HbA_{1c}, which does not take into account individual patterns of hypoglycemia, hyperglycemia, or large glucose excursions. New ideas are emerging about how to more effectively use CGM data in the clinical setting, and this in turn could possibly change the way clinicians work together with their patients.

This review describes the CGM metrics most relevant to the clinical practice of diabetes care along with the display of these metrics using the ambulatory glucose profile (AGP) to facilitate interpretation.

GLUCOSE STATISTICS AND VARIABILITY

To ensure that conclusions and therapeutic recommendations are based on appropriate CGM data, it is important to acknowledge when the data were obtained and the amount of data being reviewed. The first CGM metric to acknowledge is the date range to ensure that data are recent. Next, the number of days of available data should be assessed. Fourteen days of data, with a minimum of 10 days (or 70% of a 14-day period), is recommended for data sufficiency. It is important to note how much of the time period the CGM was active during the days the CGM is in place. If the CGM is worn for 14 days, for instance, but is only active less than 70% of the time, the accuracy of the data may be in question. In the JDRF CGM study, 14 days of CGM data was representative of 21 and even 30 days of data, so conclusions can be extrapolated from the 14 day results.[13] It may be necessary, however, to rely on a longer period of time to fully assess hypoglycemia patterns depending on the frequency of hypoglycemia. The CGM wear time is also useful for counseling patients about proper CGM use and perhaps identifying barriers to its use (skin reactions, difficulty with CGM placement, need for additional taping, and so forth).

Once satisfactory CGM data are obtained, the overall glucose statistics can be reviewed. The mean glucose is useful to help give the clinician and patient a snapshot of the period's glucose levels. Because there can be inconsistencies and confusion between estimated A_{1c} (eA_{1c}) based on the mean glucose and actual laboratory-derived HbA_{1c} values, it was recently put forward to no longer use the term, eA_{1c}, and rather use the Glucose Management Indicator (GMI).[14] GMI then conveys a similar idea to clinicians and patients about the overall glucose exposure over the time period. GMI (calculated from the CGM-derived mean glucose) is an estimate of the HbA_{1c} based on the CGM glucose levels; if the GMI is considerably different from the laboratory HbA_{1c}, it may be important to take this difference into account when setting an individual's HbA_{1c} goal. For example, if a patient's GMI is 7.0%, but laboratory-based HbA_{1c} is consistently at or approximately 8.0%, the clinician may conclude that individual tends to have a higher HbA_{1c} than the mean glucose suggests, and efforts to intensify therapy to lower the HbA_{1c} may precipitate more hypoglycemia.

Like an HbA_{1c}, however, the mean glucose and GMI do not reflect day-to-day glycemic patterns. Trying to quantify the amount of glucose variability is challenging. Several metrics are available to describe variability. In the 2017 consensus, coefficient of variation (%CV), SD, area under the curve, and low/high blood glucose indices were all proposed as suitable ways to report variability and risk for glucose excursions.[10] After further review, consensus is growing that the %CV is the more clinically useful measurement of glucose variability. Although statistical analyses may be challenging to both patients and diabetes care teams, %CV can be defined as the SD divided by the mean glucose, allowing for a more meaningful measurement when the mean glucose is lower. For instance, if the SD is 40 mg/dL (2.2 mmol/L), that deviation around a mean glucose of 100 mg/dL (5.6 mmol/L) portends more risk for hypoglycemia than the same SD around a mean glucose of 150 mg/dL (8.3 mmol/L). Although studies have not confirmed the precise %CV target, recent consensus groups suggest a %CV of less than or equal to 36% indicates reasonable variability, whereas a %CV 37% or higher may put variability at a higher priority for adjusting treatment plans.[15]

TIME IN RANGES

Although HbA_{1c} and GMI can give a high-level impression of overall glucose management, the richness of CGM data allows for more nuanced evaluation. The time a patient spends in different ranges of glycemia next becomes an immensely useful tool. Conveniently, it is a metric patients understand and find useful as well, as was shown by Runge and colleagues.[16] In a survey of patients with both T1D and T2D, TIR was more important than HbA_{1c} for patients with T1D (and T2D on insulin) with regard to the impact it has on their daily lives with diabetes.

To define specific ranges is challenging, because the consequences of transitioning from normoglycemia to hypoglycemia do not dramatically change going from a glucose of 70 mg/dL to a glucose of 69 mg/dL, for instance. Nonetheless, for the sake of a standardized approach that can be used in clinical practice, as well as in research and by regulatory agencies, it is best to have clearly defined cutoffs. To establish these ranges, a TIR consensus group was convened in early 2019. Out of this group came the following recommendations for clinically useful ranges (see **Fig. 2**): 2 hypoglycemia ranges (<54 mg/dL [<3.0 mg/dL] and <70 mg/dL [< 3.9 mmol/L]), TIR of 70 mg/dL to 180 mg/dL (or 3.9–10.0 mmol/L), and 2 hyperglycemia ranges (>180 mg/dL [>10.0 mmol/L] and >250 mg/dL [>13.9 mmol/L]). To further qualify these ranges, recommended targets also were established for each range type.[15] For instance, a TIR (70–180 mg/dL [3.9–10.0 mmol/L]) of more than 70% is considered an optimal target of time spent in this range. Although data from large randomized controlled trials are lacking to prove this target, it has been observed from studies of automated insulin delivery devices (hybrid closed-loop systems) that a TIR of approximately 70% is achievable for patients on these systems, which to date are the most advanced systems of insulin delivery. The target for TIR will likely increase and be modified as technology, medications, and insulin delivery systems improve. Ranges and targets also may differ for individuals based on their medical history and therapeutic goals.

Although HbA_{1c} continues to be attached to outcomes, and in some instances the payments made to hospitals, clinics, and even individual clinicians, it will be important to try to correlate HbA_{1c} to TIR, and more studies will be needed to address this. Just like HbA_{1c} can be associated with a wide range of mean glucose values, so too can TIR correspond to a wide range of possible HbA_{1c} values.[17,18] Yet, there is a pattern emerging between HbA_{1c} and TIR, such that it is reasonable to conclude that a TIR of 70% corresponds roughly to an HbA_{1c} of approximately 7%. Furthermore, a change of 10% in the TIR approximately corresponds to a change in HbA_{1c} by 0.5% to 0.8%, which can help clinicians and patients have an approximate idea of how TIR and HbA_{1c} correlate (**Table 2**). Because a HbA_{1c} change of 0.5% generally is considered the threshold for clinical significance of a given therapy,[19] a change in TIR of just 5% corresponds to a change in HbA_{1c} of approximately 0.3% to 0.4%, and, therefore, may be considered a clinically meaningful change.

The TIR consensus group also promoted targets for the various time in ranges for specific populations (**Table 3**). These notions of ranges and targets for time spent in them are an ever-evolving idea. Certainly there is much to learn about subgroups of patients, such as inpatients, chronic kidney disease patients, and perhaps those not on insulin therapy, to name a few. As CGM technology advances, these targets likely will change as well, so the suggestions put forth to date should be understood in the context of a rapidly changing landscape of diabetes care.

Table 2
Comparison of time in range (70–180 mg/dL [3.9–10.0 mmol/L]) and estimates of hemoglobin A_{1c} based on recent publications

Time in Range (%)	Hemoglobin A_{1c} Estimate (Vigersky & McMahon,[17] 2019)	Hemoglobin A_{1c} Estimate (%), Baseline[a] (Beck et al,[18] 2019)	Hemoglobin A_{1c} Estimate (%), Month 6[a] (Beck et al,[18] 2019)
0	12.1	NA	NA
10	11.4	NA	NA
20	10.6	9.4	8.8
30	9.8	8.9	8.4
40	9.0	8.4	8.0
50	8.3	7.9	7.6
60	7.5	7.4	7.2
70	6.7	7.0	6.8
80	5.9	6.5	6.4
90	5.1	6.0	6.0
100	4.3	NA	NA

[a] The study from Beck et al used data from CGM intervention studies, with data from both baseline and after a 6-month study period.

Data from Vigersky RA, McMahon C. The relationship of hemoglobin A1C to time-in-range in patients with diabetes. Diabetes Technol Ther. 2019; 21(2):81-5 and Beck RW, Bergenstal RM, Cheng P, et al. The relationships between time in range, hyperglycemia metrics, and HbA1c. J Diabetes Sci Technol. 2019; 13(4):614-626.

Table 3
Recommended targets for percent time spent in glucose ranges based on international time in range consensus group

Diabetes Group	Glucose Range: Target Percentage Time in Each Range	Hypoglycemia Glucose Range(s): Target Percentage Time in Each Range
People with diabetes (T1D and T2D)	70–180 mg/dL: >70% time	<70 mg/dL: <4% time <54 mg/dL: <1% time
Older/high-risk: Type 1& Type 2 Diabetes (T1D and T2D)	70–180 mg/dL: >50% time	<70 mg/dL: <1% time
T1D pregnancy	63–140 mg/dL: >70% time	<63 mg/dL: <4% time <54 mg/dL: <1% time
T2D pregnancy/gestational[a]	63–140 mg/dL: targets not established	<63 mg/dL: targets not established <54 mg/dL: targets not established

Conversion formula: mmol/L = mg/dL/18.

[a] The "target percent" for this group has not been firmly established due to limited number of publications. A TIR of approximately 85-90% is currently a reasonable clinical target in this population.

Adapted from Battelino T, Danne T, Bergenstal RM, et al. Clinical targets for continuous glucose monitoring data interpretation: recommendations from the international consensus on time in range. Diabetes Care 2019;42(8):1593-603.

THE AMBULATORY GLUCOSE PROFILE

In addition to standardizing the CGM metrics, it also is important to have a standardized method of data visualization. The AGP is a standardized, single-page glucose report designed to simplify visualization and interpretation of downloaded CGM data[20] (**Fig. 1**). The AGP was endorsed in 2012 by a consensus of experts[21] and was again recommended as the standard visualization tool by the 2017 consensus

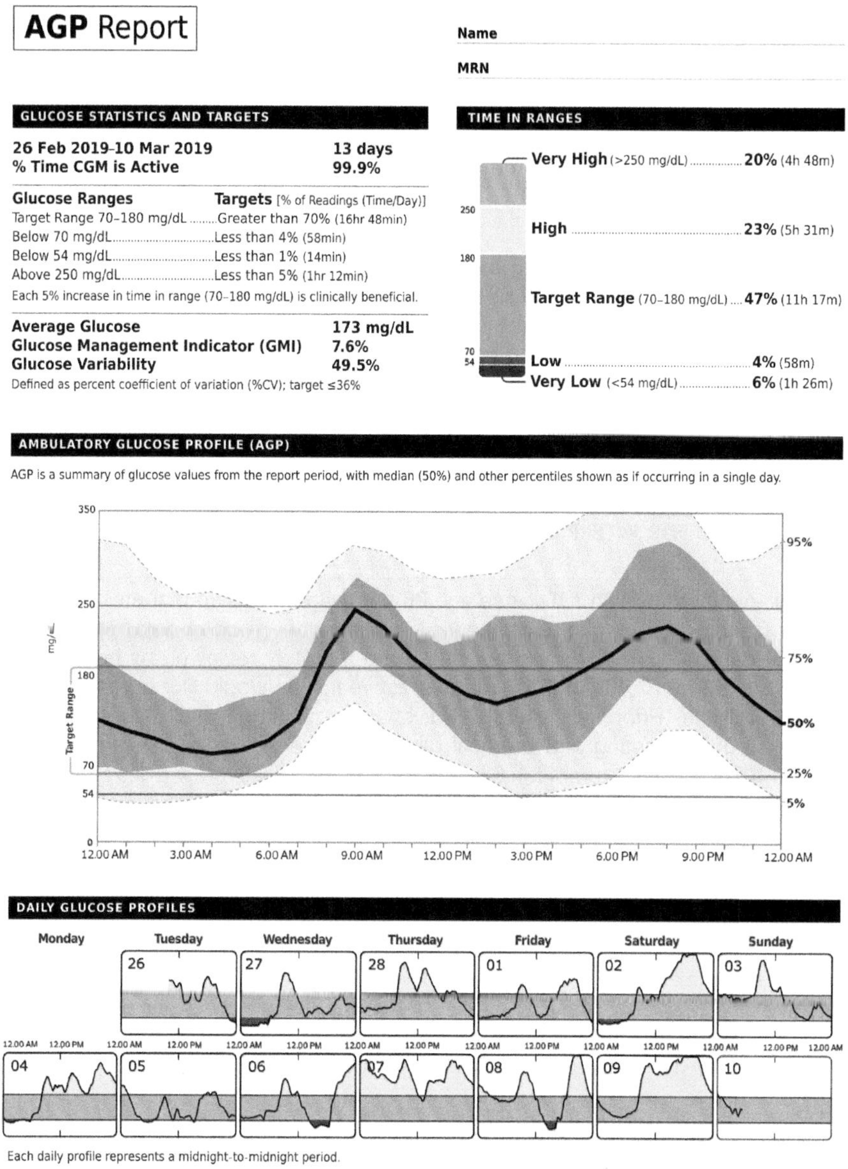

Fig. 1. The Ambulatory Glucose Profile (AGP). (© 2019 International Diabetes Center at Park Nicollet, Minneapolis, MN. Used with permission. See AGPreport.org for more information.)

group.[10] The most current version of the AGP has 4 main components: glucose statistics and targets, time in ranges, the AGP, and the daily profiles.

PUTTING CONTINUOUS GLUCOSE MONITORING AND AMBULATORY GLUCOSE PROFILE INTO CLINICAL USE

CGM can be used both personally by patients in real time (personal CGM) or owned by the clinic and used intermittently either blinded or unblinded to the patient (professional CGM). The placement, education, and removal of the professional CGM are reimbursable by most insurance plans, as is the interpretation of the CGM data (either personal or professional) by a health care professional (physician, nurse practitioner, or physician assistant). There are no universal requirements from health plans regarding what the contents of a CGM interpretation must have to be billable; however, the interpretation must be based on at least 72 hours of data (and documented accordingly). Based on CGM metrics and the AGP interpretation, the authors have previously proposed a basic strategy to CGM interpretation and documentation.[22] Such interpretations should document time in ranges, patterns of hypoglycemia/hyperglycemia, and glucose variability. Identifying these patterns over the 24-hour modal day period and correlating them to factors, such as timing of medications, meals, activity, and other daily patterns, help facilitate patient-centered decisions about lifestyle and/or therapy adjustments. If possible, capturing the AGP and its data into the electronic medical record can help readily draw comparisons when a patient is next seen for follow up. Because CGM interpretation does not need to be face-to-face for billing purposes, some clinicians are now choosing to remotely review cloud-based CGM data (by email, medical chart messages, or telehealth), allowing for a patient's treatment plan to be updated between routine office visits.

CASE EXAMPLES FOR INTERPRETATION

Case 1

A 58-year-old woman with T1D since age 26 and with no known diabetes complications is reached by phone for a phone visit to review her glucose data. She wears a CGM that can be downloaded to the cloud and remotely reviewed by her clinician. Her HbA_{1c} has been 7.4% to 7.6% for the past year. She would like to reach a lower HbA_{1c} if possible. Prior to starting CGM, she did not know her glucose patterns because all of her fasting and premeal glucoses were in the recommended target range (<140 mg/dL [<7.8 mmol/L]). Since starting CGM, however, she has seen a large spike in glucose after breakfast (**Fig. 2**). She is able to see that this spike occurs on some, but not all, days. She quickly identifies those days as ones where she has a very high carbohydrate breakfast cereal, whereas there is no spike on the other days when she does not have this type of meal. She sees her TIR is 82%, with 0% in the hypoglycemia range, so she is reassured there is no pattern of low glucose. By using the CGM, she is able to readily see how her diet choices affect the glucose, and after a few weeks of avoiding that type of meal, the 2 hours to 3 hours spent in hyperglycemia (approximately 8%–12% of the day) were now in target range. The visit, because it was done remotely by phone, can in some cases be billed for and required only a simple visualization, which did not necessitate an in-person visit.

Case 2

An 86-year-old man with T2D presents to clinic for a routine visit. He has been on multiple daily injections of insulin for the past 8 years. He has chronic kidney disease and mild cognitive impairment. He does not check any capillary self-monitored blood

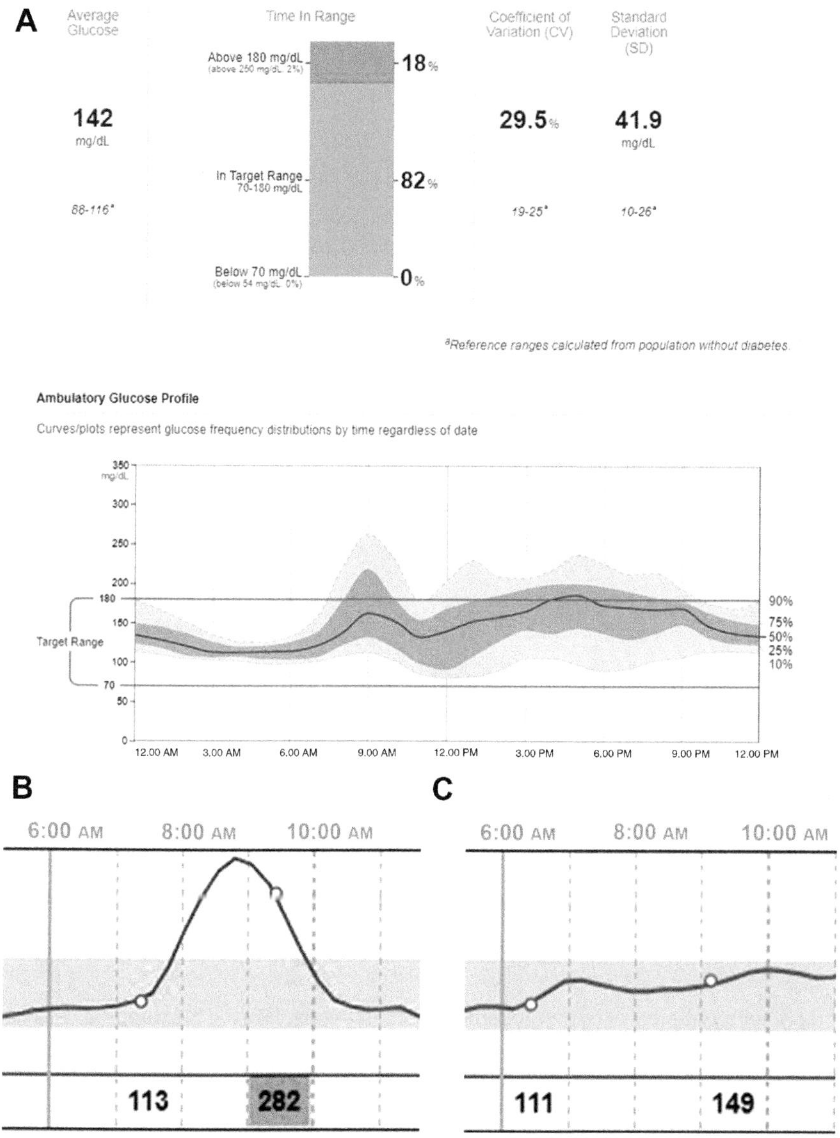

Fig. 2. (*A*) Case 1. AGP showing a frequent glucose spike at approximately 9:00 AM. (*B*) One day when she did have a high-carbohydrate breakfast and (*C*) another day where she limited the carbohydrate amount at breakfast.

glucose values because they are painful and difficult for him to perform on his own, but his daughter does perform them on occasion before dinner, and they usually are approximately 180 mg/dL to 200 mg/dL (10.0–11.1 mmol/L). His HbA_{1c} is consistently high, approximately 9%. He denies any symptoms of hypoglycemia and his daughter has not noticed anything unusual. Given the lack of glucose data and need to titrate his insulin based on the high HbA_{1c}, a blinded CGM is placed (**Fig. 3**). On return 2 weeks later, his AGP shows significant nocturnal hypoglycemia, 8% (or approximately 2 hours

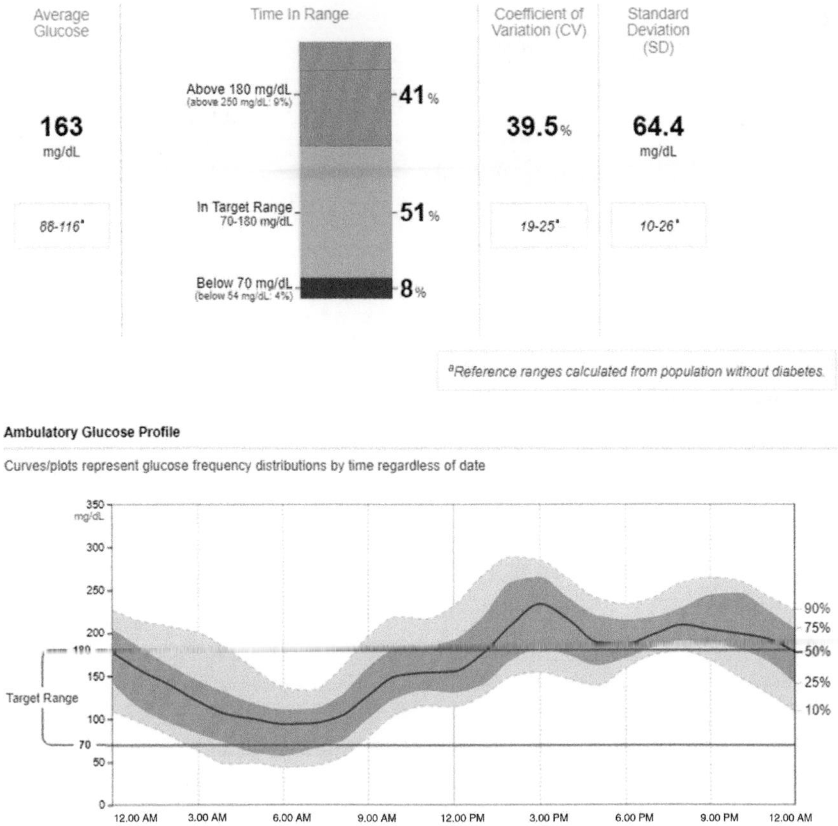

Fig. 3. Case 2. TIR report highlighting 8% of time below range (glucose <70 mg/dL), despite a high amount of time above range (glucose >180 mg/dL) and high glucose variability. AGP further showing the timing of these excursions, with a significant amount of time spent in the hypoglycemia range during the early morning time period when the patient is asleep, whereas most of the time in hyperglycemia range is during the daytime waking hours.

per day), with patterns of hyperglycemia after his meals. He and his daughter are surprised by this but by looking at the AGP they understand the pattern. They agree to lowering his basal insulin by 10% and increasing his mealtime insulins at each meal and also agree to a personal CGM to alert him to potentially dangerous glucose trends. His HbA_{1c} of 10% does not allow for an assessment of his hypoglycemia risk, and, given his lack of symptoms, it would be reasonable for a clinician to think that increasing both background and bolus insulin would be appropriate, which in this case could potentially precipitate more frequent or severe hypoglycemia. Furthermore, his TIR of 51% would be expected to correlate with a lower HbA_{1c}, and his calculated GMI is 7.2%. Seeing the discrepancy in GMI compared with the HbA_{1c} and the large amount of hypoglycemia at night allows for a more tailored and individualized recommendation for his insulin adjustments.

LIMITATIONS AND FUTURE DIRECTIONS OF CONTINUOUS GLUCOSE MONITORING

Although the future has never been brighter for people living with diabetes, many obstacles remain for many patients. It is worth acknowledging that despite advances in technology, CGM use was by only 38% of people with T1D in the T1D Exchange Registry in 2018.[23] The cost of new technologies also must be considered, and efforts are needed to ensure that all patients, no matter socioeconomic status or other demographic factors, have access to technology. Furthermore, a clinician's ability to readily view, interpret, communicate, and follow-up CGM data is largely tied to the electronic medical record, and how best to integrate CGM and AGP into this workflow has not been established.

The TIR consensus group identified subgroups of patients for whom unique times in range are recommended. More studies are needed in other groups, however, such as pediatric groups, elderly patients with diabetes, and those with impaired awareness of hypoglycemia, to name a few.

SUMMARY

Like in other areas of medicine, standardization can ease the burden of training, interpretation, and dissemination. Similar to the electrocardiogram in cardiology, having precise metrics readily available both in the clinical setting as well as in research can help unify the broader medical community and hopefully improve how outcomes are measured and tracked. CGM metrics and their standardization is a step toward this goal. Using key metrics, including TIR, GMI, and time in hypoglycemia ranges, furthers the ability to tailor treatments to individuals living with diabetes. Rather than relying solely on the HbA_{1c} to guide decisions, these CGM standards provide detailed information about a patient's daily glucose patterns and facilitates shared decision making. The AGP as a standardized visualization display also promotes a universal interpretation of glucose data. Although advancements in automated insulin delivery, CGM technology, and care delivery models will revolutionize diabetes care in the next several years, it is important to recognize these ideas of CGM metrics and visualization too will have to adapt over time, and ongoing work to drive consensus will be needed.

DISCLOSURE

Research support: Abbott and Dexcom; research support and consulting: Eli Lilly, Medtronic, Novo Nordisk, and Sanofi; consulting: Sensionics (A.L. Carlson). Research support: Abbott, Dexcom, Medtronic, and Novo Nordisk; consulting: Sensionics (A.B. Criego). Research support: Abbott, Dexcom, Medtronic, and Novo Nordisk (T.W. Martens). Research support and consulting: Abbott, Dexcom, Eli Lilly, Hygieia, Johnson & Johnson, Medtronic, Novo Nordisk, and Roche, Sanofi; consulting: Onduo, Sensionics, and United Healthcare (R.M. Bergenstal).

REFERENCES

1. Karamanou M, Protogerou A, Tsoucalas G, et al. Milestones in the history of diabetes mellitus: the main contributors. World J Diabetes 2016;7(1):1–7.
2. UK Prospective Diabetes Study (UKPDS) Group. Effect of intensive blood-glucose control with metformin on complications in overweight patients with type 2 diabetes (UKPDS 34). Lancet 1998;352(9131):854–65.
3. Diabetes Control, Complications Trial Research Group. The effect of intensive treatment of diabetes on the development and progression of long-term complications in insulin-dependent diabetes mellitus. N Engl J Med 1993;329(14): 977–86.

4. Li FR, Zhang XR, Zhong WF, et al. Glycated hemoglobin and all-cause and cause-specific mortality among adults with and without diabetes. J Clin Endocrinol Metab 2019;104(8):3345–54.
5. American Diabetes Association. Standards of medical care in diabetes - 2019. Diabetes Care 2019;42:S81.
6. Garber AJ, Abrahamson MJ, Barzilay JI, et al. AACE/ACE comprehensive diabetes management algorithm 2015. Endocr Pract 2015;21(4):438–47.
7. Hanas R, John G. 2010 consensus statement on the worldwide standardization of the hemoglobin A1C measurement. Clin Chem Lab Med 2010;48(6):775–6.
8. Beck RW, Connor CG, Mullen DM, et al. The fallacy of average: how using HbA1c alone to assess glycemic control can be misleading. Diabetes Care 2017;40(8):994–9.
9. Agiostratidou G, Anhalt H, Ball D, et al. Standardizing clinically meaningful outcome measures beyond HbA1c for type 1 diabetes: a consensus report of the American Association of Clinical Endocrinologists, the American Association of Diabetes Educators, the American Diabetes Association, the Endocrine Society, JDRF International, The Leona M. and Harry B. Helmsley Charitable Trust, the Pediatric Endocrine Society, and the T1D Exchange. Diabetes Care 2017;40(12):1622–30.
10. Danne T, Nimri R, Battelino T, et al. International consensus on use of continuous glucose monitoring. Diabetes Care 2017;40(12):1631–40.
11. Lu J, Ma X, Zhou J, et al. Association of time in range, as assessed by continuous glucose monitoring, with diabetic retinopathy in type 2 diabetes. Diabetes Care 2018;41(11):2370–6.
12. Beck RW, Bergenstal RM, Riddlesworth TD, et al. Validation of time in range as an outcome measure for diabetes clinical trials. Diabetes Care 2019;42(3):400–5.
13. Riddlesworth TD, Beck RW, Gal RL, et al. Optimal sampling duration for continuous glucose monitoring to determine long-term glycemic control. Diabetes Technol Ther 2018;20(4):314–6.
14. Bergenstal RM, Beck RW, Close KL, et al. Glucose management indicator (GMI): a new term for estimating A1C from continuous glucose monitoring. Diabetes Care 2018;41(11):2275–80.
15. Battelino T, Danne T, Bergenstal RM, et al. Clinical targets for continuous glucose monitoring data interpretation: recommendations from the international consensus on time in range. Diabetes Care 2019;42(8):1593–603.
16. Runge AS, Kennedy L, Brown AS, et al. Does time-in-range matter? Perspectives from people with diabetes on the success of current therapies and the drivers of improved outcomes. Clin Diabetes 2018;36(2):112–9.
17. Vigersky RA, McMahon C. The relationship of hemoglobin A1C to time-in-range in patients with diabetes. Diabetes Technol Ther 2019;21(2):81–5.
18. Beck RW, Bergenstal RM, Cheng P, et al. The relationships between time in range, hyperglycemia metrics, and HbA1c. J Diabetes Sci Technol 2019;13(4):614–26.
19. Centre for Clinical Practice at NICE (UK). Type 2 diabetes: newer agents for blood glucose control in type 2 diabetes. London: National Institute for Health and Clinical Excellence (UK); 2009.
20. Mazze RS, Strock E, Wesley D, et al. Characterizing glucose exposure for individuals with normal glucose tolerance using continuous glucose monitoring and ambulatory glucose profile analysis. Diabetes Technol Ther 2008;10(3):149–59.

21. Bergenstal RM, Ahmann AJ, Bailey T, et al. Recommendations for standardizing glucose reporting and analysis to optimize clinical decision making in diabetes: the Ambulatory Glucose Profile (AGP). J Diabetes Sci Technol 2013;7(2):562–78.
22. Carlson AL, Mullen DM, Bergenstal RM. Clinical use of continuous glucose monitoring in adults with type 2 diabetes. Diabetes Technol Ther 2017; 19(S2):S4–11.
23. Foster NC, Beck RW, Miller KM, et al. State of type 1 diabetes management and outcomes from the T1D Exchange in 2016–2018. Diabetes Technol Ther 2019; 21(2):66–72.

Diabetes Technology and Exercise

Michael C. Riddell, PhD[a,b,c,*], Rubin Pooni, MSc[a,c], Federico Y. Fontana, PhD[d,e], Sam N. Scott, PhD[e,f]

KEYWORDS

• Type 1 diabetes • Exercise • Technology • Physical activity • Closed loop • Automated insulin delivery • Glucose monitor • Diabetes

KEY POINTS

- Regular physical activity and planned exercise sessions are important for people living with diabetes for a variety of health and fitness reasons.
- However, the challenges around managing blood glucose concentrations mean that many people with diabetes lead a sedentary lifestyle.
- Rapid advances in technologies are already helping many individuals with diabetes reach their physical activity goals more safely and more easily.
- However, although these technological advances are exciting, there are limitations that need to be addressed with further research.
- This article provides an overview of recently developed technologies designed to help patients with diabetes to be more physically active, while also trying to improve glucose control around exercise.

INTRODUCTION

Regular physical activity (PA) is important for people living with type 1 diabetes for a variety of health and fitness reasons.[1] However, because of the challenges around managing blood glucose concentrations, many people with type 1 diabetes lead a sedentary life.[2] Advances in technologies, including continuous glucose monitoring

[a] School of Kinesiology and Health Science, York University, Toronto, ON M3J 1P3, Canada; [b] LMC Diabetes & Endocrinology, 1929 Bayview Avenue, Toronto, ON M4G 3E8, Canada; [c] York University, 347 Bethune College, North York, Ontario M3J 1P3, Canada; [d] Department of Neurosciences, Biomedicine and Movement Sciences, University of Verona, Via Casorati, 43, 37121 Verona, Italy; [e] Team Novo Nordisk Professional Cycling Team, 2144 Hills Avenue NW, Atlanta, 30318 GA, USA; [f] Department of Diabetes, Endocrinology, Nutritional Medicine and Metabolism, Bern University Hospital, University of Bern, Freiburgstrasse 15, 3010 Bern, Switzerland
* Corresponding author. York University, 347 Bethune College, North York, Ontario M3J 1P3, Canada.
E-mail address: mriddell@yorku.ca
Twitter: @MCRiddell1 (M.C.R.); @FeedYourFlock (F.Y.F.); @SamNathanScott (S.N.S.)

Endocrinol Metab Clin N Am 49 (2020) 109–125
https://doi.org/10.1016/j.ecl.2019.10.011
endo.theclinics.com

(CGM), intermittent flash glucose monitoring (fGM), and automated insulin delivery (AID) systems, are helping many individuals with type 1 diabetes reach their PA goals more safely and more easily. The development of strategies that integrate the use of smartphone technologies and PA monitors provides users with important data metrics, such as activity levels, carbohydrate counting, and glucose monitoring, to help users make better-informed decisions. This article provides an overview of recent technologies that help engage patients with diabetes to be more physically active, while also trying to improve glucose control around exercise.

TYPES OF EXERCISE AND TERMINOLOGY

PA is defined as any body movement caused by the contraction of skeletal muscle that substantially increases energy expenditure compared with rest, whereas exercise is defined as a structured form of PA that is performed with the intent to maintain or improve health and fitness.[3] These terms are used interchangeably for this review. Numerous categories of PA exist that can tax various components of physical endurance, strength, balance, and/or flexibility. For those living with diabetes, and in particular type 1 diabetes, the exercise type, intensity, and duration all have major impacts on glucose homeostasis.[4] Aerobic exercise (eg, walking, bicycling, swimming, or jogging) involves continuous, rhythmic movements of large muscle groups, normally lasting at least 10 minutes at a time. Resistance exercise involves brief, repetitive muscle contractions with weights, weight machines, resistance bands, or the person's own body weight (eg, push-ups, pull-ups, leg press). Flexibility exercises (eg, lower back or hamstring stretching) are intended to enhance the ability to move through fuller ranges of motion with little resistance. Many types of activities, such as yoga and Pilates, incorporate elements of both resistance and flexibility exercise and use components of both aerobic and anaerobic metabolism. High-intensity interval training (HIIT) is defined as brief, intermittent periods of vigorous aerobic/anaerobic exercise, interspersed with periods of rest or recovery, and is frequently used to improve fitness. Under the umbrella term HIIT, there are several protocols that have been investigated in the literature, including aerobic interval training,[5] sprint interval training,[6] and constant-load low-volume HIIT,[7] all of which are likely to have differing effects on glycemia in people with diabetes.

BENEFITS OF REGULAR PHYSICAL ACTIVITY

Regular PA can help people with type 1 diabetes achieve a variety of goals, including increased cardiorespiratory fitness, better sleep, enhanced energy levels, improved glycemic control, decreased insulin resistance, improved blood lipid profile, enhanced blood pressure control, and the maintenance of a healthy body weight.[1] In general, both regular PA[8–10] and/or a high level of cardiorespiratory fitness[11] are associated with reductions in the incidence of cardiovascular disease and overall mortality. In addition to aerobic fitness, anaerobic fitness and/or muscular strength also have independent and additive benefits for people living with diabetes,[12] including those with type 1 diabetes.[13] The American Diabetes Association (ADA)[1] and others[4,14] recommend that adults with diabetes should engage in 150 minutes or more per week of moderate to vigorous aerobic exercise, spread over at least 3 d/wk, with no more than 2 consecutive days without activity. Moreover, the ADA points out that less PA may be sufficient (ie, minimum 75 min/wk) if the activities are more vigorous. They also recommend that strength training be done 2 to 3 times per week to help maximize the health and fitness benefits of regular PA.[1] Flexibility training and balance training are also recommended 2 to 3 times/wk.[1]

TOOLS AND TECHNIQUES FOR MEASURING PHYSICAL ACTIVITY

To assist with the challenge of achieving the PA recommendations, patients may benefit from the ability to objectively measure and record their bouts of PA. However, many health care providers do not ask about patient PA patterns, and activity monitors are seldom prescribed.[15] PA levels are often suboptimal in people living with diabetes, according to self-report[16] and accelerometry[2,17] data. Monitoring PA levels objectively using accelerometry, along with behavior change interventions, increases activity levels in inactive youth with type 1 diabetes.[18]

PA and exercise events can be measured in a variety of ways, from surveys requiring user input (eg, International Physical Activity Questionnaire, Minnesota Leisure Time Physical Activity Questionnaire)[19] to automated wearable sensors that can automatically track the movements of the user and even quantify the intensity of effort by measuring heart rate.[20] The widely used International Physical Activity Questionnaire has been used in various research settings to gauge the PA levels of individuals living with diabetes.[21,22] In smaller studies, wearable sensors, such as wrist-worn smart watches, that combine accelerometry with photoplethysmography and other sensors to measure heart rate, step count, energy expenditure, and other descriptors of movement and sleep (quality and quantity) have also been used.[23,24] Although fitness trackers and smartphone apps offer some solutions for documenting PA levels in individuals, issues of reliability and accuracy remain.[23] To date, the authors know of only 2 studies that have assessed the accuracy of these devices in individuals with diabetes during exercise, with both displaying varying results in heart rate and energy expenditure measurement accuracy.[25,26] Although many wearable sensors using photoplethysmography measure heart rate levels reasonably accurately during exercise, these devices typically show poor accuracy in measuring energy expenditure during activities of low to high intensity[23,27,28] (**Fig. 1**). In general, the accuracy of measuring heart rate and energy expenditure in many sensors decreases as exercise intensity increases.[23,27,29] Some newer wearables, such as the Garmin activity monitor with Garmin Move IQ, can automatically quantify the number of active minutes per week.

ACTIVITY MONITORS IN DIABETES SELF-MANAGEMENT

Overall, consumer-based wrist monitors, from manufacturers including Fitbit, Apple Watch, and Garmin, are reasonable at estimating heart rate, daily step count, and energy expenditure for activities of light to moderate intensity. In general, these consumer products are affordable, easy to use, and accessible for the general population and could be useful for patients with diabetes to self-monitor their PA habits. It is therefore tempting, from a technology perspective, to strive to incorporate ways of detecting, characterizing, and integrating signals from various forms of exercise so that AID systems can be adapted appropriately to limit any exercise-associated dysglycemia. However, several challenges exist when trying to accurately characterize a PA event for an AID system.[24,30] These challenges include determining the physiologic thresholds for movement/exercise based on heart rate and/or accelerometry (or some other physiologic measurement) that would trigger a change in insulin delivery rate and the complicated relationship between relative exercise intensity and the body's insulin needs (**Fig. 2**). At the least, wearable sensors and smartphone applications that document activity levels are useful for determining whether patients

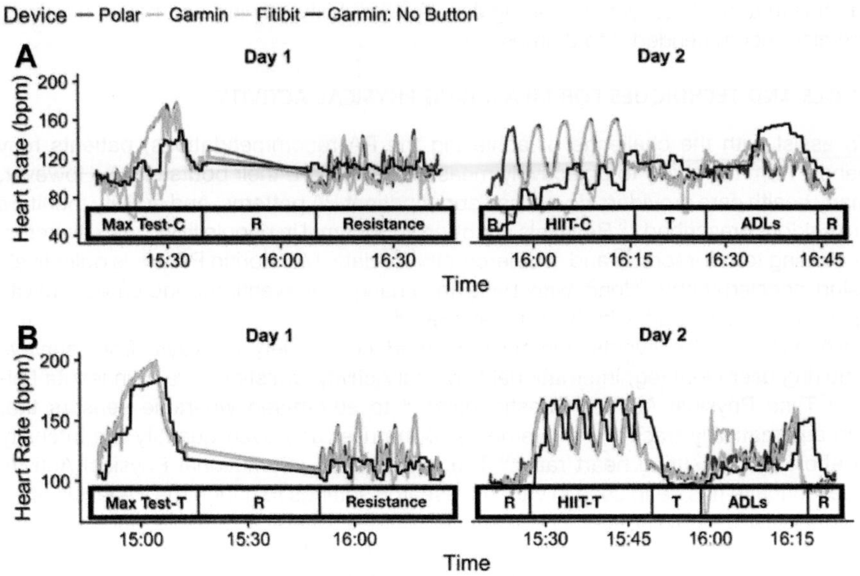

Fig. 1. Accuracy of wearable technologies during exercise and rest. (*A*) Two-day wear study protocol with R indicating rest periods and T indicating a transition period between 2 different types of activities. Data are shown from 2 different participants (*A* and *B*) wearing a Polar H10 (Polar, Kempele, Finland) heart rate chest strap (reference standard) and a Garmin vivosmart 3 (Garmin, Olathe, KS) watch and a Fitbit Charge 2 (San Francisco, CA) watch. Note, the Garmin device was worn by the participants in 2 different modes: 1 with the activity mode indicated (Garmin) and the other without (Garmin: no button). (*A*) Heart rate data during a progressive cycling test to exhaustion; (*B*) The data during a progressive treadmill running test to exhaustion. Data in (*A*) highlight the error observed during higher intensity cycling exercises in which wrist movement was less pronounced during cycle ergometer testing. (*B*) Treadmill results when the Garmin, Fitbit, and Polar data are closely matched across the exercise types. ADLs, activities of daily living; HIIT-C, high-intensity interval training–cycle ergometer; HIIT-T, high-intensity interval training–treadmill; Max Test-C, maximum test–cycle ergometer; Max Test-T, maximum test–treadmill.

are achieving their activity goals.[24] Emerging evidence suggests that wearable fitness trackers merged with smartphone technologies/apps and electronic health record systems may facilitate behavioral goal setting and improve PA monitoring in patients living with diabetes.[31]

ASSESSING PHYSICAL ACTIVITY IN PATIENTS WITH DIABETES

There is little consensus on how activity data should be described or expressed for the purposes of prescribing, tracking, or decision support around glucose management in diabetes. For example, some clinicians or researchers may simply prescribe or document the number of minutes of PA performed over a week (eg, 150 min/wk of moderate-intensity activity; 75 min/wk of vigorous-intensity activity), whereas others may express PA metrics more objectively, such as the time spent at a given metabolic equivalent (MET) for a given task (eg, 40 minutes jogging or cycling at 5 METS = 200 MET-minutes).[32] The latter approach may be preferred in certain situations of exercise prescription, because it considers the relative intensity (ie, a unit of energy expenditure relative to the individual's energy expenditure at rest) and the

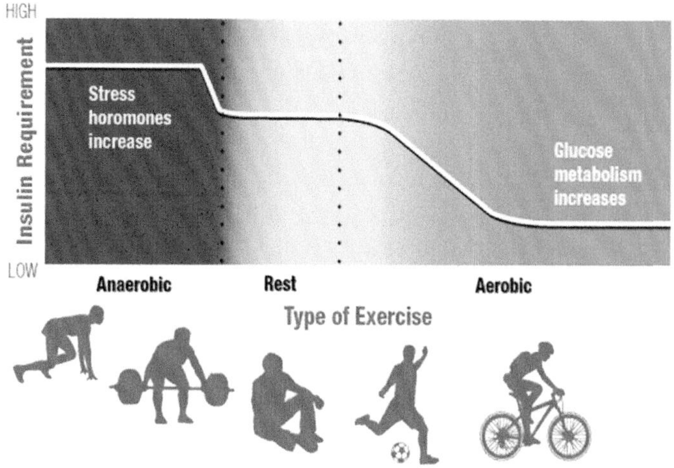

Fig. 2. Insulin needs depend on the type and intensity of physical activity performed. In general, insulin needs increase during or after intensive aerobic and anaerobic activity when stress hormone (ie, adrenaline, noradrenaline), growth hormone, and lactate levels increase. In contrast, insulin needs diminish with more prolonged mild to moderate-intensity aerobic activities when stress hormone levels are less pronounced. (*Courtesy of* Michael C. Riddell, PhD, North York, ON, Canada.)

duration of the task, although this approach may be more difficult to explain to most patients. Energy expenditure during exercise can also be expressed as kilocalories, joules, or watts, depending on the activity sensor used, whereas relative energy expenditure is often expressed relative to the individual's maximal percentage of oxygen consumption (ie, $\%Vo_{2max}$) or maximal heart rate (HR_{max}). These various technical terms used to describe PA make it cumbersome for patients, clinicians, and researchers to effectively communicate how much exercise is required, or being performed, and at what level of intensity. However, it is likely that the consideration of these terms may be necessary, because both the relative[33] and absolute[34] PA intensity influence glucose homeostasis in people living with diabetes.

For decision support with exercise, it is important to detect when spontaneous activity occurs, perhaps with accelerometry and/or heart rate. Another approach is to schedule a planned exercise event into a controller, perhaps using a smartphone application that is somehow tied to a calendar app. In any case, the relative exercise intensity and the activity duration should be considered when it comes to basal and/or bolus insulin adjustments. The relative intensity of aerobic exercise is typically gauged by estimating the $\%Vo_{2max}$ or percentage HR_{max}. Typically, as the relative exercise intensity increases, the risk for hyperglycemia increases in a J shape, whereas the risk for hypoglycemic increases in an inverted U shape, although the risk for dysglycemia depends, at least in part, on circulating insulin levels (**Fig. 3**). With very intensive aerobic/anaerobic exercise, insulin needs typically increase compared with basal conditions, whereas, with less intense exercise, insulin needs decrease markedly. Resistance-based activities can have variable effects on glycemia in type 1 diabetes.[35]

Individuals with type 1 diabetes who are in competitive events likely benefit from being able to visualize their performance and glycemia data together to better understand the relationships between glucose levels and performance. Some patients living with type 1 diabetes are very physically active and many reach the competitive

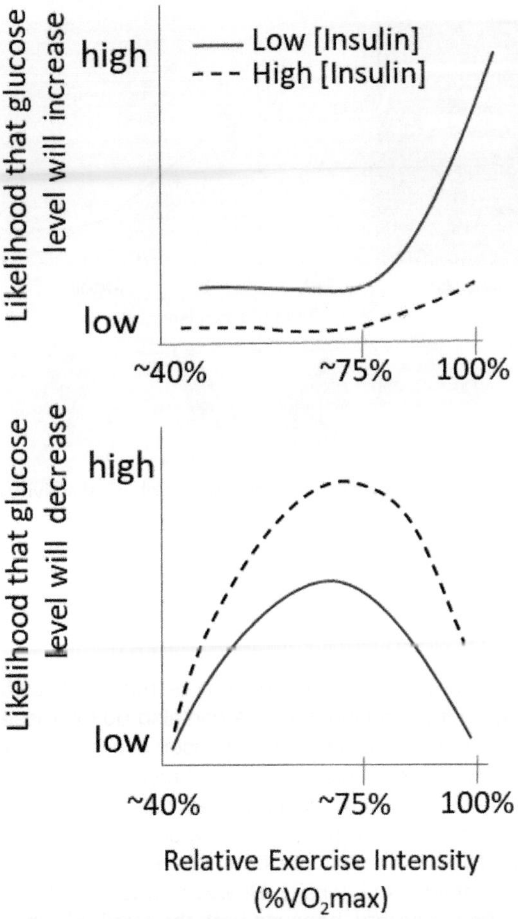

Fig. 3. Theoretic risks for exercise-related dysglycemia in type 1 diabetes. As the relative exercise intensity increases, the risk of hyperglycemia increases in a J shape, whereas the risk for hypoglycemia increases in an inverted U shape, depending on the circulating insulin levels.

or even elite level (see https://en.wikipedia.org/wiki/List_of_sportspeople_with_diabetes). Rapidly improving technologies are now enabling athletes to measure and visualize data (eg, insulin, glucose, heart rate, power output) during training or competition (**Fig. 4**) with minimal burden to the athlete. This ability facilitates communication between the athletes, their coaches, and health care providers, potentially resulting in improved time in target and performance.

EXERCISE AND GLYCEMIC TRENDS

PA comes in several forms for individuals with diabetes, all of which may affect glucose homeostasis. For example, leisure time PA (eg, walking, hiking, gardening, sport, dance) and physically demanding occupations (eg. letter carrier, general laborer, food service industry) may make glucose levels decrease and insulin dosing needs may need to be decreased and carbohydrate snacking initiated to prevent

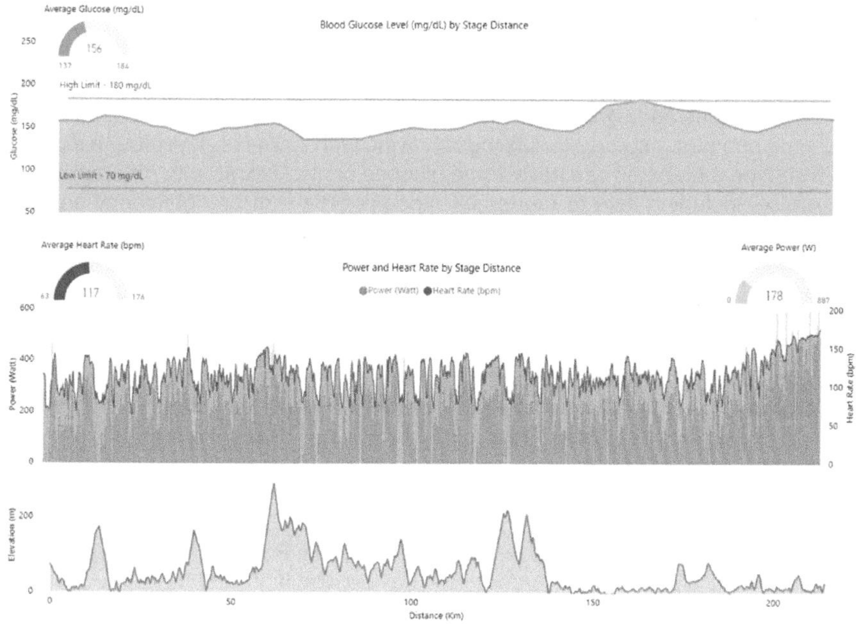

Fig. 4. Example of diabetes and physiologic performance data collection and visualization during professional cycling races. Data visualization of interstitial glucose level (Dexcom G6, Dexcom, San Diego, CA), cycling power output (Watts; Pioneer HD power meter, Long Beach, CA), heart rate in beats per minute (bpm; Wahoo TICKER chest strap), and elevation in meters (Wahoo Element cycling computer) in a 214 km professional cycling stage race. (Data courtesy of Team Novo Nordisk.)

hypoglycemia.[36] In contrast, a stressful competitive event, such as a short cross-country ski race, a swimming event, or a HIIT session, may cause glucose levels to increase rapidly,[37,38] sometimes requiring bolus insulin correction for hyperglycemia.[39] Paradoxically, symptoms of hypoglycemia, rather than hyperglycemia, ensue with intensive exercise even as glucose levels increase.[40]

Exercise duration,[41] mode,[42] relative intensity,[33] absolute intensity,[34] and fitness[34] all affect glucose homeostasis in people living with type 1 diabetes. For example, a more prolonged exercise session in an aerobically fit individual with type 1 diabetes typically increases the reliance on plasma glucose as fuel, compared with a shorter session of exercise at the same relative intensity.[41] In contrast, a brief session of very intense exercise lasting seconds to minutes tends to promote an increase in glycemia in aerobically fit individuals with type 1 diabetes,[43,44] even though a high rate of plasma glucose uptake into working muscle exists.[37] High-intensity interval-based or circuit-based exercise activities tend to have variable effects in diabetes, with some studies showing a decrease in glycemia,[45] whereas others show glucose stability[46] or an increase in glycemia.[44,47] To date, only a few investigators have attempted to use technologies that can distinguish between aerobic, anaerobic, and mixed forms of exercise for the purpose of developing more sophisticated multivariable adaptive artificial pancreas systems for PA and type 1 diabetes.[30] The inability to correctly assess the relative exercise intensity of persons with type 1 diabetes on an AID system may limit the ability of the system to make appropriate changes to insulin delivery for a range of exercise modalities.

STRATEGIES FOR IMPROVED TIME IN TARGET DURING AND AFTER EXERCISE FOR THOSE ON MULTIPLE DAILY INSULIN INJECTIONS OR OPEN-LOOP CONTINUOUS SUBCUTANEOUS INSULIN INFUSION

Various guidelines and strategies exist to help establish and maintain glucose control during and after exercise for individuals living with diabetes.[1,4] Although individuals with type 2 diabetes can have some glucose control issues with different types of exercise, including mild to moderate hypoglycemia with predominantly aerobic exercise[48] or a small increase in glycemia with intensive interval training,[49] they have less exercise dysglycemia overall compared with individuals living with type 1 diabetes. For patients with type 1 diabetes on multiple daily insulin injections (MDI)[50] or continuous subcutaneous insulin infusion (CSII),[51] reduction in prandial (bolus) insulin at the meal before prolonged aerobic exercise, by 25% to 75% depending on the intensity and duration of the exercise, helps reduce hypoglycemia risk when the activity occurs 1 to 3 hours after a meal. This strategy of reduced bolus insulin at the meal before aerobic exercise could be incorporated into AID systems for exercise if the controller, and perhaps user, takes into account a planned exercise session later in the day.

For prolonged aerobic exercise before meals (or ≥3 hours after a meal), basal insulin reductions are helpful in preventing hypoglycemia. For patients on MDI, a 20% reduction in basal insulin before an active day (ie, the night before or morning of, depending on when the basal insulin is administered) is an effective strategy to reduce hypoglycemia risk.[52] Even ultralong-acting insulin degludec can be reduced by ~20% to 25% the day before activity to help decrease hypoglycemia risk, although some additional carbohydrate intake may still be required and there may be a small increase in glucose levels at other times of the day.[53] Overall, based on limited observations, CSII may offer some improvements compared with MDI in managing postexercise hyperglycemia,[54] although postexercise hyperglycemia can be sufficiently managed in individuals on MDI via postexercise insulin bolus administration.[39,55] For those on CSII, reductions in basal insulin infusion rate by 50% to 80% set 90 minutes before exercise, carried throughout the exercise session, effectively attenuate the decrease in glucose level associated with prolonged aerobic exercise.[56] Note that not all physically active patients with type 1 diabetes want to wear insulin pumps and CGM devices. Pump and CGM discontinuation often occurs because the individual (often a child or adolescent) finds that the devices are burdensome during periods of increased PA.[57] It is possible that adding additional sensors (eg, heart rate monitors or other exercise wearables) during exercise may increase the burden for patients rather than reduce it.

Overall, the use of wearable technologies, such as step counters, accelerometers, and heart rate monitors, should help identify periods of increased activity and thus the requirement for insulin dose changes and/or carbohydrate feeding. In 1 study, automated weekly review of accelerometer, CGM, and insulin pump data was used to identify children with type 1 diabetes who had increased risk of nighttime hypoglycemia and preemptively adjust the nighttime basal insulin profile according to daytime activity.[58] Hypoglycemia during a PA session lasting 30 to 60 minutes can be predicted, to some degree, if the pre-exercise blood glucose level is less than 180 mg/dL (10 mmol/L) and heart rate level during exercise is greater than 120 beats per minute (ie, the 180/120 rule).[59] More complex random forest models may be incorporated into future AID systems or decision-support systems for type 1 diabetes.[59]

ROLE AND ACCURACY OF REAL-TIME CONTINUOUS GLUCOSE MONITORING AND FLASH GLUCOSE MONITORING FOR EXERCISE

For physically active people with diabetes, CGMs have advantages compared with self-monitoring of blood glucose level with a hand-held glucose meter and capillary sample. For example, the ability to track glucose levels in real time near continuously during prolonged aerobic exercise can be used to initiate carbohydrate feeding before hypoglycemia occurs.[60] However, exercise, in most forms, seems to significantly deteriorate the apparent accuracy of both real-time CGM (rtCGM)[61–64] and intermittent flash glucose monitoring (fGM)[65,66] devices, at least in part because of a significant lag effect. The significant rtCGM lag effect with exercise (15–30 minutes) may mean AID systems have a reduced ability to respond quickly to rapidly occurring changes in glucose concentration associated with aerobic or anaerobic activities. Emerging real-time intradermal CGM technologies using microneedles may help to reduce the time delay associated with exercise and other common physiologic stimuli.[67]

CLOSED-LOOP AND EXERCISE

Advances in CGM technologies, rapid-acting insulin analogues, programmable smart pumps, and smart decision-making algorithms all contribute to the possibility that glucose control can be enhanced with exercise in people living with type 1 diabetes. The recent emergence of hybrid AID systems is showing that glycemic control can be improved overall while reducing the burden on patients around self-management.[68] Current AID systems automate basal insulin delivery rate using intelligent algorithms that receive information from an interstitial glucose sensor. These systems that suspend insulin delivery before hypoglycemia ensues, based on a predicted hypoglycemic event (either during or after), show efficacy compared with standard sensor-augmented pumps (SAPs) in some exercise settings.[69] However, hypoglycemia can still occur with these approaches, particularly if prandial insulin is in circulation. Prototypes and future closed-loop systems may use other signals, such as exercise sensors, and possibly infuse other hormones, such as glucagon, to help improve glucose time in target during times of increased PA or during and after an acute exercise session. The need to reduce basal insulin delivery well in advance of prolonged aerobic exercise to get levels down in circulation by the start of exercise is a major hurdle for the use of AID systems. This hurdle could be overcome by patient preplanning either manually or with the use of a smartphone-based controller that could be set up well in advance of the activity using a calendar tool (eg, Loop-JOJO application on iOS).

Basal insulin suspension at the onset of aerobic exercise offers limited protection against the decrease in glucose concentration.[56,70,71] It is currently unclear whether insulin-only closed-loop AID systems will be sufficient for moderate to vigorous aerobic exercise, because it is difficult to decrease insulin levels in circulation rapidly if the insulin is infused subcutaneously.[72] In one insulin-only AID study by Elleri and colleagues,[73] adolescents with type 1 diabetes still developed significant hypoglycemia with unannounced exercise. However, compared with SAPs, single-hormone closed-loop systems have shown improved time in target and less hypoglycemia in a variety of exercise and post-exercise settings in which hypoglycemia is particularly common.[74–79] It is worth noting that many of these studies examined AID efficacy in exercise settings of predominantly aerobic-based activity, in which insulin needs typically decrease. As mentioned earlier, most AID systems simply increase the glucose target in their exercise modes to reduce insulin infusion rates. As expected, based on recent open-loop exercise research,[56,80] setting the AID system in exercise mode or to temp target mode well before the start of exercise seems to be more effective than setting the system at exercise start time.

In general, closed-loop systems are reasonably safe and effective for improving time in range and reducing hypoglycemia during unannounced exercise sessions in young, active people with type 1 diabetes.[74,81] These technologies generally rely on setting a temporarily higher glycemic target during exercise to pull back on basal insulin delivery, although this is an oversimplification because even if a higher glycemic target is set, glucose levels during the exercise session may still decrease to less than the set target.[82] Perhaps the most challenging exercise-related task will be creating a closed-loop system capable of adapting to all types and durations of PA for a wide range of individuals, although considerable progress is being made.

One strategy that should improve the capacity of AID systems to cope with exercise is to simultaneously measure additional physiologic variables, such as heart rate or other signals, that could be used to gauge the relative intensity of exercise and then use this information in a multivariable adaptive AID system.[83,84] The use of various exercise signals (accelerometer and heart rate) to gauge the onset of increased activity and its intensity does improve estimation (prediction) of a change in glucose in silico.[85] The addition of heart rate signals alone to a glucose dynamic model improves glucose prediction accuracy.[84] Using heart rate as an input signal should help AID systems automatically switch to an algorithm that is more conservative in insulin delivery for aerobic exercise as insulin sensitivity increases.[84] Heart rate is a reasonably accurate way to track the body's response to activity, providing objective personalized data that account for age and fitness level and reflect exercise intensity regardless of the type of exercise performed.[86] Of all the exercise signals, heart rate may be the best gauge of aerobic exercise, although these data may be better expressed as a percentage of heart rate reserve for a given individual to help account for age-related and fitness-related differences in the heart rate to work rate (ie, relative intensity) relationships.

The integration of other signals in addition to heart rate, such as ventilation rate, accelerometry, near body temperature, galvanic skin response, interstitial lactate, or interstitial ketone sensing, may help to discriminate between exercise artifacts (eg, heart rate increases caused by stress or caffeine) and various modes and intensities of exercise. However, with the current mode of insulin delivery (subcutaneous) and pharmacokinetic profile, an exercise sensor, such as a detection of an increase in heart rate, may not trigger a change in set point for the glycemic target or reduce basal insulin delivery soon enough to prevent a decrease in glycemia during predominantly aerobic exercise.[87] In the future, implantable AID systems with rapid insulin delivery (or rapidly reduced insulin delivery) directly into the intraperitoneal space may improve glucose control around exercise.

Several research groups are currently pursuing dual-hormone approaches for prolonged aerobic exercise. In general, dual-hormone approaches outperform SAP during continuous aerobic and interval-type exercise in adults with type 1 diabetes.[88] The addition of glucagon delivery to a closed-loop system with automated exercise detection reduces, but does not eliminate, hypoglycemia in physically active adults with type 1 diabetes.[89] Adjusting insulin and glucagon delivery at exercise onset within a dual-hormone closed-loop system significantly reduces hypoglycemia compared with no adjustment during prolonged aerobic exercise and performs similarly to SAP therapy when insulin is adjusted before exercise.[90] The failure to eliminate hypoglycemia during aerobic exercise in dual-hormone systems may be because the insulin levels in circulation do not decrease fast enough when the insulin delivery on the

AID decreases and perhaps because the glucagon delivery is not triggered soon enough with the current algorithms. Another approach may be to administer a small dose of glucagon (150–200 μg) just before prolonged aerobic exercise to help eliminate hypoglycemia risk.[91,92] However, future studies are needed to determine whether administration of glucagon before very intensive exercise may exaggerate hyperglycemia and possibly increase ketone production.

SUMMARY AND FUTURE DIRECTIONS

The rapid developments in wearable sensors, glucose sensors, insulins, AID systems, and other technologies are helping many people with diabetes to be more physically active, with some patients even competing at the Olympic and/or professional level. Activity wearables and mobile apps help to keep track of activity levels and provide feedback on whether the individuals are achieving their activity goals. Increasingly accurate and reliable rtCGM and fGM devices provide convenient and near-instantaneous information on glycemia during exercise and in the recovery period to facilitate decision making to reduce the risk of hypoglycemia or hyperglycemia. Advances in artificial pancreas systems that link CGM to the user's insulin pump, potentially with the addition of solubilized glucagon, through intelligent hormone dosing algorithms have the potential to ease the burden of exercise management in type 1 diabetes. The integration with automated exercise detection tools in these closed-loop systems may help to discriminate between exercise artifacts (eg, heart rate increases caused by stress or caffeine) and various modes and intensities of exercise to further reduce user input. Within elite-level sport and type 1 diabetes, data from multiple technologies, including CGM, smart insulin pens, and power meters, are now being combined to facilitate communication between the athletes, their coaches, and health care professionals. These technologies are intended to improve time in glycemic target range, and, ultimately, improve the health and performance of the athletes. Although these technologies are exciting, there are limitations that need to be addressed with further research. At present, optimal use of these technologies depends largely on patient and family motivation, competence, and adherence to daily diabetes care requirements.

DISCLOSURE

M.C. Riddell has received speaker's honoraria from Medtronic Diabetes, Insulet Corporation, Ascensia Diabetes, Novo Nordisk (via JDRF PEAK Program), Xeris Pharmaceuticals, Lilly Diabetes, and Lilly Innovation. F.Y. Fontana and S.N. Scott are employed by Team Novo Nordisk. No other authors have any conflicts of interest to declare.

REFERENCES

1. Colberg SR, Sigal RJ, Yardley JE, et al. Physical activity/exercise and diabetes: a position statement of the American Diabetes Association. Diabetes Care 2016; 39(11):2065–79.
2. Matson RIB, Leary SD, Cooper AR, et al. Objective measurement of physical activity in adults with newly diagnosed type 1 diabetes and healthy individuals. Front Public Health 2018;6:360.
3. Howley ET. Type of activity: resistance, aerobic and leisure versus occupational physical activity. Med Sci Sports Exerc 2001;33(6 Suppl):S364–9 [discussion: S419–20].

4. Riddell MC, Gallen IW, Smart CE, et al. Exercise management in type 1 diabetes: a consensus statement. Lancet Diabetes Endocrinol 2017;5(5):377–90.
5. Wisløff U, Støylen A, Loennechen JP, et al. Superior cardiovascular effect of aerobic interval training versus moderate continuous training in heart failure patients: a randomized study. Circulation 2007;115(24):3086–94.
6. Burgomaster KA, Hughes SC, Heigenhauser GJF, et al. Six sessions of sprint interval training increases muscle oxidative potential and cycle endurance capacity in humans. J Appl Physiol (1985) 2005;98(6):1985–90.
7. Little JP, Gillen JB, Percival ME, et al. Low-volume high-intensity interval training reduces hyperglycemia and increases muscle mitochondrial capacity in patients with type 2 diabetes. J Appl Physiol (1985) 2011;111(6):1554–60.
8. Hu G, Jousilahti P, Barengo NC, et al. Physical activity, cardiovascular risk factors, and mortality among Finnish adults with diabetes. Diabetes Care 2005; 28(4):799–805.
9. Moy CS, Songer TJ, LaPorte RE, et al. Insulin-dependent diabetes mellitus, physical activity, and death. Am J Epidemiol 1993;137(1):74–81.
10. Tikkanen-Dolenc H, Wadén J, Forsblom C, et al. Physical activity reduces risk of premature mortality in patients with type 1 diabetes with and without kidney disease. Diabetes Care 2017;40(12):1727–32.
11. Nielsen PJ, Hafdahl AR, Conn VS, et al. Meta-analysis of the effect of exercise interventions on fitness outcomes among adults with type 1 and type 2 diabetes. Diabetes Res Clin Pract 2006;74(2):111–20.
12. Sampath Kumar A, Maiya AG, Shastry BA, et al. Exercise and insulin resistance in type 2 diabetes mellitus: a systematic review and meta-analysis. Ann Phys Rehabil Med 2019;62(2):98–103.
13. Yardley JE, Hay J, Abou-Setta AM, et al. A systematic review and meta-analysis of exercise interventions in adults with type 1 diabetes. Diabetes Res Clin Pract 2014;106(3):393–400.
14. Diabetes Canada Clinical Practice Guidelines Expert Committee, Sigal RJ, Armstrong MJ, Bacon SL, et al. Physical activity and diabetes. Can J Diabetes 2018;42(Suppl 1):S54–63.
15. Bellicha A, Macé S, Oppert J-M. Prescribing of electronic activity monitors in cardiometabolic diseases: qualitative interview-based study. J Med Internet Res 2017;19(9):e328.
16. McCarthy MM, Whittemore R, Grey M. Physical activity in adults with type 1 diabetes. Diabetes Educ 2016;42(1):108–15.
17. Hult A, Johansson J, Nordström P, et al. Objectively measured physical activity in older adults with and without diabetes. Clin Diabetes 2019;37(2):142–9.
18. Mitchell F, Wilkie L, Robertson K, et al. Feasibility and pilot study of an intervention to support active lifestyles in youth with type 1 diabetes: the ActivPals study. Pediatr Diabetes 2018;19(3):443–9.
19. van Poppel MNM, Chinapaw MJM, Mokkink LB, et al. Physical activity questionnaires for adults: a systematic review of measurement properties. Sports Med 2010;40(7):565–600.
20. Ludwig M, Hoffmann K, Endler S, et al. Measurement, prediction, and control of individual heart rate responses to exercise-basics and options for wearable devices. Front Physiol 2018;9:778.
21. Nolan RC, Raynor AJ, Berry NM, et al. Self-reported physical activity using the International Physical Activity Questionnaire (IPAQ) in Australian adults with type 2 diabetes, with and without peripheral neuropathy. Can J Diabetes 2016; 40(6):576–9.

22. Hui SS-C, Hui GP-S, Xie YJ. Association between physical activity knowledge and levels of physical activity in chinese adults with type 2 diabetes. PLoS One 2014; 9(12):e115098.
23. Reddy RK, Pooni R, Zaharieva DP, et al. Accuracy of wrist-worn activity monitors during common daily physical activities and types of structured exercise: evaluation study. JMIR Mhealth Uhealth 2018;6(12):e10338.
24. Schwartz FL, Marling CR, Bunescu RC. The promise and perils of wearable physiological sensors for diabetes management. J Diabetes Sci Technol 2018;12(3): 587–91.
25. Machač S, Procházka M, Radvanský J, et al. Validation of physical activity monitors in individuals with diabetes: energy expenditure estimation by the multisensor SenseWear Armband Pro3 and the step counter omron HJ-720 against indirect calorimetry during walking. Diabetes Technol Ther 2013;15(5):413–8.
26. Yavelberg L, Zaharieva D, Cinar A, et al. A pilot study validating select research-grade and consumer-based wearables throughout a range of dynamic exercise intensities in persons with and without type 1 diabetes: a novel approach. J Diabetes Sci Technol 2018;12(3):569–76.
27. Wallen MP, Gomersall SR, Keating SE, et al. Accuracy of heart rate watches: implications for weight management. Calbet JAL. PLoS One 2016;11(5):e0154420.
28. Shcherbina A, Mattsson C, Waggott D, et al. Accuracy in wrist-worn, sensor-based measurements of heart rate and energy expenditure in a diverse cohort. J Pers Med 2017;7(2):3.
29. Kendall B, Bellovary B, Gothe NP. Validity of wearable activity monitors for tracking steps and estimating energy expenditure during a graded maximal treadmill test. J Sports Sci 2019;37(1):42–9.
30. Turksoy K, Paulino TML, Zaharieva DP, et al. Classification of physical activity: information to artificial pancreas control systems in real time. J Diabetes Sci Technol 2015;9(6):1200–7.
31. Wang J, Coleman DC, Kanter J, et al. Connecting smartphone and wearable fitness tracker data with a nationally used electronic health record system for diabetes education to facilitate behavioral goal monitoring in diabetes care: protocol for a pragmatic multi-site randomized trial. JMIR Res Protoc 2018;7(4):e10009.
32. Jetté M, Sidney K, Blümchen G. Metabolic equivalents (METS) in exercise testing, exercise prescription, and evaluation of functional capacity. Clin Cardiol 1990;13(8):555–65.
33. Shetty VB, Fournier PA, Davey RJ, et al. Effect of exercise intensity on glucose requirements to maintain euglycemia during exercise in type 1 diabetes. J Clin Endocrinol Metab 2016;101(3):972–80.
34. Al Khalifah RA, Suppère C, Haidar A, et al. Association of aerobic fitness level with exercise-induced hypoglycaemia in Type 1 diabetes. Diabet Med 2016; 33(12):1686–90.
35. Yardley JE, Sigal RJ, Perkins BA, et al. Resistance exercise in type 1 diabetes. Can J Diabetes 2013;37(6):420–6.
36. Buoite Stella A, Assaloni R, Tonutti L, et al. Strategies used by patients with type 1 diabetes to avoid hypoglycemia in a 24×1-hour marathon: comparison with the amounts of carbohydrates estimated by a customizable algorithm. Can J Diabetes 2017;41(2):184–9.
37. Marliss EB, Vranic M. Intense exercise has unique effects on both insulin release and its roles in glucoregulation: implications for diabetes. Diabetes 2002; 51(Suppl 1):S271–83.

38. Harmer AR, Chisholm DJ, McKenna MJ, et al. High-intensity training improves plasma glucose and acid-base regulation during intermittent maximal exercise in type 1 diabetes. Diabetes Care 2007;30(5):1269–71.
39. Aronson R, Brown RE, Li A, et al. Optimal insulin correction factor in post-high-intensity exercise hyperglycemia in adults with type 1 diabetes: the FIT study. Diabetes Care 2019;42(1):10–6.
40. Potashner D, Brown RE, Li A, et al. Paradoxical rise in hypoglycemia symptoms with development of hyperglycemia during high-intensity interval training in type 1 diabetes. Diabetes Care 2019;42(10):2011–4.
41. Shetty VB, Fournier PA, Davey RJ, et al. The time lag prior to the rise in glucose requirements to maintain stable glycaemia during moderate exercise in a fasted insulinaemic state is of short duration and unaffected by the level at which glycaemia is maintained in Type 1 diabetes. Diabet Med 2018;35(10):1404–11.
42. Guelfi KJ, Ratnam N, Smythe GA, et al. Effect of intermittent high-intensity compared with continuous moderate exercise on glucose production and utilization in individuals with type 1 diabetes. Am J Physiol Endocrinol Metab 2007;292(3):E865–70.
43. Fahey AJ, Paramalingam N, Davey RJ, et al. The effect of a short sprint on post-exercise whole-body glucose production and utilization rates in individuals with type 1 diabetes mellitus. J Clin Endocrinol Metab 2012;97(11):4193–200.
44. Riddell MC, Pooni R, Yavelberg L, et al. Reproducibility in the cardiometabolic responses to high-intensity interval exercise in adults with type 1 diabetes. Diabetes Res Clin Pract 2019;148:137–43.
45. Iscoe KE, Riddell MC. Continuous moderate-intensity exercise with or without intermittent high-intensity work: effects on acute and late glycaemia in athletes with Type 1 diabetes mellitus. Diabet Med 2011;28(7):824–32.
46. Scott SN, Cocks M, Andrews RC, et al. Hit improves aerobic capacity without a detrimental decline in blood glucose in people with type 1 diabetes. J Clin Endocrinol Metab 2019;104(2):604–12.
47. Harmer AR, Ruell PA, Hunter SK, et al. Effects of type 1 diabetes, sprint training and sex on skeletal muscle sarcoplasmic reticulum Ca2+ uptake and Ca2+-ATPase activity. J Physiol 2014;592(3):523–35.
48. Ferland A, Brassard P, Lemieux S, et al. Impact of high-fat/low-carbohydrate, high-, low-glycaemic index or low-caloric meals on glucose regulation during aerobic exercise in Type 2 diabetes. Diabet Med 2009;26(6):589–95.
49. Savikj M, Gabriel BM, Alm PS, et al. Afternoon exercise is more efficacious than morning exercise at improving blood glucose levels in individuals with type 2 diabetes: a randomised crossover trial. Diabetologia 2019;62(2):233–7.
50. Campbell MD, Walker M, Trenell MI, et al. Metabolic implications when employing heavy pre- and post-exercise rapid-acting insulin reductions to prevent hypoglycaemia in type 1 diabetes patients: a randomised clinical trial. PLoS One 2014;9(5):e97143.
51. Rabasa-Lhoret R, Bourque J, Ducros F, et al. Guidelines for premeal insulin dose reduction for postprandial exercise of different intensities and durations in type 1 diabetic subjects treated intensively with a basal-bolus insulin regimen (ultralente-lispro). Diabetes Care 2001;24(4):625–30.
52. Campbell MD, Walker M, Bracken RM, et al. Insulin therapy and dietary adjustments to normalize glycemia and prevent nocturnal hypoglycemia after evening exercise in type 1 diabetes: a randomized controlled trial. BMJ Open Diabetes Res Care 2015;3(1):e000085.

53. Moser O, Eckstein ML, Mueller A, et al. Pre-exercise blood glucose levels determine the amount of orally administered carbohydrates during physical exercise in individuals with type 1 diabetes-a randomized cross-over trial. Nutrients 2019; 11(6) [pii:E1287].
54. Yardley JE, Iscoe KE, Sigal RJ, et al. Insulin pump therapy is associated with less post-exercise hyperglycemia than multiple daily injections: an observational study of physically active type 1 diabetes patients. Diabetes Technol Ther 2013;15(1):84–8.
55. Turner D, Luzio S, Gray BJ, et al. Algorithm that delivers an individualized rapid-acting insulin dose after morning resistance exercise counters post-exercise hyperglycaemia in people with Type 1 diabetes. Diabet Med 2016;33(4):506–10.
56. Zaharieva DP, McGaugh S, Pooni R, et al. Improved open-loop glucose control with basal insulin reduction 90 minutes before aerobic exercise in patients with type 1 diabetes on continuous subcutaneous insulin infusion. Diabetes Care 2019;42(5):824–31.
57. Binek A, Rembierz-Knoll A, Polańska J, et al. Reasons for the discontinuation of therapy of personal insulin pump in children with type 1 diabetes. Pediatr Endocrinol Diabetes Metab 2016;21(2):65–9.
58. Ortiz-Rubio P, Oladunjoye A, Agus MSD, et al. Adjusting Insulin Delivery to Activity (AIDA) clinical trial: effects of activity-based insulin profiles on glucose control in children with type 1 diabetes. Pediatr Diabetes 2018;19(8):1451–8.
59. Reddy R, Resalat N, Wilson LM, et al. Prediction of hypoglycemia during aerobic exercise in adults with type 1 diabetes. J Diabetes Sci Technol 2019;13(5): 919–27.
60. Riddell MC, Milliken J. Preventing exercise-induced hypoglycemia in type 1 diabetes using real-time continuous glucose monitoring and a new carbohydrate intake algorithm: an observational field study. Diabetes Technol Ther 2011; 13(8):819–25.
61. Zaharieva DP, Turksoy K, McGaugh SM, et al. Lag time remains with newer real-time continuous glucose monitoring technology during aerobic exercise in adults living with type 1 diabetes. Diabetes Technol Ther 2019;21(6):313–21.
62. Biagi L, Bertachi A, Quirós C, et al. Accuracy of continuous glucose monitoring before, during, and after aerobic and anaerobic exercise in patients with type 1 diabetes mellitus. Biosensors (Basel) 2018;8(1) [pii:E22].
63. Moser O, Mader JK, Tschakert G, et al. Accuracy of Continuous Glucose Monitoring (CGM) during continuous and high-intensity interval exercise in patients with type 1 diabetes mellitus. Nutrients 2016;8(8) [pii:E489].
64. Li A, Riddell MC, Potashner D, et al. Time lag and accuracy of continuous glucose monitoring during high intensity interval training in adults with type 1 diabetes. Diabetes Technol Ther 2019;21(5):286–94.
65. Zaharieva DP, Riddell MC, Henske J. The accuracy of continuous glucose monitoring and flash glucose monitoring during aerobic exercise in type 1 diabetes. J Diabetes Sci Technol 2019;13(1):140–1.
66. Moser O, Eckstein ML, Mueller A, et al. Impact of physical exercise on sensor performance of the FreeStyle Libre intermittently viewed continuous glucose monitoring system in people with Type 1 diabetes: a randomized crossover trial. Diabet Med 2019;36(5):606–11.
67. Ribet F, Stemme G, Roxhed N. Real-time intradermal continuous glucose monitoring using a minimally invasive microneedle-based system. Biomed Microdevices 2018;20(4):101.

68. Boughton CK, Hovorka R. Is an artificial pancreas (closed-loop system) for Type 1 diabetes effective? Diabet Med 2019;36(3):279–86.
69. Bally L, Thabit H. Closing the loop on exercise in type 1 diabetes | Bentham Science. Current Diabetes Reviews 2018;14(3):257–65.
70. Diabetes Research in Children Network (DirecNet) Study Group, Tsalikian E, Kollman C, Tamborlane WB, et al. Prevention of hypoglycemia during exercise in children with type 1 diabetes by suspending basal insulin. Diabetes Care 2006;29(10):2200–4.
71. Franc S, Daoudi A, Pochat A, et al. Insulin-based strategies to prevent hypoglycaemia during and after exercise in adult patients with type 1 diabetes on pump therapy: the DIABRASPORT randomized study. Diabetes Obes Metab 2015; 17(12):1150–7.
72. Tagougui S, Taleb N, Rabasa-Lhoret R. The benefits and limits of technological advances in glucose management around physical activity in patients type 1 diabetes. Front Endocrinol (Lausanne) 2018;9:818.
73. Elleri D, Allen JM, Kumareswaran K, et al. Closed-loop basal insulin delivery over 36 hours in adolescents with type 1 diabetes: randomized clinical trial. Diabetes Care 2013;36(4):838–44.
74. Ekhlaspour L, Forlenza GP, Chernavvsky D, et al. Closed loop control in adolescents and children during winter sports: Use of the Tandem Control-IQ AP system. Pediatr Diabetes 2019;20(6):759–68.
75. Forlenza GP, Buckingham BA, Christiansen MP, et al. Performance of omnipod personalized model predictive control algorithm with moderate intensity exercise in adults with type 1 diabetes. Diabetes Technol Ther 2019;21(5):265–72.
76. Pinsker JE, Laguna Sanz AJ, Lee JB, et al. Evaluation of an artificial pancreas with enhanced model predictive control and a glucose prediction trust index with unannounced exercise. Diabetes Technol Ther 2018;20(7):455–64.
77. Breton MD, Cherñavvsky DR, Forlenza GP, et al. Closed-loop control during intense prolonged outdoor exercise in adolescents with type 1 diabetes: the artificial pancreas Ski study. Diabetes Care 2017;40(12):1644–50.
78. Petruzelkova L, Pickova K, Sumnik Z, et al. Effectiveness of SmartGuard technology in the prevention of nocturnal hypoglycemia after prolonged physical activity. Diabetes Technol Ther 2017;19(5):299–304.
79. Huyett LM, Ly TT, Forlenza GP, et al. Outpatient closed-loop control with unannounced moderate exercise in adolescents using zone model predictive control. Diabetes Technol Ther 2017;19(6):331–9.
80. McAuley SA, Horsburgh JC, Ward GM, et al. Insulin pump basal adjustment for exercise in type 1 diabetes: a randomised crossover study. Diabetologia 2016; 59(8):1636–44.
81. Dovc K, Macedoni M, Bratina N, et al. Closed-loop glucose control in young people with type 1 diabetes during and after unannounced physical activity: a randomised controlled crossover trial. Diabetologia 2017;60(11):2157–67.
82. Petruzelkova L, Soupal J, Plasova V, et al. Excellent glycemic control maintained by open-source hybrid closed-loop AndroidAPS during and after sustained physical activity. Diabetes Technol Ther 2018;20(11):744–50.
83. Turksoy K, Hajizadeh I, Hobbs N, et al. Multivariable artificial pancreas for various exercise types and intensities. Diabetes Technol Ther 2018;20(10):662–71.
84. Hobbs N, Hajizadeh I, Rashid M, et al. Improving glucose prediction accuracy in physically active adolescents with type 1 diabetes. J Diabetes Sci Technol 2019; 13(4):718–27.

85. Jacobs PG, Resalat N, El Youssef J, et al. Incorporating an exercise detection, grading, and hormone dosing algorithm into the artificial pancreas using accelerometry and heart rate. J Diabetes Sci Technol 2015;9(6):1175–84.
86. Zisko N, Skjerve KN, Tari AR, et al. Personal Activity Intelligence (PAI), sedentary behavior and cardiovascular risk factor clustering – the HUNT study. Prog Cardiovasc Dis 2017;60(1):89–95.
87. Stenerson M, Cameron F, Payne SR, et al. The impact of accelerometer use in exercise-associated hypoglycemia prevention in type 1 diabetes. J Diabetes Sci Technol 2015;9(1):80–5.
88. Taleb N, Emami A, Suppere C, et al. Efficacy of single-hormone and dual-hormone artificial pancreas during continuous and interval exercise in adult patients with type 1 diabetes: randomised controlled crossover trial. Diabetologia 2016;59(12):2561–71.
89. Castle JR, El Youssef J, Wilson LM, et al. Randomized outpatient trial of single- and dual-hormone closed-loop systems that adapt to exercise using wearable sensors. Diabetes Care 2018;41(7):1471–7.
90. Jacobs PG, El Youssef J, Reddy R, et al. Randomized trial of a dual-hormone artificial pancreas with dosing adjustment during exercise compared with no adjustment and sensor-augmented pump therapy. Diabetes Obes Metab 2016;18(11):1110–9.
91. Rickels MR, DuBose SN, Toschi E, et al. Mini-Dose glucagon as a novel approach to prevent exercise-induced hypoglycemia in type 1 diabetes. Diabetes Care 2018;41(9):1909–16.
92. Steineck IK, Ranjan A, Schmidt S, et al. Preserved glucose response to low-dose glucagon after exercise in insulin-pump-treated individuals with type 1 diabetes: a randomised crossover study. Diabetologia 2019;62(4):582–92.

Psychosocial Aspects of Diabetes Technology Use

The Child and Family Perspective

Jaclyn Lennon Papadakis, PhD[a,*], Lindsay M. Anderson, PhD[a], Kimberly Garza, MPH[b], Marissa A. Feldman, PhD[c], Jenna B. Shapiro, PhD[a], Meredyth Evans, PhD[a,d], Laurie Gayes Thompson, PhD[a,d], Jill Weissberg-Benchell, PhD, CDE[a,d]

KEYWORDS

• Pediatric • Psychosocial • Technology • Type 1 diabetes

KEY POINTS

- Existing research on youth with type 1 diabetes and their families has found associations between diabetes technology use and psychosocial constructs, such as quality of life, depression, fear of hypoglycemia, self-management, sleep quality, caregiver burden, and more.
- The current literature suggests that there are positive and negative aspects to diabetes technology use among youth with type 1 diabetes and their families. However, some findings are inconsistent or contradictory. Therefore, it is difficult to draw robust conclusions.
- Rigorous research is needed, with primary outcomes focused on the psychosocial impact of technology use on youth with type 1 diabetes and their families.

INTRODUCTION

Current national and international guidelines recommend treating youth with type 1 diabetes (T1D) with intensive insulin regimens and continuous glucose monitoring (CGM), and considering use of automated insulin delivery systems to promote optimal glycemic outcomes.[1,2] Rates of diabetes technology use in pediatric T1D are difficult to estimate, yet continue to rise. Recent estimates suggest that 56% of youth in the

[a] Pritzker Department of Psychiatry and Behavioral Health, Ann & Robert H. Lurie Children's Hospital of Chicago, 225 East Chicago Avenue, Box 10, Chicago, IL 60611, USA; [b] Department of Anthropology, University of Illinois at Chicago, 1007 West Harrison Street, M/C 027, Chicago, IL 60607, USA; [c] Child Development and Rehabilitation Center, Johns Hopkins All Children's Hospital, 880 6th Street South, #170, Saint Petersburg, FL 33701, USA; [d] Department of Psychiatry and Behavioral Sciences, Northwestern University Feinberg School of Medicine, 446 East Ontario Street, #7-200, Chicago, IL 60611, USA
* Corresponding author.
E-mail address: jpapadakis@luriechildrens.org

Endocrinol Metab Clin N Am 49 (2020) 127–141
https://doi.org/10.1016/j.ecl.2019.10.004
endo.theclinics.com

German/Austrian DPV (Prospective Diabetes Follow-Up Registry) and 64% of youth in the US T1D Exchange Registry use continuous subcutaneous insulin infusion (CSII), and between 18.4% and 21.7% of youth use CGM or intermittently scanned ("flash") glucose monitoring, with even higher use among very young children (28%–41% of youth <6 years).[3,4] In addition, several clinical trials for hybrid closed loop and automated insulin delivery systems are underway,[5] with growing interest from youth, caregivers, and families for these systems.[6,7]

The impact of technology on adherence and glycemic control has been well-studied, with benefits including greater adherence with recommended insulin regimens, improved glycemic outcomes, fewer episodes of severe hypoglycemia, and reduction in diabetic ketoacidosis and associated hospital admissions.[1,3] Furthermore, technologies allow for additional metrics of glycemic outcomes (eg, time in range when using CGM),[1,8] and real-time adjustments to insulin delivery (eg, temporary basal or glucose suspend when using CSII) that can have a positive impact on glycemic outcomes.

Despite these well-documented benefits to glycemic control, the impact of technology on psychosocial outcomes in youth and their families is less understood. Given that technology is imperfect and may increase perceived burden,[1,9] the psychosocial impact of technology on youth and families is an important consideration in clinical practice. Furthermore, psychosocial factors may impact uptake and continued use, making them relevant for clinical decision-making. Only recently has there been a strong push to include psychosocial assessment and patient-reported outcomes when evaluating new technologies, and therefore data are limited.[10] Nevertheless, the evaluation of psychosocial outcomes is growing[11] and critical given the well-documented relationship between psychosocial difficulties, such as depression, distress, and diabetes-related family conflict and health outcomes.[12,13]

This article provides a summary of the psychosocial aspects of different technologies available for use among youth with T1D and their families by examining the current literature via systematic review. We further discuss clinical implications and recommendations for practice, limitations of the current data, and areas for future inquiry.

METHOD

Fig. 1 provides an explanation of the methods used.

RESULTS

Four authors (JLP, LMA, KG, JW-B) independently screened all titles and abstracts for eligibility. Articles identified in the initial screen were then reviewed independently by all authors, examining full text (see **Fig. 1** for systematic search results). Fifty-six articles met inclusion criteria, 11 of which were randomized controlled trials. Thirty-two studies focused on CSII, 17 studies were focused on CGM, 2 studies on predictive low-glucose suspend, and 10 studies on artificial pancreas (AP) systems (five studies were focused on CSII and CGM). Twenty-eight studies reported psychosocial data on youth only, 6 studies reported data on parents/caregivers only, and 22 studies reported data on youth and their parents/caregivers. Discussion of results, organized by type of diabetes technology, follows.

Continuous Subcutaneous Insulin Infusion

Quality of life (QoL) was the most studied psychosocial construct related to CSII. QoL was generally higher in CSII users compared with youth using multiple daily injections

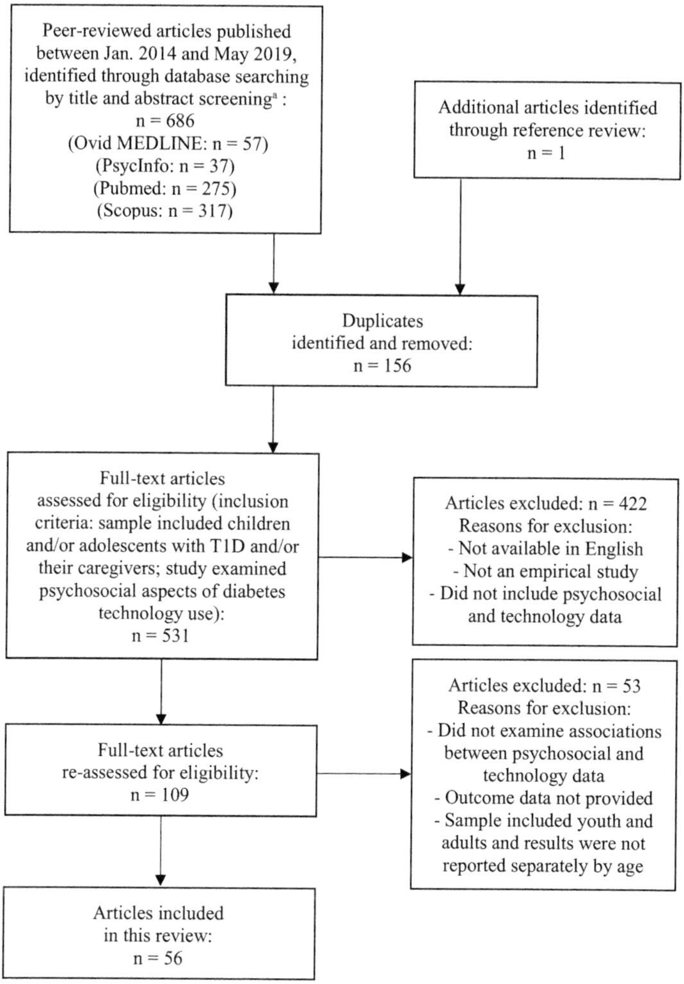

Fig. 1. Method and search results of systematic review of psychosocial aspects of diabetes technology use in children and adolescents with T1D and their families. [a] Search terms: diabetes AND (pediatr OR child OR adolescen OR fam) AND [(insulin pump OR continuous subcutaneous insulin infusion OR CSII OR insulin infusion system OR Tslim OR Omnipod) OR (continuous glucose monitor OR CGM OR Eversense OR Dexcom OR Flash Monitoring OR Libre OR Medtronic OR Nightscout) OR (artificial pancreas OR open APS OR bionic pancreas OR automatic insulin delivery OR automated insulin delivery OR closed loop) OR (predictive low-glucose suspend OR sensor augmented pump)].

(MDI).[14–21] However, one study noted that overall QoL was not higher among CSII users with comorbid celiac disease,[22] and another indicated no differences in QoL compared with MDI or less intensive regimens.[23] There were also no differences in QoL between early (within 30 days of diagnosis) and late (greater than 12 months after diagnosis) adopters of pump therapy.[24]

Depression and anxiety have also been examined in youth with T1D who use CSII. Across two studies, 17% to 21% of CSII users experienced clinically elevated depressive symptoms.[25,26] In contrast, Adler and colleagues[27] found no differences in depressive symptoms based on insulin delivery method. Another study found that higher depressive scores preceded a switch from CSII to MDI, and a switch from MDI to CSII resulted in a trending decrease in depressive symptoms. This highlights that depressive symptoms may be associated with the transitioning of insulin delivery method in general.[28] Regarding anxiety, youth and their caregivers report lower fear of hypoglycemia (FOH) and overall anxiety with CSII compared with MDI.[20,29] However, young children (ie, 6–10 years) and their caregivers endorsed greater fear of injections with CSII than MDI.[30]

The psychosocial impact of CSII on caregivers yields mixed results. One study found no difference in caregiver burden,[31] whereas another study found that caregiver burden, FOH, and parenting stress were reduced after switching from MDI to CSII.[20] Caregiver QoL and family conflict were similar between the two groups.[20]

Findings related to sleep among CSII users are inconsistent. One study found no differences in sleep-related difficulties or sleep quality.[32] Another study found that children using CSII experienced more difficulties with initiating and maintaining sleep when compared with children using MDI, whereas no differences in adolescents were observed.[27]

In regards to self-management and related factors, one study found no significant differences in self-management, self-efficacy, disease knowledge, or distress when compared with other insulin delivery methods.[33] Another study found that there were no significant differences in illness beliefs or coping strategies, but those using CSII reported a greater sense of treatment control when compared with youth using pens.[34] Importantly, compared with youth using MDI, CSII users and their caregivers reported greater expectations for independence with diabetes self-care[35] without a negative impact on child-parent collaboration.[36]

Studies on the uptake and continued use of CSII have found that anxiety was associated with discontinuation among youth, with up to 44% of youth citing fear or anxiety as a reason for discontinuation.[37,38] In addition to practical concerns (ie, wearability, difficulties with sports), 63% of youth who discontinued use reported worse well-being while using CSII.[37] Skin problems (eg, pain, irritation, itching) from infusion sites can have a negative emotional impact (eg, difficulty concentrating, increased conflict about use, worry or distress),[39] which may also affect discontinuation rates. Factors predicting continued use include engaging in more support seeking, using adaptive coping strategies, and feeling as if parents understand their diabetes.[40]

In qualitative studies examining youth and caregiver perspectives, CSII use was described as increasing flexibility and well-being,[41] and facilitating youth's ability to listen and respond to cues from their body about glycemic level.[42] Caregivers of very young children (ie, <2 years) found CSII to be challenging but facilitating a feeling of being in control.[43] In a study assessing youth, caregivers, and health care provider perspectives, positive (eg, flexibility, ease of use) and negative (eg, cost/insurance coverage, visible sign of diabetes) aspects of CSII use were identified as needing consideration before starting that technology.[44] In a study assessing provider perspectives only, CSII was perceived as valued by families, able to facilitate behavior change, and likely to improve a family's well-being, whereas at the same time CSII was perceived as challenging for families because of high user demands and poor systemic support (ie, through school, funding agencies).[45]

Continuous Glucose Monitor

QoL has consistently been rated as higher among youth using CGM compared with self-monitoring of blood glucose via glucose meter, particularly among youth who consistently use CGM.[46] Qualitative reports from caregivers of children using CGM reported increased child independence,[47,48] with some caregivers reporting that CGM "gave their child their life back."[49] In addition, adolescents initiating intermittently scanned CGM reported decreased FOH and worry and improved QoL.[50]

Other studies have examined the relative influence of CGM on caregiver functioning. Caregivers of youth using CGM and remote monitoring report decreased parental worry or stress,[47,51] and that CGM brought "peace of mind and sense of security."[47] However, parents of youth using CGM have also reported that diabetes has a higher negative impact on family life (ie, through areas of school, work, and finances) compared with parents of non-CGM users.[31]

There are mixed findings on the impact of CGM on sleep, which is often evaluated alongside FOH. Caregivers report experiencing increased sleep disturbances after CGM initiation,[52] with 38% experiencing disrupted sleep because of alarms and 19% because of FOH.[53] Similarly, in parents of young children, parental worries about hypoglycemia during sleep were higher in CGM users than in nonusers.[54] In contrast, CGM with remote monitoring has also been associated with improved sleep quality, improved FOH, and improved QoL for parents using CGM.[51] Although sleep disruption in youth using CGM (specifically with regards to sleep initiation and maintenance) was found in one study,[27] there was no association between CGM and child sleep quality or duration in another sample.[32]

Studies have also examined factors related to CGM use and discontinuation. Compared with disinterested youth, those interested in using CGM and their parents reported greater adherence, less diabetes-specific family conflict, and higher youth QoL, but no differences in parent involvement in diabetes management.[55] It has also been found that youth reporting higher CGM self-efficacy use their CGM more frequently,[56] whereas youth reporting more conflict related to blood glucose monitoring use it less.[40] A study assessing consistency in use of CGM found that, compared with youth who used their CGM 3 to 7 days each week, those who used it only 0 to 2 days reported greater depressive symptoms, diabetes burden, and lower QoL.[57] Focus group data suggest that skin irritation from CGM negatively affected continued use because of disturbed concentration, parental guilt, family conflict, and concerns regarding the future.[39]

Predictive Low-Glucose Suspend Feature

Few studies have examined the impact of predictive low-glucose management among youth, a feature that suspends insulin delivery when hypoglycemia is either predicted or detected. Abraham and colleagues[58] conducted a randomized controlled trial of adolescents comparing the effectiveness of "suspend before low" with sensor augmented pump therapy (SAP) alone and found no differences in QoL, hypoglycemia awareness, or FOH among adolescents or their parents. In a study examining how families with more than one child with diabetes would adapt to using SAP with an automated insulin suspend feature,[59] families reported that the first 2 weeks were stressful and overwhelming, but by the end of the study 80% reported they would continue using SAP.

Artificial Pancreas

Compared with studies on CSII and CGM, few articles have assessed the psychosocial aspects of AP systems among youth with T1D. Both youth and their parents expressed hope that using an AP would lead to improvements in worry, burden, stress, and family dynamics.[6] In a study assessing children and adults, many expressed interest in an implantable closed-loop, with expected improvements in mood, relaxation, and QoL.[60] However, some concerns were also reported regarding the potential size of the AP, the method of implanting the system, and being able to trust the system.[60] Additional views combined across children and adults include concerns with trust and management burden with AP; desired features and adaptability of AP; and hope for improvements in stress, conflict, and social and school-related situations.[61]

Studies of youth who have used AP systems suggest positive psychosocial benefits, including that reduced FOH,[62,63] reduced worry about hyperglycemia,[64] and less burden with the daily demands of the diabetes regimen.[62] Qualitative findings suggest that youth think about diabetes less when using AP, engage more in activities, experience increased flexibility when making food choices,[62] feel less worried about high blood sugars and glycemic control,[62,65] spend less time on the daily diabetes management tasks,[65] experience improved sleep,[64,65] and feel better overall.[66] No differences have been identified in youth's self-reported diabetes distress[62] or QoL[67] compared with those using CSII or SAP, and no differences in sleep compared with those using predictive low-glucose suspend features.[68] Studies assessing the impact of AP systems on caregivers have found parents to report improvements in their own anxiety, confidence in the technology, and sleep.[64,66]

DISCUSSION

The current review summarizes psychosocial aspects of diabetes technology use among youth with T1D and their families by systematically reviewing the research literature published over the past 5 years. This review focused on the most recently published literature given the pace at which advancements in technology occur; indeed, certain models/devices that were used years ago may no longer be the same devices that youth with diabetes are using today. Most studies focus on CSII, followed by CGM, AP systems, and other types of technology (eg, predictive low-glucose suspend); this largely reflects the number of studies in general on these technologies. There are strengths to the current literature, including the examination of a broad array of psychosocial constructs, use of mixed methods, focus on youth with diabetes and their caregivers, and the international scope of the literature. However, it is currently difficult to draw robust conclusions about the relationship between diabetes technology and psychosocial outcomes given that these studies have produced contradictory findings. For example, one study found that parents' sleep was negatively impacted by CGM (ie, because of alarms and FOH),[53] whereas another study found parents experienced improve sleep quality.[51]

Overall, the literature indicates that there are positive and negative psychosocial aspects to diabetes technology use among youth and their families. The strongest evidence for benefits of technology seem to be on QoL. The use of diabetes technology seems to lead to either no differences or improved QoL in youth. Child anxiety and FOH also tend to improve with technology use; however, an undesirable consequence of CSII may be increased fear of injections, perhaps because exposure to injections is reduced.[30] Some studies also suggest that technology improves self-management and self-efficacy, whereas others have found no differences. More consistently, studies have found technology to lead to an increased sense of control and independence. For caregivers, technology either leads to no differences in psychosocial outcomes or decreases in burden, stress, and anxiety/worry.

Several findings suggested complex or mixed impact of technology on psychosocial outcomes. For instance, the association between technology use and depression is unclear, and has only been examined in studies on CSII and CGM. Specifically, it seems that the initiation or discontinuation of technology is related to depressive symptoms, and how consistently one uses the technology. Sleep was examined in studies on CSII, CGM, and AP systems, and produced similarly contradictory findings, in that it seems technology can improve sleep (eg, decrease FOH in middle of the night) while also disrupting it (eg, because of alarms). Few studies have looked at the impact on the family unit; those that have, found it either had no impact or a negative impact on the family. This suggests that although technology may ease the management of T1D, it does not fully eliminate distress, nor does technology eliminate the daily requirements of families to ensure children's diabetes is properly managed.

Lastly, across technology groups, studies have looked at the expectations that families have about how technology will positively or negatively affect their lives, what leads to starting technology, and continued use. These aspects are specific to the type of technology and its features. It may be that the benefits of technology are attenuated when there is less satisfaction with the specific features of the technology. For example, skin problems and their associated emotional consequences seem to be a common reason for discontinuation of CSII and CGM, whereas negative experiences of AP systems have included issues related to equipment size, connectivity, and calibration.[39,66]

Future Research

Although the research in this area is promising, there are several gaps that future studies should aim to fill. First, compared with the larger body of literature on diabetes technology use, the number of studies that examine psychosocial aspects is low. This review found that when psychosocial factors were examined, it was a secondary objective rather than the primary interest of the study. The small number of studies makes it difficult to draw conclusions, particularly in the context of conflicting findings.

Future studies on diabetes technology should include assessment of psychosocial factors, because such aspects are vital to how youth and their families engage with technology, psychosocial factors impact diabetes management and glycemic outcomes,[69] and because youth with T1D and their parents may be at risk for psychosocial difficulties.[70] Although a variety of psychosocial constructs have been assessed, the literature would benefit from a harmonization of constructs to allow for drawing stronger conclusions across the literature. Focus should be on constructs that have been linked with metabolic outcomes in youth with T1D (eg, depression, diabetes distress, diabetes-specific family conflict).[69,71]

As with all pediatric research, special consideration needs to be given to developmental issues when studying children and adolescents. First, efforts should be made to design longitudinal studies to track developmental trajectories and better understand causal factors. Most studies in this review used cross-sectional data. For example, one study found that parents of youth using CGM reported that diabetes has a higher negative impact on family life (ie, through areas of school, work, and finances) compared with parents of non-CGM users.[31] Because these data are cross-sectional, it cannot be determined whether families who perceive a greater diabetes impact turn to technology or whether technology use negatively impacts family life. In contrast, Bomba and colleagues[59] used a longitudinal design to capture the nuances of everyday adjustment (eg, fluctuations in feeling stressed, overwhelmed) over a 6-month period by parents and adolescents using SAP.

Second, future studies should give greater consideration to age and development level when deciding participant inclusion criteria and statistical treatment (eg, controlling for age or evaluating age as a moderator). Some existing studies included a wide age range, even including children and adults in the same sample. Developmental stages matter, as is evidenced by the well documented decline in metabolic control

Table 1
Considerations when discussing diabetes technology with youth with T1D and their families, based on current research evidence

Positive Aspects of Use	Mixed/Neutral Findings	Negative Aspects of Use
All Technology		
• Many contradictions in the literature exist, which may be because diabetes management preferences are highly individual • Patient preferences are paramount when considering how technology may impact a particular youth and their family • More longitudinal research is needed to assess developmental changes		
Continuous Subcutaneous Insulin Infusion		
• Decreased anxiety and FOH • Self-management: greater sense of control, greater expectations for youth independence • Parental impact: decreased stress • Factors that contribute to initiation: flexibility, ease of use • Factors that contribute to continued use: support seeking, using adaptive coping strategies, feeling as if parents understand their diabetes	• QoL: better or no differences • Depression: no differences • Self-management: no differences in self-management or self-efficacy • Sleep: no differences • Parental impact: decreased or no differences in caregiver burden • Family impact: no differences	• Depression: higher depressive symptoms when transitioning to/from CSII • Anxiety: may have higher fear of injections compared with MDI • Sleep: younger users may have difficulties initiating/maintaining sleep • Factors that deter initiation: visible signs of diabetes, cost • Factors that contribute to discontinuation: anxiety, skin problems that led to distress
Continuous glucose monitoring		
• Improved QoL • Less depression for those who used it more • Anxiety: decreased worry and FOH • Self-management: increased independence, self-efficacy linked to more frequent use • Parental impact: decreased parental worry and stress • Factors that contribute to initiation: initiators report better adherence, less diabetes-specific family conflict, and higher youth QoL, but not differences in parent involvement	• Sleep: mixed findings for youth and caregivers	• Family impact: negative impact on family life through interferences with school, work, and finances • Factors that contribute to less use/ discontinuation: conflict related to blood glucose monitoring, skin problems and their impact on parental guilt and family conflict

Predictive low-glucose suspend feature		
• Most chose to continue use	• QoL: no differences compared with SAP • Hypoglycemia awareness: no differences compared with SAP • FOH: no differences compared with SAP	• Initial use may be stressful/overwhelming
Artificial pancreas system		
• Anxiety: reduced worry, FOH • Self-management: increased flexibility in food choices, less time on management • Sleep: improved sleep • Parental impact: decreased anxiety, increased confidence in technology, improved sleep • Other: less diabetes burden, better engagement in activities	• Families have positive and negative expectations about use • QoL: no differences compared with CSII/SAP • Diabetes distress: no differences compared with CSII/SAP • Sleep: no differences compared with predictive low-glucose suspend feature	• No current literature

Abbreviations: CSII, continuous subcutaneous insulin infusion; FOH, fear of hypoglycemia; MDI, multiple daily injections; PLGS, predictive low glucose suspend; SAP, sensor augmented pump; QOL, quality of life.

(ie, hemoglobin A_{1c}) during adolescence,[72] and risk for psychosocial difficulties varies across development (eg, anxiety in early childhood, depression in adolescence). Lastly, future studies on youth and their families should examine how they collaborate in their use of technology to manage diabetes,[48] because parental involvement is a key aspect of effective diabetes management.[73]

Future research should also consider how psychosocial factors interact with the economic aspects of technology use. Indeed, sociodemographic factors (eg, socioeconomic status, insurance type) influence a family's access to technology.[28] Although consideration of these factors was outside the scope of this review, it is clear from the research on health disparities among individuals with diabetes that such factors have important implications for health and psychosocial outcomes,[74] and are likely to impact how families engage with and use technology.

Clinical Implications and Summary

This review highlights implications for how health care providers can collaborate with families to discuss and manage diabetes technology. **Table 1** highlights key points for discussion with patients and their families when discussing diabetes technology. Providing youth and parents/caregivers anticipatory guidance on what they can expect when using technology is crucial, and this includes discussion on how youth and their caregivers will work together to use technology for diabetes management (eg, who will have access to shared CGM data). Families may also benefit from behavioral health consultation to address challenges with technology.

Findings from this systematic review should be considered with the following limitations in mind. First, this review included studies published over the last 5 years, because of concern that older findings are related to older technologies. Second, generalizability of study findings is limited given methodologic limitations, including sample restrictions (eg, lack of ethnic/racial diversity, small sample sizes) and construct/measurement challenges (eg, single-rater, subjective reports, operationalization of variables). Overall, consideration of psychosocial aspects of diabetes technology use will promote optimal functioning and outcomes for youth with T1D and their families.

DISCLOSURE

The authors have nothing to disclose.

REFERENCES

1. Sherr JL, Tauschmann M, Battelino T, et al. ISPAD clinical practice consensus guidelines 2018: diabetes technologies. Pediatr Diabetes 2018;19(Suppl 27):302–25.
2. Chiang JL, Maahs DM, Garvey KC, et al. Type 1 diabetes in children and adolescents: a position statement by the American Diabetes Association. Diabetes Care 2018;41(9):2026–44.
3. DeSalvo DJ, Miller KM, Hermann JM, et al. Continuous glucose monitoring and glycemic control among youth with type 1 diabetes: international comparison from the T1D Exchange and DPV Initiative. Pediatr Diabetes 2018;19(7):1271–5.
4. Heinemann L, Fleming GA, Petrie JR, et al. Insulin pump risks and benefits: a clinical appraisal of pump safety standards, adverse event reporting, and research needs: a joint statement of the European Association for the Study of Diabetes and the American Diabetes Association Diabetes Technology Working Group. Diabetes Care 2015;38(4):716–22.

5. Musolino G, Allen JM, Hartnell S, et al. Assessing the efficacy, safety and utility of 6 month day-and-night automated closed-loop insulin delivery under free living conditions compared to insulin pump therapy in children and adolescents with type 1 diabetes: an open-label, multi-centre, multi-national, single-period, randomised, parallel group study protocol. BMJ Open 2019;9(6):e027856.
6. Garza KP, Jedraszko A, Weil LEG, et al. Automated insulin delivery systems: hopes and expectations of family members. Diabetes Technol Ther 2018;20(3): 222–8.
7. Iturralde E, Tanenbaum ML, Hanes SJ, et al. Expectations and attitudes of individuals with type 1 diabetes after using a hybrid closed loop system. Diabetes Educ 2017;43(2):223–32.
8. Agiostratidou G, Anhalt H, Ball D, et al. Standardizing clinically meaningful outcome measures beyond HbA1c for type 1 diabetes: a consensus report of the American Association of Clinical Endocrinologists, the American Association of Diabetes Educators, the American Diabetes Association, the Endocrine Society, JDRF International, The Leona M. and Harry B. Helmsley Charitable Trust, the Pediatric Endocrine Society, and the T1D Exchange. Diabetes Care 2017;40(12): 1622–30.
9. Alcantara-Aragon V. Improving patient self-care using diabetes technologies. Ther Adv Endocrinol Metab 2019;10. 2042018818824215.
10. Petrie JR, Peters AL, Bergenstal RM, et al. Improving the clinical value and utility of CGM systems: issues and recommendations a joint statement of the European Association for the Study of Diabetes and the American Diabetes Association Diabetes Technology Working Group. Diabetes Care 2017;40:1614–21.
11. Naranjo D, Tanenbaum ML, Iturralde E, et al. Diabetes technology: uptake, outcomes, barriers, and the intersection with distress. J Diabetes Sci Technol 2016;10(4):852–8.
12. Hood KK, Beavers DP, Yi-Frazier J, et al. Psychosocial burden and glycemic control during the first 6 years of diabetes: results from the SEARCH for diabetes in youth study. J Adolesc Health 2014;55(4):498–504.
13. McGrady ME, Laffel L, Drotar D, et al. Depressive symptoms and glycemic control in adolescents with type 1 diabetes: mediational role of blood glucose monitoring. Diabetes care 2009;32(5):804–6.
14. Bayrakdar A, Noureddine S, Farhood L, et al. Comparison of quality of life in a group of Lebanese type 1 diabetics on insulin pump and those on multiple daily injections. J Med Liban 2014;62(1):22–6.
15. Birkebaek NH, Kristensen LJ, Mose AH, et al. Quality of life in Danish children and adolescents with type 1 diabetes treated with continuous subcutaneous insulin infusion or multiple daily injections. Diabetes Res Clin Pract 2014;106(3):474–80.
16. Blair J, McKay A, Ridyard C, et al. Continuous subcutaneous insulin infusion versus multiple daily injections in children and young people at diagnosis of type 1 diabetes: the SCIPI RCT. Health Technol Assess 2018;22(42):1–112.
17. Cherubini V, Gesuita R, Bonfanti R, et al. Health-related quality of life and treatment preferences in adolescents with type 1 diabetes. The VIPKIDS study. Acta Diabetol 2014;51(1):43–51.
18. Lukács A, Mayer K, Sasvári P, et al. Health-related quality of life of adolescents with type 1 diabetes in the context of resilience. Pediatr Diabetes 2018;19(8):1481–6.
19. Lukács A, Varga B, Kiss-Tóth Ek, et al. Factors influencing the diabetes-specific health-related quality of life in children and adolescents with type 1 diabetes mellitus. J Child Health Care 2014;18(3):253–61.

20. Mueller-Godeffroy E, Vonthein R, Ludwig-Seibold C, et al. Psychosocial benefits of insulin pump therapy in children with diabetes type 1 and their families: the pumpkin multicenter randomized controlled trial. Pediatr Diabetes 2018;19(8): 1471–80.
21. Stahl-Pehe A, Strassburger K, Castillo K, et al. Quality of life in intensively treated youths with early-onset type 1 diabetes: a population-based survey. Pediatr Diabetes 2014;15(6):436–43.
22. Pham-Short A, Donaghue KC, Ambler G, et al. Quality of life in type 1 diabetes and celiac disease: role of the gluten-free diet. J Pediatr 2016;179:131–1380.
23. Keller M, Attia R, Beltrand J, et al. Insulin regimens, diabetes knowledge, quality of life, and HbA1c in children and adolescents with type 1 diabetes. Pediatr Diabetes 2017;18(5):340–7.
24. Lang EG, King BR, Miller MN, et al. Initiation of insulin pump therapy in children at diagnosis of type 1 diabetes resulted in improved long-term glycemic control. Pediatr Diabetes 2017;18(1):26–32.
25. McGill DE, Volkening LK, Pober DM, et al. Depressive symptoms at critical times in youth with type 1 diabetes: following type 1 diabetes diagnosis and insulin pump initiation. J Adolesc Health 2018;62(2):219–26.
26. Zdunczyk B, Sendela J, Szypowska A. High prevalence of depressive symptoms in well-controlled adolescents with type 1 diabetes treated with continuous subcutaneous insulin infusion. Diabetes Metab Res Rev 2014;30(4):333–8.
27. Adler A, Gavan MY, Tauman R, et al. Do children, adolescents, and young adults with type 1 diabetes have increased prevalence of sleep disorders? Pediatr Diabetes 2017;18(6):450–8.
28. Wong JC, Dolan LM, Yang TT, et al. Insulin pump use and glycemic control in adolescents with type 1 diabetes: predictors of change in method of insulin delivery across two years. Pediatr Diabetes 2015;16(8):592–9.
29. Al Hayek AA, Robert AA, Braham RB, et al. Predictive risk factors for fear of hypoglycemia and anxiety-related emotional disorders among adolescents with type 1 diabetes. Med Princ Pract 2015;24(3):222–30.
30. Cemeroglu AP, Can A, Davis AT, et al. Fear of needles in children with type 1 diabetes mellitus on multiple daily injections and continuous subcutaneous insulin infusion. Endocr Pract 2015;21(1):46–53.
31. Harrington KR, Boyle CT, Miller KM, et al. Management and family burdens endorsed by parents of youth <7 years old with type 1 diabetes. J Diabetes Sci Technol 2017; 11(5):980–7.
32. Jaser SS, Foster NC, Nelson BA, et al. Sleep in children with type 1 diabetes and their parents in the T1D exchange. Sleep Med 2017;39:108–16.
33. Perry L, James S, Steinbeck K, et al. Young people with type 1 diabetes mellitus: attitudes, perceptions, and experiences of diabetes management and continuous subcutaneous insulin infusion therapy. J Eval Clin Pract 2017;23(3):554–61.
34. Wisting L, Bang L, Skrivarhaug T, et al. Psychological barriers to optimal insulin therapy: more concerns in adolescent females than males. BMJ Open Diabetes Res Care 2016;4(1):e000203.
35. Cemeroglu AP, Can A, Davis AT, et al. Comparison of the expectations of caregivers and children with type 1 diabetes mellitus for independence in diabetes care-related tasks. Endocr Pract 2014;20(7):629–37.
36. Cemeroglu AP, Timmer S, Turfe Z, et al. Differences in parental involvement in the care of children and adolescents with type 1 diabetes mellitus on multiple daily insulin injections versus continuous subcutaneous insulin infusion. J Pediatr Endocrinol Metab 2016;29(3):265–72.

37. Binek A, Rembierz-Knoll A, Polanska J, et al. Reasons for the discontinuation of therapy of personal insulin pump in children with type 1 diabetes. Pediatr Endocrinol Diabetes Metab 2016;21(2):65–9.
38. Wong JC, Boyle C, DiMeglio LA, et al. Evaluation of pump discontinuation and associated factors in the T1D exchange clinic registry. J Diabetes Sci Technol 2017;11(2):224–32.
39. Berg AK, Simonsen AB, Svensson J. Perception and possible causes of skin problems to insulin pump and glucose sensor: results from pediatric focus groups. Diabetes Technol Ther 2018;20(8):566–70.
40. Neylon OM, Skinner TC, O'Connell MA, et al. A novel tool to predict youth who will show recommended usage of diabetes technologies. Pediatr Diabetes 2016; 17(3):174–83.
41. Alsaleh FM, Smith FJ, Thompson R, et al. Insulin pump therapy: impact on the lives of children/young people with diabetes mellitus and their parents. Int J Clin Pharm 2014;36(5):1023–30.
42. Ferrari M, McIlwain DJF, Ambler G. A qualitative comparison of needles and insulin pump use in children with type 1 diabetes. J Health Psychol 2018;23(10): 1332–42.
43. Forsner M, Berggren J, Masaba J, et al. Parents' experiences of caring for a child younger than two years of age treated with continuous subcutaneous insulin infusion. Eur Diabetes Nurs 2014;11(1):7–13.
44. Wysocki T, Hirschfeld F, Miller L, et al. Consideration of insulin pumps or continuous glucose monitors by adolescents with type 1 diabetes and their parents: stakeholder engagement in the design of web-based decision aids. Diabetes Educ 2016;42(4):395–408.
45. Shulman R, Miller FA, Daneman D, et al. Valuing technology: a qualitative interview study with physicians about insulin pump therapy for children with type 1 diabetes. Health Policy 2016;120(1):64–71.
46. Giani E, Snelgrove R, Volkening LK, et al. Continuous glucose monitoring (CGM) adherence in youth with type 1 diabetes: associations with biomedical and psychosocial variables. J Diabetes Sci Technol 2017;11(3):476–83.
47. Erie C, Van Name MA, Weyman K, et al. Schooling diabetes: use of continuous glucose monitoring and remote monitors in the home and school settings. Pediatr Diabetes 2018;19(1):92–7.
48. Litchman ML, Allen NA, Colicchio VD, et al. A qualitative analysis of real-time continuous glucose monitoring data sharing with care partners: to share or not to share? Diabetes Technol Ther 2018;20(1):25–31.
49. Pickup JC, Ford Holloway M, Samsi K. Real-time continuous glucose monitoring in type 1 diabetes: a qualitative framework analysis of patient narratives. Diabetes Care 2015;38(4):544–50.
50. Al Hayek AA, Robert AA, Al Dawish MA. Evaluation of FreeStyle Libre flash glucose monitoring system on glycemic control, health-related quality of life, and fear of hypoglycemia in patients with type 1 diabetes. Clin Med Insights Endocrinol Diabetes 2017;10. 1179551417746957.
51. Burckhardt MA, Roberts A, Smith GJ, et al. The use of continuous glucose monitoring with remote monitoring improves psychosocial measures in parents of children with type 1 diabetes: a randomized crossover trial. Diabetes Care 2018; 41(12):2641–3.
52. Landau Z, Rachmiel M, Pinhas-Hamiel O, et al. Parental sleep quality and continuous glucose monitoring system use in children with type 1 diabetes. Acta Diabetol 2014;51(3):499–503.

53. Barnard K, Crabtree V, Adolfsson P, et al. Impact of type 1 diabetes technology on family members/significant others of people with diabetes. J Diabetes Sci Technol 2016;10(4):824–30.
54. Van Name MA, Hilliard ME, Boyle CT, et al. Nighttime is the worst time: parental fear of hypoglycemia in young children with type 1 diabetes. Pediatr Diabetes 2018;19(1):114–20.
55. Telo GH, Volkening LK, Butler DA, et al. Salient characteristics of youth with type 1 diabetes initiating continuous glucose monitoring. Diabetes Technol Ther 2015; 17(6):373–8.
56. Rasbach LE, Volkening LK, Markowitz JT, et al. Youth and parent measures of self-efficacy for continuous glucose monitoring: survey psychometric properties. Diabetes Technol Ther 2015;17(5):327–34.
57. McGill DE, Volkening LK, Butler DA, et al. Baseline psychosocial characteristics predict frequency of continuous glucose monitoring in youth with type 1 diabetes. Diabetes Technol Ther 2018;20(6):434–9.
58. Abraham MB, Nicholas JA, Smith GJ, et al. Reduction in hypoglycemia with the predictive low-glucose management system: a long-term randomized controlled trial in adolescents with type 1 diabetes. Diabetes Care 2018;41(2):303–10.
59. Bomba F, Muller-Godeffroy E, von Sengbusch S. Experiences in sensor-augmented pump therapy in families with two children with type 1 diabetes: a qualitative study. Exp Clin Endocrinol Diabetes 2018;126(3):162–7.
60. Taylor MJ, Gregory R, Mitchell H, et al. Insulin pump users would not rule out using an implantable artificial pancreas. Practical Diabetes 2014;31(1):18–23a.
61. Naranjo D, Suttiratana SC, Iturralde E, et al. What end users and stakeholders want from automated insulin delivery systems. Diabetes Care 2017;40(11): 1453–61.
62. Weissberg-Benchell J, Hessler D, Polonsky WH, et al. Psychosocial impact of the bionic pancreas during summer camp. J Diabetes Sci Technol 2016;10(4):840–4.
63. Ziegler C, Liberman A, Nimri R, et al. Reduced worries of hypoglycaemia, high satisfaction, and increased perceived ease of use after experiencing four nights of MD-Logic Artificial Pancreas at Home (DREAM4). J Diabetes Res 2015;590308. https://doi.org/10.1155/2015/590308.
64. Barnard KD, Wysocki T, Allen JM, et al. Closing the loop overnight at home setting: psychosocial impact for adolescents with type 1 diabetes and their parents. BMJ Open Diabetes Res Care 2014;2(1):e000025.
65. Tauschmann M, Allen JM, Wilinska ME, et al. Home use of day-and-night hybrid closed-loop insulin delivery in suboptimally controlled adolescents with type 1 diabetes: a 3-week, free-living, randomized crossover trial. Diabetes Care 2016;39(11):2019–25.
66. Barnard KD, Wysocki T, Ully V, et al. Closing the loop in adults, children and adolescents with suboptimally controlled type 1 diabetes under free living conditions: a psychosocial substudy. J Diabetes Sci Technol 2017;11(6):1080–8.
67. Tauschmann M, Thabit H, Bally L, et al, APCam11 Consortium. Closed-loop insulin delivery in suboptimally controlled type 1 diabetes: a multicentre, 12-week randomised trial. Lancet 2018;392(10155):1321–9.
68. Sharifi A, De Bock MI, Jayawardene D, et al. Glycemia, treatment satisfaction, cognition, and sleep quality in adults and adolescents with type 1 diabetes when using a closed-loop system overnight versus sensor-augmented pump with low-glucose suspend function: a randomized crossover study. Diabetes Technol Ther 2016;18(12):772–83.

69. Hegelson VS, Siminerio L, Escobar O, et al. Predictors of metabolic control among adolescents with diabetes: a 4-year longitudinal study. J Pediatr Psychol 2009;34(3):254–70.
70. Jaser SS. Psychological problems in adolescents with diabetes. Adolesc Med State Art Rev 2010;21(1):138–51, x–xi.
71. Delamater AM, Patiño-Fernández AM, Smith KE, et al. Measurement of diabetes stress in older children and adolescents with type 1 diabetes mellitus. Pediatr Diabetes 2013;14(1):50–6.
72. Clements MA, Foster NC, Maahs DM, et al. Hemoglobin A1c (HbA1c) changes over time among adolescent and young adult participants in the T1D exchange clinic registry. Pediatr Diabetes 2016;17(5):327–36.
73. King PS, Berg CA, Butner J, et al. Longitudinal trajectories of parental involvement in type 1 diabetes and adolescents' adherence. Health Psychol 2014;33(5):424–32.
74. Borschuk AP, Everhart RS. Health disparities among youth with type 1 diabetes: a systematic review of the current literature. Fam Syst Health 2015;33(3):297–313.

Psychosocial Aspects of Diabetes Technology

Adult Perspective

William H. Polonsky, PhD[a,b,*]

KEYWORDS

• CGM • CSII • Psychosocial • Technology • Adults

KEY POINTS

- Across most studies, treatment satisfaction increases significantly following the introduction of real-time continuous glucose monitoring (CGM) and/or continuous subcutaneous insulin infusion (CSII).
- Surprisingly, the observed impact of real-time CGM and/or CSII on quality of life (QOL) in RCTs has been observed to be minimal.
- To date, longitudinal studies to evaluate the impact of QOL have not included any of the newer CSII or real-time CGM systems.
- For many patients, comprehensive education and personalized support at the outset may be key to their acceptance and ongoing use of CGM and/or CSII systems.

The premise underlying the accelerating growth in innovative diabetes technology is that new devices and other new support tools allow users with both type 1 diabetes (T1D) and type 2 diabetes (T2D) to more effectively and/or more easily achieve adequate (or excellent) glycemic control while also enhancing (or at least not reducing) quality of life (QOL). Critically, the success of such innovations, be it devices for real-time continuous glucose monitoring (RT-CGM) or continuous subcutaneous insulin infusion (CSII), devices that combine both technologies (sensor-augmented insulin pumps [SAPs]), or the array of new digital support tools, depends on the buy-in by the end users (ie, the individuals with diabetes). To what degree will people with diabetes accept diabetes technology (ie, choose to initiate its use) and make good use of it over time? None of the diabetes self-care tools can be effective if the end users are not engaging with that tool in an effective manner. For example, RT-CGM leads to minimal glycemic benefits if the individual wears it only infrequently[1]; similarly, blood glucose monitoring is of no glycemic value when no one is making good use of the resulting data.[2,3]

[a] Behavioral Diabetes Institute, 5405 Oberlin Drive, Suite 100, San Diego, CA 92121, USA; [b] University of California, San Diego, San Diego, CA, USA
* Behavioral Diabetes Institute, 5405 Oberlin Drive, Suite 100, San Diego, CA 92121.
E-mail address: whp@behavioraldiabetes.org

Endocrinol Metab Clin N Am 49 (2020) 143–155
https://doi.org/10.1016/j.ecl.2019.10.003
endo.theclinics.com

It is, therefore, the psychosocial perspective of end users that must be carefully considered as researchers evaluate current diabetes technology and as developers work to develop more patient-friendly technological solutions. Toward this end, this article focuses on the experiences of adults and discusses what is known regarding how diabetes technology affects QOL and how such technology is perceived by the users (and potential users), with special attention to the perceived benefits and costs. It also considers the psychosocial predictors of who is likely to accept and make good use of such technology, and puts forward a series of strategies for encouraging technology acceptance. Given the wide differences in the currently available types and uses of diabetes technology, this narrative review is limited to an examination of wearable technology, and focuses on the 3 major forms: RT-CGM, CSII, and SAP. There remain many more distal technological tools (including health care system–directed telehealth, text messaging and patient portals, and social platforms, and more self-directed tools such as automated decision-support systems and a plethora of diabetes apps)[4,5] as well as new, more proximal tools that are now beginning to emerge (eg, so-called smart pens that track insulin injection data and recommend doses), but these are beyond the scope of the current review.

CONTINUOUS GLUCOSE MONITORING

There is little doubt that RT-CGM has begun to change almost everything for people living with diabetes. For example, patients with RT-CGM now have the opportunity to see not only what their glucose levels (GLs) are in the current moment but also how their GLs are changing. For the first time, they have the opportunity to see in the immediate moment how foods, activity, and stress affect GLs. In addition, RT-CGM alerts and alarms provide the opportunity to catch and respond to hypoglycemic events before GLs become dangerously low. In short, it provides patients (and their families) with the potential to be more in control and, perhaps even more importantly, to feel safer. To date, most RT-CGM research has focused on patients with T1D, and retrospective surveys, qualitative interview , and real-world observational evidence indicate that patients' experiences with RT-CGM are overwhelmingly positive, with multiple aspects of QOL reportedly enhanced.[6–9]

These encouraging data stand seemingly in contrast with the more sobering results emerging from randomized controlled trials (RCTs), in which the impact of RT-CGM use on measures of QOL, both generic and diabetes specific, compared with self-monitoring of blood glucose has been observed to be minimal, in both T1D[1,10–12] and T2D populations.[13–16] However, it is perhaps noteworthy that several of the most recent RCTs have reported a positive influence on specific elements of diabetes-specific QOL.[17–19] The QOL findings from all RCTs to date are detailed in **Table 1** (generic QOL) and **Table 2** (diabetes-specific QOL).

Three factors may help to explain these disparate findings and thereby encourage new approaches for QOL evaluation in future trials. First, the choice of QOL measure may be critical. Qualitative data suggest that RT-CGM may influence only certain and fairly limited QOL dimensions, such as enhancing the sense of confidence that severe hypoglycemia can be avoided or reducing the overall sense of diabetes burden (ie, diabetes distress), and have little impact on other (typically broader) dimensions, such as overall health status. The available RCT data are generally supportive of these findings, suggesting that measures of hypoglycemic confidence[18,19] and, perhaps, diabetes distress[18] may be of particular value. Of note, there now exists a T1D-specific diabetes distress scale (T1-DDS[20]) that seems likely to be of greater value in assessing this key QOL aspect, although this has not yet been examined in any

Table 1
Generic quality-of-life outcomes following the introduction of continuous glucose monitoring

Study	Number Enrolled	Study Subjects	Insulin Method	CGM Studied	QOL Measure	Findings[a]
JDRF CGM Study Group,[1] 2010	451	Children and adults with T1D	CSII, MDI	All available	SF-12	Modest positive impact on SF-12 physical component subscale
Riveline et al,[10] 2012	178	Children and adults with T1D	CSII, MDI	FreeStyle Navigator	SF-36	Modest positive impact on SF-36 physical component subscale
Lind et al,[19] 2017	161	Adults with T1D	MDI	Dexcom G4	WHO-5	Modest positive impact
van Beers et al,[17] 2016	52	Adults with T1D with impaired hypoglycemic awareness	CSII, MDI	Medtronic Enlite	WHO-5 EQ-5D	No significant group differences
Polonsky et al,[18] 2017	158	Adults with T1D	MDI	Dexcom G4	WHO-5 EQ-5D	No significant group differences
Beck et al,[14] 2017	158	Adults with T2D	MDI	Dexcom G4	WHO-5 EQ-5D	No significant group differences

Abbreviations: CGM, continuous glucose monitoring; EQ, EuroQol; JDRF, Juvenile Diabetes Research Foundation; MDI, multiple daily injections; SF, short form; WHO, World Health Organization.

[a] Compared with self-monitoring of blood glucose (SMBG).

Data from Refs.[1,10,14, 7–19]

Table 2
Diabetes-specific quality-of-life outcomes following the introduction of continuous glucose monitoring

Study	Number Enrolled	Study Subjects	Insulin Method	CGM Studied	QOL Measure	Findings[a]
JDRF CGM Study Group,[1] 2010	451	Children and adults with T1D	CSII, MDI	DexCom SEVEN, MiniMed Paradigm, FreeStyle Navigator	PAID HFS	Modest positive impact on HFS total and HFS behavior subscale
Riveline et al,[10] 2012	178	Children and adults with T1D	CSII, MDI	FreeStyle Navigator	DQOL	No significant group differences
Bolinder et al,[11] 2016	239	Adults with T1D	CSII, MDI	FreeStyle Libre	DDS DQOL HFS	No significant group differences[b]
Yaron et al,[16] 2019	101	Adults with T1D	MDI	FreeStyle Libre	ADDQoL	No significant group differences
Little et al,[12] 2014	96	Adults with T1D	CSII, MDI	Medtronic Enlite	HFS	No significant group differences
van Beers et al,[17] 2016	52	Adults with T1D with impaired hypoglycemic awareness	CSII, MDI	Medtronic Enlite	PAID-5 HFS CIDS	Modest positive impact on HFS worry subscale
Polonsky et al,[18] 2017	158	Adults with T1D	MDI	Dexcom G4	DDS HFS HCS	Modest positive impact on DDS and HCS
Lind et al,[19] 2017	161	Adults with T1D	MDI	Dexcom G4	PAID HFS worry HCS	Modest positive impact on HCS
Beck et al,[14] 2017	158	Adults with T2D	MDI	Dexcom G4	DDS HFS HCS	No significant group differences
Haak et al,[15] 2017	224	Adults with T2D	CSII, MDI	FreeStyle Libre	DDS DQOL	No significant group differences
Vigersky et al,[13] 2012	100	Adults with T2D	No prandial insulin	Dexcom SEVEN	PAID	No significant group differences

Abbreviations: ADDQoL, audit of diabetes dependent quality of life questionnaire; CIDSS, confidence in diabetes self-care scale; DDS, diabetes distress scale; DQOL, Diabetes QOL; HFS, hypoglycemic fear survey; PAID, problem areas in diabetes survey.

[a] Compared with SMBG.

[b] ... in DQOL in the CGM group versus control group.

RT-CGM trial. Second, the choice of RT-CGM device may be critical. For example, the positive (but modest) QOL findings in the DIAMOND and GOLD studies[18,19] stand in contrast with almost all of the other RCT findings, which may be at least partly caused by the higher degree of accuracy and reliability of the type of RT-CGM used in those 2 studies (Dexcom G4). In addition, although the latest generation of CGM technology delivers even greater accuracy and reliability, includes valuable new features (eg, predictive low-glucose and high-glucose alarms), and reduces the burden even further on the users (eg, elimination of the need for confirmatory finger sticks), there are as yet no published data regarding possible QOL benefits in, for example, Dexcom G5 or G6 users. Third, subject selection may also be critical. For example, enhancing hypoglycemic confidence may be easier in a T1D population (who are at greater risk of severe hypoglycemia) than a T2D population.[18,19] Alleviating diabetes distress among patients with T1D may be harder to achieve in CSII users (in whom substantial distress benefits may have already accrued[21]) than in multiple daily injection (MDI) users, especially if hypoglycemic concerns are not predominant.[9]

CONTINUOUS SUBCUTANEOUS INSULIN INFUSION

Thanks to innovations in pump technology, including temporary basal rates and a range of bolus delivery options, insulin users have the ability to take control of their own GLs in a manner that has been all but impossible with MDI. It is therefore not surprising that the evidence, although limited, suggests that CSII use in adults with T1D contributes to marked diabetes-specific QOL improvements. This finding includes observational evidence[22,23] as well as RCTs.[24–26] Of note, most of these studies are dated, and only 1 of the RCTs, relative effectiveness of pumps over MDI and structured education (REPOSE), evaluated a newer CSII system (Paradigm Veo). In REPOSE, all subjects received structured education in flexible intensive insulin management, then were randomized to CSII or a determir-based MDI regimen. Although there were few significant group differences on any generic or diabetes-specific QOL measures over 24 months, the CSII group did show significantly better gains on 2 of the diabetes-specific QOL (DSQOL)[27] subscales: diet restrictions and daily hassle.[26]

The QOL findings from all RCTs to date are detailed in **Table 3**.

CSII technology has advanced considerably over the years (eg, tubeless pumps, bolus calculators, innovations in data downloading), but aside from REPOSE there have been few investigations of the potential impact of these newer CSII systems on QOL. One recent exception is a randomized crossover study in adults with T2D that examined an innovative insulin bolus patch pump versus pen; subjects scored significantly higher on 2 of the DSQOL subscales (diet restrictions and daily functions) while on the patch pump compared with MDI.[29] In addition, a recent survey of one of the newer CSII systems (Omnipod) suggests that broad QOL-related benefits may be common.[21] Most of the 1245 responding adults indicated positive changes in overall well-being (53.5%), perceived control over diabetes (72.5%), hypoglycemic safety (50.6%), and diabetes distress (69.6%) since beginning Omnipod use. Taken together, although the available data regarding newer CSII systems are limited, CSII does seem to have a positive impact on QOL.

Further studies are needed, and, as with RT-CGM, the same 3 factors should be given careful consideration: the appropriate selection of QOL instruments, the choice of CSII devices to be assessed, and careful subject selection. The results to date suggest that the critical QOL value of CSII lies in its ability to help patients feel less burdened and/or constrained by the day-to-day demands of diabetes. The best

Table 3
Generic and diabetes-specific quality-of-life outcomes following the introduction of continuous subcutaneous insulin infusion

Study	Number Enrolled	Study Subjects	CSII System Studied	QOL Measure	Findings
Tsui et al,[28] 2001	27	Adults with T1D	MiniMed 507	DQOL	No significant group differences[a]
DeVries et al,[25] 2002	79	Adults with T1D	Disetronic H-TRONplus V100	SF-36	Modest positive impact on the general health and mental health subscales[a]
Hoogma et al,[24] 2005	272	Adults with T1D	Disetronic H-TRON V100, Disetronic H-TRONplus V100	DQOL SF-12	Modest positive impact on DQOL and on SF-12 mental health subscale[a]
Heller et al,[26] 2017	260	Adults with T1D	MiniMed Paradigm Veo	Sf-12 WHOQOL-BREF EQ-5D HADS DSQOL	Modest positive impact on DSQOL diet restrictions and daily hassle subscales[b]
Bergenstal et al,[29] 2019	278	Adults with T2D	Calibra bolus patch	DSQOL	Modest positive impact on 2 of the 7 DSQOL subscales[c]

Abbreviations: HADS, Hospital Anxiety and Depression Scale; WHOQOL-BREF, World Health Organization Quality of Life Abbreviated Questionnaire.
[a] Compared with neutral protamine Hagedorn–based MDI.
[b] Compared with determir-based MDI.
[c] Compared with bolus insulin via pen.
Data from Refs.[24–26,28,29]

QOL target may therefore be diabetes distress (eg, the T1-DDS[20]) or any of the broader scales that examine how diabetes-specific hassles influence QOL.[30] The choice of CSII device may also be critical, especially if potentially influential features are considered, such as differences between systems in ease of use, the presence or absence of tubes, and RT-CGM connectivity. It is reasonable to surmise that QOL benefits could now be more common,[21] especially given the recent advancements in CSII technology.[31] In addition, consideration must be given to subject selection. It may be more reasonable to expect QOL benefits to accrue following CSII initiation in those populations in which MDI has proved to be insufficient[31] and/or there is impaired QOL at baseline (eg, high levels of hypoglycemic fear). Furthermore, there have been no studies examining the impact of CSII on QOL in the T2D population; such research is sorely needed.

SENSOR-AUGMENTED INSULIN PUMPS

The marriage of RT-CGM and CSII has begun, with several promising new products now on the market, including the first hybrid closed-loop system (Medtronic 670G). Despite many positive anecdotes regarding the impact of SAP use on QOL, good-quality evidence has been lacking. In the most well-known RCT investigating SAP technology, STAR 3 (Sensor-Augmented Pump Therapy for A1C Reduction 3), researchers compared SAP with MDI (plus blinded CGM) over 12 months and observed a significant positive impact in the adult subgroup on QOL (reduced hypoglycemic fear).[32] Hermanides and colleagues,[33] using a similar study design, also found a significant QOL benefit (a reduction in diabetes distress) in the SAP group versus the MDI group. However, given the comparators, it is unknown whether the observed positive QOL improvements in the two studies were caused by 1 or more of the individual components of the SAP (RT-CGM or CSII) or by the SAP system itself. More recently, researchers examined one of the key elements of these integrated systems, the low glucose suspend (LGS) feature. LGS did contribute to a significant decrease in nocturnal hypoglycemia (compared with SAP use with the LGS feature disabled), but there was no significant difference in QOL outcomes.[34]

In summary, the current data point to a promising trend, but remain too limited to allow any solid conclusions. Furthermore, there are no published QOL findings with regard to any of the currently available systems: the Medtronic 670G, sensor-augmented Tandem pump, and the variety of do-it-yourself artificial pancreas (looping) systems.[35] In addition, little is known about how recent innovative device features, such as the ability to easily share personal glucose and insulin use data in real time with others, may influence QOL.[36] Anecdotally, the perceived benefits of the newest SAP systems include improved sleep quality (secondary to the marked cutback in nighttime hypoglycemia) and a reduction in daily self-management efforts. Future studies might therefore benefit by focusing on measures of sleep quality as an important QOL outcome as well as on the key QOL measures specific to T1D as highlighted earlier, diabetes distress, and hypoglycemic concerns.

BENEFITS VERSUS COSTS

The glycemic benefits arising from the use of CGM, CSII, and SAP systems, especially in the reduction of hypoglycemic and hyperglycemic excursions, are generally (although not always) recognized to be substantial. This view is consistent with the overwhelmingly positive experiences elucidated by adults with T1D in survey studies and from observational evidence, especially regarding RT-CGM and CSII. Perhaps not surprisingly, across many of the current studies, treatment satisfaction has increased significantly following the introduction of RT-CGM,[11,15,19] CSII,[12,26] and SAP.[33,37] Clinicians see how lives are being changed every day by these technologies, with many patients becoming inspired to engage more fully with their own diabetes care, while at the same time feeling less restricted by the daily demands of the disease and gaining confidence in their ability to avoid and address hypoglycemia. However, the available RCT data point to only a small QOL benefit at best, and most adults with T1D have yet to adopt RT-CGM or CSII systems (although the recent increase in technology adoption, as seen in the T1D Registry, is impressive).[38] What then is the disconnect?

Even with newer, better, and more reliable technology, it seems that the perceived negatives of CGM and CSII still outweigh the potential positives for many people, which would explain why the majority have not (yet) embraced such technological solutions. For example, out-of-pocket costs remain a crucial deterrent for large numbers of patients, both with T1D and T2D.[39,40] The wearability factor also looms large; in 1 recent T1D survey, a large fraction of respondents indicated that the "hassle of wearing devices" (47% of respondents) and "not liking devices on one's body" (35%) were significant barriers.[41] Aside from cost concerns, wearability issues were the most common concerns reported, which is understandable. First, wearing a diabetes device may be off-putting because it can make the diabetes seemingly visible to the whole world. For many individuals, the need to keep diabetes private is paramount, especially if there is a perceived sense of stigma associated with the disease.[41] Patients fear that they will be viewed, or judged, by others as different, less attractive, or damaged in some manner. Second, wearing a device may be aversive because it is, or represents, a constant reminder of diabetes. Especially for patients with T1D, the ongoing need to stay vigilant and attentive to diabetes-related needs can be exhausting[20]; therefore, there is often a desire to have a mental break from diabetes or, at the least, an opportunity to have some period of time when T1D elements are not omnipresent (ie, not attached to the body). Even among patients with T2D, the urge to not be repeatedly reminded about the diabetes is reported as one of the chief reasons for avoiding blood glucose monitoring.[42]

For those using or who have quit using RT-CGM, CSII, or SAP systems, there are other critical negatives that can surface; perhaps most important is a sense of frustration and/or mistrust with device operations. For example, consider that CSII malfunctions are reported by approximately half of users,[43] annoyance about incessant alarms (so-called alarm fatigue) are common,[44] and there is often disappointment that the expected results (be they realistic or not) are not achieved.[43,45,46]

PSYCHOSOCIAL PREDICTORS

Despite the common aggravations described earlier, it seems that more and more technology users are persevering,[47] they continue to achieve good results, and the numbers of patients who are adopting diabetes technology continue to grow.[38] What personal traits contribute to individuals embracing these new devices and their subsequent glycemic success? In cross-sectional studies, CSII-using patients with T1D who felt more personally responsible for their diabetes (scoring higher on measures of internal locus of control) achieved better glycemic control than those who felt less responsible (eg, ascribing diabetes outcomes to chance).[48,49] This finding suggests that individuals who are more actively engaging with the device, are able to tolerate the frustrations of an imperfect technology, and are active problem solvers in response to obstacles are more likely to be successful. Qualitative data suggest that these same traits may also apply to success with RT-CGM.[50]

As a group, these traits underscore the central importance of patient behavior as a critical variable in achieving success with diabetes technology. These tools are, after all, for the patients. It has been shown, for example, that glycemic outcomes with RT-CGM are better when the device is worn more frequently.[1] Furthermore, it is the users' consistent and appropriate use of the technology that is mostly likely to generate glycemic success: timely and accurate bolusing with the CSII system, frequent viewing and appropriate response to the RT-CGM data,[51] and more. As seen in the clinical setting, early adopters of diabetes technology have tended to be those individuals who are the more engaged, active, problem solvers, but there are now more and more potential technology users who do not excel in these areas. Therefore, education, skill development, and ongoing support are likely to become increasingly critical.[47]

STRATEGIES FOR ENCOURAGING TECHNOLOGY ACCEPTANCE

As diabetes technology continues to advance, clinicians will be recommending RT-CGM, CSII, and SAP systems more often, but what about reluctant or ambivalent patients? Individuals with T1D and/or T2D may be more willing to begin using an RT-CGM or perhaps switch to an SAP system, for example, when they come to believe it is worthwhile, meaning that perceived benefits (eg, better glycemic control, less nocturnal hypoglycemia, greater ease in managing the complex tasks of diabetes) are thought to outweigh the perceived negatives (eg, intrusiveness of the device, concerns about malfunction, out-of-pocket costs, mistrust in the accuracy and/or reliability of the system). As out-of-pocket costs decrease and/or as systems become smaller, more accurate, and easier to use, this may be enough to shift the thinking of many patients to believe that adoption is worthwhile. The recent evidence from the T1D Registry, pointing to a sharp increase in RT-CGM and CSII use, suggests that this may already be happening.[38] However, this will not be sufficient for everyone. Clinicians could further encourage this shift by considering the following 3 strategies:

1. If possible, recommend a limited trial period. Many patients are interested in the possibility of technology adoption, but worry that the device may be a disappointment and that the decision to begin using it will be irreversible. Will this device be as intrusive as they might fear? Will friends, family members, and coworkers be put off by this starkly visible emblem of diabetes? Will the demands of the device be more trouble than it is worth? Can this technology be trusted? By providing a structure so that individuals maintain a sense of control over the decision (ie, by reassuring them that, after the trial period, if it seems as unpleasant as they fear, they can choose to discontinue), they may be more likely to give it a try.
2. Provide the right mindset. For people who are already feeling constrained by T1D or T2D in some manner (eg, feeling limited in their activities, feeling judged by health care professionals, or feeling an undue pressure to immediately respond to all out-of-range glucose values), the addition of a device can seem like 1 more demand being placed on them (eg, it may seem to patients that they are working for the RT-CGM more than it is working for them). Therefore, when introducing a new device, it can useful to discuss such concerns and to highlight ways in which the device would support, not hinder, their independence; how CSII or RT-CGM, for example, can potentially help individuals to gain a greater sense of personal control over diabetes.[18,21] Also important is to remind users that they are not permanently wedded to the device; that it is completely acceptable, when done safely, to take pump or RT-CGM "vacations" as needed, especially if it is beginning to feel overwhelming or too intrusive.

3. Offer comprehensive education and personalized support. There is often insufficient guidance when CSII or RT-CGM is initiated (which may explain why the glycemic benefits achieved in recent clinical trials are not as dramatic as might have been hoped).[52] To experience the greatest benefits, both QOL as well as glycemic, from diabetes technology, many patients benefit from proactive education, guidance, and support at the outset. This point may be especially important for patients who are not technologically inclined and/or are not curious, active problem solvers. Also needed is ongoing support. For example, when patients with RT-CGM data can retrospectively review their own glucose data over time with a trusted health care professional, thereby learning how to interpret and better respond to their own glucose patterns and gaining understanding with regard to how their own personal actions are influencing those patterns, greater glycemic benefits and consequent greater satisfaction are more likely.[52,53] In total, this means that it is especially important not to abandon struggling patients with their new devices. This strategy may be the most potent for enhancing the perceived worthwhileness of the newly adopted technology.

SUMMARY

The success of current and future diabetes technologies depends on the attitudes and behavior of the individuals who choose to adopt them. The need is therefore to develop systems that are patient friendly, and this means that careful attention must be paid to the perspectives, experiences, and concerns of end users. The available data suggest that RT-CGM, CSII, and SAP systems may positively affect diabetes-related QOL, although the influence on QOL outcomes seems to be modest at best and the results from RCTs are limited and controversial. This finding seems surprising, given the consistently positive responses emerging from observational data.[6–9,22,23] What seems most likely is that these systems, especially the newer generations of devices (none of which are included in any of the currently available RCT data), do hold the promise for alleviating diabetes distress, helping patients to feel more in control of their diabetes, and enhancing confidence that severe hypoglycemia can be avoided or addressed, but perhaps not for everyone. It needs to be appreciated that, from the patients' perspectives, diabetes technology offers potential minuses as well as pluses, that this balance between pluses and minuses differs from one individual to the next, and that it would be beneficial if the hopes and concerns that result from these viewpoints could be fully aired and discussed before initiating a new device. Especially for patients who may be less enthused or less engaged with their new systems at the outset, appropriate training and ongoing support are likely to be the key to successful uptake.

DISCLOSURE

The author has served as a consultant for Dexcom, Insulet and Abbott Diabetes Care.

REFERENCES

1. The Juvenile Diabetes Research Foundation Continuous Glucose Monitoring Study Group. Quality of life measures in children and adults with type 1 diabetes. Diabetes Care 2010;33:2175–7.
2. Polonsky WH, Fisher L. When does personalized feedback make a difference? A narrative review of recent findings and their implications for promoting better diabetes self-care. Curr Diab Rep 2015;15:620–7.

3. Polonsky WH, Fisher L. Right answer, but wrong question: self-monitoring of blood glucose can be clinically valuable for noninsulin users. Diabetes Care 2013;36: 179–82.
4. Duke DC, Barry S, Wagner DV, et al. Distal technologies and type 1 diabetes management. Lancet Diabetes Endocrinol 2018;6:143–56.
5. Hunt CW. Technology and diabetes self-management: an integrative review. World J Diabetes 2015;6:225–33.
6. Polonsky WH, Hessler D. What are the quality of life-related benefits and losses associated with real-time continuous glucose monitoring? A survey of current users. Diabetes Technol Ther 2013;15:295–301.
7. Pickup JC, Ford Holloway M, Samsi K. Real-time continuous glucose monitoring in type 1 diabetes: a qualitative framework analysis of patient narratives. Diabetes Care 2015;38:544–50.
8. Polonsky W, Peters AL, Hessler D. The impact of real-time continuous glucose monitoring in patients 65 years and older. J Diabetes Sci Technol 2016;10:892–7.
9. Charleer S, Mathieu C, Nobels F, et al. Effect of continuous glucose monitoring on glycemic control, acute admissions, and quality of life: a real-world study. J Clin Endocrinol Metab 2018;103:1224–32.
10. Riveline JP, Schaepelynck P, Chaillous L, et al. Assessment of patient-led or physician-driven continuous glucose monitoring in patients with poorly controlled type 1 diabetes using basal-bolus insulin regimens: a 1-year multicenter study. Diabetes Care 2012;35:965–71.
11. Bolinder J, Antuna R, Geelhoed-Duijvestijn P, et al. Novel glucose-sensing technology and hypoglycaemia in type 1 diabetes: a multicentre, non-masked, randomised controlled trial. Lancet 2016;388:2254–63.
12. Little SA, Leelarathna L, Walkinshaw E, et al. Recovery of hypoglycemia awareness in long-standing type 1 diabetes: a multicenter 2 × 2 factorial randomized controlled trial comparing insulin pump with multiple daily injections and continuous with conventional glucose self-monitoring (HypoCOMPaSS). Diabetes Care 2014;37:2114–22.
13. Vigersky RA, Fonda SJ, Chellappa M, et al. Short- and long-term effects of real-time continuous glucose monitoring in patients with type 2 diabetes. Diabetes Care 2012;35:32–8.
14. Beck RW, Riddlesworth TD, Ruedy K, et al. Continuous glucose monitoring versus usual care in patients with type 2 diabetes receiving multiple daily insulin injections: a randomized trial. Ann Intern Med 2017;167:365–74.
15. Haak T, Hanaire H, Ajjan R, et al. Use of flash glucose-sensing technology for 12 months as a replacement for blood glucose monitoring in insulin-treated type 2 diabetes. Diabetes Ther 2017;8:573–86.
16. Yaron M, Roitman E, Aharon-Hananel G, et al. Effect of flash glucose monitoring technology on glycemic control and treatment satisfaction in patients with type 2 diabetes. Diabetes Care 2019. https://doi.org/10.2337/dc18-0166.
17. van Beers CA, DeVries JH, Kleijer SJ, et al. Continuous glucose monitoring for patients with type 1 diabetes and impaired awareness of hypoglycaemia (IN CONTROL): a randomised, open-label, crossover trial. Lancet Diabetes Endocrinol 2016;4:893–902.
18. Polonsky WH, Hessler D, Ruedy KJ, et al. The impact of continuous glucose monitoring on markers of quality of life in adults with type 1 diabetes: further findings from the DIAMOND randomized clinical trial. Diabetes Care 2017;40:736–41.
19. Lind M, Polonsky W, Hirsch IB, et al. Continuous glucose monitoring vs conventional therapy for glycemic control in adults with type 1 diabetes treated with

multiple daily insulin injections: the GOLD randomized clinical trial. JAMA 2017;317:379–87.
20. Fisher L, Polonsky WH, Hessler DM, et al. Understanding the sources of diabetes distress in adults with type 1 diabetes. J Diabetes Complications 2015;29:572–7.
21. Polonsky WH, Hessler D, Layne JE, et al. Impact of the Omnipod insulin management system on quality of life: a survey of current users. Diabetes Technol Ther 2016;18:664–70.
22. Linkeschova R, Raoul M, Bott U, et al. Less severe hypoglycaemia, better metabolic control, and improved quality of life in Type 1 diabetes mellitus with continuous subcutaneous insulin infusion (CSII) therapy; an observational study of 100 consecutive patients followed for a mean of 2 years. Diabet Med 2002;19:746–51.
23. EQuality1 Study Group–Evaluation of QUALITY of Life and Costs in Diabetes Type 1, Nicolucci A, Maione A, Franciosi M, et al. Quality of life and treatment satisfaction in adults with Type 1 diabetes: a comparison between continuous subcutaneous insulin infusion and multiple daily injections. Diabet Med 2008;25:213–20.
24. Hoogma RP, de Vries JH, Michels RP, et al. Continuous subcutaneous insulin infusion is sometimes a good choice in case of poorly regulated diabetes mellitus type I. Ned Tijdschr Geneeskd 2005;149:2261–4.
25. DeVries JH, Snoek FJ, Kostense PJ, et al. A randomized trial of continuous subcutaneous insulin infusion and intensive injection therapy in type 1 diabetes for patients with long-standing poor glycemic control. Diabetes Care 2002;25:2074–80.
26. Heller S, White D, Lee E, et al. A cluster randomised trial, cost-effectiveness analysis and psychosocial evaluation of insulin pump therapy compared with multiple injections during flexible intensive insulin therapy for type 1 diabetes: the REPOSE Trial. Health Technol Assess 2017;21:1–278.
27. Bott U, Muhlhauser I, Overmann H, et al. Validation of a diabetes-specific quality-of-life scale for patients with type 1 diabetes. Diabetes Care 1998;21:757–69.
28. Tsui E, Barnie A, Ross S, et al. Intensive insulin therapy with insulin lispro: a randomized trial of continuous subcutaneous insulin infusion versus multiple daily insulin injection. Diabetes Care 2001;24:1722–7.
29. Bergenstal RM, Peyrot M, Dreon DM, et al. Implementation of Basal–bolus therapy in type 2 diabetes: a randomized controlled trial comparing bolus insulin delivery using an insulin patch with an insulin pen. Diabetes Technol Ther 2019;21:273–85.
30. Tang TS, Yusuf FLA, Polonsky WH, et al. Assessing quality of life in diabetes: II. Deconstructing measures into a simple framework. Diabetes Res Clin Pract 2017;126:286–302.
31. Pickup JC. Management of diabetes mellitus: is the pump mightier than the pen? Nat Rev Endocrinol 2012;28:425–33.
32. Rubin RR, Peyrot M, STAR 3 Study Group. Health-related quality of life and treatment satisfaction in the Sensor-Augmented Pump Therapy for A1C Reduction 3 (STAR 3) trial. Diabetes Technol Ther 2012;14:143–51.
33. Hermanides J, Nørgaard K, Bruttomesso D, et al. Sensor-augmented pump therapy lowers HbA(1c) in suboptimally controlled Type 1 diabetes; a randomized controlled trial. Diabet Med 2011;28:1158–67.
34. Bergenstal RM, Klonoff DC, Garg SK, et al. Threshold-based insulin-pump interruption for reduction of hypoglycemia. N Engl J Med 2013;369:224–32.
35. Barnard KD, Ziegler R, Klonoff DC, et al. Open source closed-loop insulin delivery systems: a clash of cultures or merging of diverse approaches? J Diabetes Sci Technol 2018;12:1223–6.

36. Litchman ML, Allen NA, Colicchio VD, et al. A qualitative analysis of real-time continuous glucose monitoring data sharing with care partners: to share or not to share? Diabetes Technol Ther 2018;20:25–31.
37. Schmidt S, Nørgaard K. Sensor-augmented pump therapy at 36 months. Diabetes Technol Ther 2012;14:1174–7.
38. Foster NC, Beck RW, Miller KM, et al. State of type 1 diabetes management and outcomes from the T1D exchange in 2016-2018. Diabetes Technol Ther 2019;21: 66–72.
39. Engler R, Routh TL, Lucisano JY. Adoption barriers for continuous glucose monitoring and their potential reduction with a fully implanted system: results from patient preference surveys. Clin Diabetes 2018;36:50–8.
40. Tanenbaum ML, Hanes SJ, Miller KM, et al. Diabetes device use in adults with type 1 diabetes: barriers to uptake and potential intervention targets. Diabetes Care 2017;40:181–7.
41. Tanenbaum ML, Adams RN, Iturralde E, et al. From wary wearers to d-embracers: personas of readiness to use diabetes devices. J Diabetes Sci Technol 2018;12: 1101–7.
42. Polonsky WH, Fisher L, Hessler D, et al. What is so tough about self-monitoring of blood glucose? Perceived obstacles among patients with Type 2 diabetes. Diabet Med 2014;31:40–6.
43. Pickup JC, Yemane N, Brackenridge A, et al. Nonmetabolic complications of continuous subcutaneous insulin infusion: a patient survey. Diabetes Technol Ther 2014;16:145–9.
44. Polonsky WH, Hessler D. Perceived accuracy in continuous glucose monitoring: understanding the impact on patients. J Diabetes Sci Technol 2015;9:339–41.
45. Kubiak T, Mann CG, Barnard KC, et al. Psychosocial aspects of continuous glucose monitoring: connecting to the patients' experience. J Diabetes Sci Technol 2016;10:859–63.
46. Choudhary P, Amiel SA. Hypoglycaemia in type 1 diabetes: technological treatments, their limitations and the place of psychology. Diabetologia 2018;61:761–9.
47. Pickup JC. Is insulin pump therapy effective in Type 1 diabetes? Diabet Med 2019;36:269–78.
48. Indelicato L, Mariano V, Galasso S, et al. Influence of health locus of control and fear of hypoglycaemia on glycaemic control and treatment satisfaction in people with type 1 diabetes on insulin pump therapy. Diabet Med 2017;34:691–7.
49. Aberle I, Scholz BU, Bach-Kliegel CB, et al. Psychological aspects in continuous subcutaneous insulin infusion: a retrospective study. J Psychol 2009;143:147–60.
50. Ritholz MD, Atakov-Castillo A, Beste M, et al. Psychosocial factors associated with use of continuous glucose monitoring. Diabet Med 2010;27:1060–5.
51. Pettus J, Edelman SV. Use of glucose rate of change arrows to adjust insulin therapy among individuals with type 1 diabetes who use continuous glucose monitoring. Diabetes Technol Ther 2016;18(Suppl 2):S234–42.
52. Ehrmann D, Kulzer B, Schipfer M, et al. Efficacy of an education program for people with diabetes and insulin pump treatment (INPUT): results from a randomized controlled trial. Diabetes Care 2018;41:2453–62.
53. Hermanns N, Ehrmann D, Schipfer M, et al. The impact of a structured education and treatment programme (FLASH) for people with diabetes using a flash sensor-based glucose monitoring system: results of a randomized controlled trial. Diabetes Res Clin Pract 2019;150:111–21.

Automated Insulin Delivery in Children with Type 1 Diabetes

Eda Cengiz, MD, MHS[a,b,*]

KEYWORDS

• Diabetes • Insulin • Children • Insulin pump

KEY POINTS

- The advent of insulin pump therapy marked an important milestone in diabetes treatment and has become the tipping point for automated insulin delivery (AID).
- Continuous glucose monitor (CGM)-integrated insulin pump treatment made the real-time optimization of diabetes mellitus control possible and introduced us to the smart insulin pump systems with a dynamic treatment response.
- The aim of this review is to summarize evidence from AID studies conducted in children with type 1 diabetes and discuss the outlook for future generation AID systems from a pediatric treatment perspective.

INTRODUCTION

The advent of insulin pump therapy marked an important milestone in diabetes treatment several decades ago and has since become the tipping point for automated insulin delivery (AID) development. AID had been an unattainable treatment method until another important milestone in diabetes management, indirect measurement of blood glucose by real time continuous glucose monitor (CGM), became available. CGM-integrated insulin pump treatment made the real-time optimization of glucose control possible and introduced us to smart insulin pump systems with dynamic treatment response.

Managing diabetes in children presents unique challenges and demands a customized, highly dynamic, and engaging system to sustain glycemic control. The physiologic and developmental changes that occur through childhood make insulin treatment and glycemic control a moving target requiring frequent treatment adjustments and customized therapy. Consequently, the pediatric population with type 1 diabetes (T1D) has the highest mean HbA1c within the T1D patient population; this,

[a] Yale School of Medicine, 333 Cedar Street, PO Box 208064, New Haven, CT 06520, USA; [b] Bahçeşehir Üniversitesi, Istanbul, Turkey
* 333 Cedar Street, PO Box 208064, New Haven, CT 06520.
E-mail address: Eda.Cengiz@yale.edu

Endocrinol Metab Clin N Am 49 (2020) 157–166
https://doi.org/10.1016/j.ecl.2019.10.012

in turn, increases their risk for developing short-term and long-term complications. AID addresses the unmet clinical need for improved glucose control while reducing the burden of diabetes management; therefore, the pediatric population with T1D for whom achievement of ideal glucose control is most difficult, would most likely be the one to most benefit from the fine-tuned, customizable AID systems.

The aim of this review was to summarize evidence from AID studies conducted in children with T1D and discuss the outlook for future generation AID systems from a pediatric treatment perspective.

EVOLUTION OF AUTOMATED INSULIN DELIVERY AND TREATMENT OUTCOMES

Standalone external insulin pump systems have evolved over the course of several years and have been replaced by modern high-technology insulin pumps with CGM interface. Pairing insulin pump with CGM, that is, the sensor augmented pump (SAP), enhanced safety and eased some of the diabetes treatment stress by alerting the user concerning low and high glucose levels in real-time allowing them to intervene and modify their insulin doses accordingly. The paradigm shift in AID occurred when CGM-augmented smart insulin pump systems were introduced. Such systems have been equipped with insulin delivery decision-making algorithms augmented by CGM trends and allow real-time adjustment of insulin delivery.

Fear of hypoglycemia has been a major barrier to insulin treatment intensification leading to suboptimal glycemic control and a major source of stress and anxiety for families and caregivers, affecting quality of life and psychological well-being of children with T1D and their families.[1]

Prevention of nocturnal hypoglycemia has been particularly challenging given that more than 50% of severe hypoglycemic episodes in children and adolescents occur during sleep. First-generation sensor-augmented pumps were designed to alleviate hypoglycemia and enhanced treatment safety by automatically suspending insulin infusion during hypoglycemia for up to 2 hours, when hypoglycemia is detected, and the hypoglycemia-driven alarm is not acknowledged.[2] A large multicenter randomized-controlled clinical trial (RCT) demonstrated a reduced frequency and duration of nocturnal hypoglycemia and proved benefits of a low-glucose suspend system in hypoglycemia-prone subjects aged 16 years and older.[3]

Newer generations of sensor-augmented insulin pumps have taken the low-glucose suspend feature a step further by regulating insulin delivery based on predicted sensor glucose values, thus enabling detection of glucose values that are anticipated to fall outside the lower limit of the target range. A randomized crossover clinical study with subjects as young as 6 years of age has demonstrated a 31% reduction in the time less than 70 mg/dL (3.9 mmol/L) without an increase in mean glucose concentration or percentage of time spent greater than 180 mg/dL (10.0 mmol/L),[4] indicating that it was possible to reduce the time spent in hypoglycemia without rebound hyperglycemia by smart insulin algorithm delivery systems. These systems addressed the nocturnal and daytime hypoglycemia challenge that are one of the critical issues in management of children with T1D and overcame a significant barrier for intensification of diabetes treatment.

The ultimate goal of AID has been to implement a fully automated insulin treatment ecosystem during which the devices and digital systems do all the tracking, observation, estimating, and treatment both automatically and passively. This was the rationale behind the development of automated glucose-responsive insulin delivery systems. These automated systems, broadly referred to as artificial pancreas (AP) or closed loop (CL) systems could be categorized in 2 major groups as single-hormone (insulin only) and multiple-hormone (insulin + glucagon or other hormones) AP systems. Dual-hormone systems most commonly infuse glucagon and insulin. The glucagon has been added to counteract the relatively long duration of action of subcutaneously infused insulin, therefore to reduce hypoglycemia risk; however, it also increases system complexity, device footprint, and cost.[5,6]

Although full automated AP systems have been the main aim, an incremental step approach to achieve full automated AP has been implemented. The Juvenile Diabetes Research Foundation (JDRF) Artificial Pancreas Project established in 2005 has been an important milestone in AP research by providing a roadmap for the AP project and ensured that safety and efficacy of AP systems are thoroughly investigated in the pediatric population throughout the developmental stages of AP systems. First-generation investigational AP systems have been tested at the research setting and focused on nighttime glycemic control. Randomized crossover studies in children with T1D showed that AP insulin delivery overnight was able to significantly increase the percentage of time spent within the target glucose range and reduce time in hypoglycemia.[7–13] Although frequency of hypoglycemia (blood glucose <70 mg/dL or 3.9 mmol/L) was well-controlled, daytime post-meal blood glucose targets could not be attained without a pre-meal insulin bolus. Counting the carbohydrate amount of the meal and manually entering the meal carbohydrate information into the pump has been the prerequisite to determine the amount of meal insulin bolus. Although fully automated AP systems without the need for meal announcement is the ultimate treatment goal to ease the burden of diabetes treatment, findings indicating suboptimal post-meal glycemic control during fully automated AP treatment made it apparent that pre-meal announcement was essential. Subsequently, meal announcement feature with full or partial bolus triggered by the patient was implemented to improve postprandial glucose control, thereby trading-off autonomy for performance. The semiautomated insulin treatment system, the Hybrid AP, was introduced as the preceding step toward the full automated AP treatment to optimize after meal glycemia.[14] The Hybrid AP system requires the user's input for meal announcement, which consists of the carbohydrate amount or qualitative information (ie, small, medium, or large meal) to deliver a meal bolus with background insulin dose adjustments dictated by the algorithm based on CGM values. The MiniMed 670G Hybrid AP system has become the first AP system with Food and Drug Administration approval and is currently used to treat children with T1D ages ≥7 years.[15]

The treatment efficacy and safety of MiniMed 670G were shown by a 3-month clinical trial during which both adult and adolescent subjects experienced an improvement in HbA1c and multiple other glycemic metrics. The adolescent subject group (mean age ±SD: 16.5 ± 2.3 years) clearly declared their stark differences from adult patients with T1D as indicated by higher baseline hyperglycemia, glucose variability, and HbA1c levels. The HbA1c reduction from baseline was slightly greater for the adolescent group than the adult cohort (0.6% vs 0.5% respectively, $P < .001$ in both groups). Hybrid AP use increased the amount of time spent in the target range (TIR, 70–180 mg/dL or 3.9–10.0 mmol/L) to greater than 70% for the day and night period, and 75% of the nocturnal period alone. The amount of time in hyperglycemia was also decreased. The results were fairly consistent across age groups, although adults saw more benefit in hypoglycemia reduction, whereas adolescents saw more benefit in reducing hyperglycemia.[16]

Auto Mode usage decreased from 87.0% to 71.8% by the end of 3 months in a subgroup of adolescent and young adult population[17] and subjects encountered exits from Auto Mode frequently (5–6 exits/week). The most common reasons for Auto

Mode exits have been safe basal alerts and overt hyperglycemia. Time spent in Auto Mode significantly contributed to the improvement of time spent in target range.

A follow-on study using the same Hybrid AP system in subjects ages 7 to 13 reported and average sensor glucose of 161.7 ± 12.4 mg/dL (9.0 ± 0.7 mmol/L), with 65.0% ± 7.7% TIR, 3.0% to 1.6% time less than 70 mg/dL (3.9 mmol/L) and median Auto Mode use of 81% of the time. The HbA1c reduction was 0.4% (*P*<.01) from baseline.[18–20]

Multiple other AP system studies have been conducted since the approval of the Hybrid AP system.[21,22] Moreover, new metrics of glycemic control beyond HbA1c, such as time in target glucose range, time in hypoglycemia and hyperglycemia, and glycemic variability[19,20] have been accepted as measures of treatment success and safety given that an AP system may benefit individual patients in unique ways that would not be reflected in HbA1c improvements alone. It is notable that many of these studies have been undertaken in free-living conditions given the wealth of data indicating the safety of investigational AP systems.

The Diabetes Assistant Hybrid AP system use compared with SAP has demonstrated improved glycemic control (mean sensor glucose 152 mg/dL vs 190 mg/dL [8.4 mmol/L vs 10.6 mmol/L], *P* < .001) among children 5 to 8 years old in a randomized clinical, crossover clinical trial. Subjects had activity trackers, and sensor glucose data analyses were adjusted for activity to account for the impact of activity on glucose utilization. Hybrid AP system use resulted in an increase in time in the range (73% vs 47%) of 70 to 180 mg/dL (3.9–10.0 mmol/L) without increased hypoglycemia, addressing 2 main obstacles to improved glycemic control in this age group.[20]

A recently published randomized clinical trial examined the use of an investigational AP system (Control IQ) in school-aged children with T1D and compared it with the sensor augmented insulin pump treatment. Study participants using the Tandem t:slim X2 with Control-IQ Hybrid AP system at home had significantly greater improvement of time in target range (71.0% ± 6.6% vs 52.8% ± 13.5%; *P* = .001) and mean sensor glucose (153.6 ± 13.5 vs 180.2 ± 23.1 mg/dL [8.5 ± 0.8 vs 10.0 + 1.3 mmol/L]; *P* = .003) without increasing hypoglycemia time (<70 mg/dL, or <3.9 mmol/L). The decrease in average sensor glucose was 27 mg/dL (1.5 mmol/L) for the full day and 42 mg/dL (2.3 mmol/L) overnight reflective of the increase in TIR by 4.4 hours per day. It is notable that the Hybrid AP system was active for 94.4% and subjects reported that use of the system was associated with less time thinking about diabetes, decreased worry about blood sugars, and decreased burden in managing diabetes.

Diluted insulin has been used to treat young children with T1D in clinical practice and a recently published study examined its use in a randomized crossover study. Subjects were 1 to 7 years of age (interquartile range 3–6 years) and used U-20 (diluted insulin) and U-100 insulin during a 21-day Hybrid AP treatment period for each insulin type with a washout period in between. The glycemic and safety metrics were similar, suggesting that there is no tangible difference between using regular concentration insulin and diluted insulin during AP treatment.[24]

Challenging the Artificial Pancreas System

Managing diabetes in the pediatric population presents unique challenges. Children have unpredictable dietary habits and daily activity patterns, and have dynamic growth and developmental physiologic changes from birth until age 18.[25] Cognitive and verbal immaturity at younger ages limits the ability to identify, report, and treat hypoglycemia. Adolescence marks another challenging time in diabetes care. It is a period of change, including growth development and hormonal changes, some of which lead to insulin resistance. In addition, adolescence naturally is a time of increasing independence and self-assertiveness and of risk-taking. Consequently, pediatric patients with T1D require a customized, highly dynamic and engaging system to sustain glycemic control and tackle multiple disruptors of daily life. As scientists gained more experience with AP systems, the next logical step was to ascertain AP systems' response to challenging conditions and potential disruptors that might be experienced during daily life. Scientists initiated multiple clinical trials to determine whether AP systems could handle diabetes management in the setting of suboptimal glycemic control, missed insulin boluses and intense activity.[26–31]

Type 1 Diabetes with Suboptimal Control

Data from the T1D Exchange registry confronted us with the inconvenient truth regarding the striking percentage of patients in suboptimal glycemic control.[32] Notably, pediatric participants have the highest mean Hba1c values, therefore it is fair to say that the most challenging group of subjects with AIDSs has been children with diabetes. An open-label, multicenter, multinational, single-period, parallel RCT assessed the effectiveness of day and night hybrid AP insulin delivery compared with sensor-augmented pump therapy in participants with suboptimally controlled T1D aged 6 years and older.[29] At the end of the study period, reductions in HbA1c percentages were significantly greater in the AP group compared with the control group (mean difference in change 0.36%, 95% confidence interval [CI] 0.19–0.53; $P<.0001$). The proportion of time that glucose concentration was within the target range was significantly higher in the AP group (65%) compared with the control group (54%) (mean difference in change −10.8% points, 95% CI 8.2–13.5; $P<0\cdot0001$). In the AP group, HbA1c was reduced from a baseline value of 8.3% (67 mmol/mol) to 8.0% (64 mmol/mol) after the 4-week run-in, and to 7.4% (57 mmol/mol) after the 12-week intervention period ($P<.001$).

The time spent with glucose concentrations less than 70 mg/dL or 3.9 mmol/L (mean difference in change −0.83% points, −1.40 to −0.16; $P = .0013$) and more than 180 mg/dL or 10.0 mmol/L (mean difference in change −10.3% points, −13.2 to −7.5; $P < .0001$) was shorter in the AP group than the control group. The coefficient of variation of sensor-measured glucose was not different between interventions (mean difference in change −0.4%, 95% CI −1.4% to 0.7%; $P = .50$). Similarly, total daily insulin dose was not different (mean difference in change 0.031 U/kg per day, 95% CI −0.005 to 0.067; $P = .09$) and body weight did not differ (mean difference in change 0.68 kg, 95% CI −0.34 to 1.69; $P = .1$). In summary, AP use increased time in range and reduced hypoglycemia for subjects in suboptimal glycemic control, including the pediatric cohort.

Missed and Underestimated Insulin Bolus

Poor treatment compliance due to missed and underestimated meal boluses has been well recognized particularly among adolescents with T1D. Postprandial glycemic control after a missed and an underestimated meal bolus during AP treatment has been examined by a clinical study among 16 adolescents with T1D. Subjects were studied for 2 days AP versus home insulin pump treatment with a 1-day wash out in between each treatment. Subjects were given a snack with 30 g of carbohydrates at 9 AM with no insulin bolus and an 80-g of carbohydrate lunch meal at 1 PM with only 75% of the calculated insulin pre-meal bolus on each day. The mean blood glucose was lower (197 ± 10 vs 235 ± 14 mg/dL [10.9 ± 0.6 vs 13.1 ± 0.8 mmol/L]) and time in range 70 to 180 mg/dL (3.9–10.0 mmol/L) was higher (43% ± 7% vs 19% ± 7%) (both $P < .05$) on the AP day compared with the home insulin pump treatment indicating that AP was able to mitigate hyperglycemia better than the conventional treatment after a missed or underestimated insulin bolus.[27]

Exercise and Camp

Despite well-known benefits of exercise, fear of hypoglycemia often results in avoidance of physical activity or overtreatment with carbohydrates. Unpredictable activity patterns during childhood adds to the glycemic guessing game of diabetes management. AP studies using multiple different systems have been conducted at the diabetes camp setting under supervision. In general, AP treatment resulted in better glycemic control with a significant reduction of hypoglycemic episodes during both day and night when compared with conventional insulin treatment and established the safety and the feasibility of AP treatment in the pediatric population at diabetes camp setting with and without exercise announcement.[33–36]

Attaining target glycemic control has been more challenging in the younger age group. AP system use in a randomized crossover diabetes camp study with 30 children (5–9 years old) resulted in a significant reduction of hypoglycemic episodes during both day and night (time spent in hypoglycemia: 6.7% with open loop vs 2.0% with AP; $P<.001$), but it was associated with a higher mean glucose value with the AP.[35,36]

AP treatment was stress-tested during unannounced exercise and extreme sports conditions. Ten adolescents with T1D underwent 72 hours of AP in a hotel setting and exercised twice daily without announcement of exercise to the AP system. Unrestricted meals during the study added another level of stress to the AP system. Increased percent time within target sensor glucose range (70–180 mg/dL or 3.9–10.0 mmol/L) CL 71% versus 57% SAP (P = .012) and lower percent time in hypoglycemic range (<70 mg/dL or < 3.9 mmol/L) during overnight AP 0% versus 1.1% SAP (P = NS) have been reported. Results from the study suggested that AP insulin delivery was safe both during and after unannounced exercise in the in-hospital environment, maintaining glucose values mostly within the target range without an increased risk of hypoglycemia.[34]

A notable amount of research has proven AID's treatment efficacy and safety during and after exercise. The University of Virginia AP research group challenged their AP system by an extremely intense sports activity during a 5-day ski camp during which the participants skied on average 5 hours a day. Thirty-two adolescents (age 10–16 years) with T1D were studied when using AP versus sensor augmented pump treatment. Compared with physician-monitored open loop, percent time in range (70–180 mg/dL or 3.9–10.0 mmol/L) improved using hybrid AP system 71.3 versus 64.7% (+6.6% [95% CI 1–12]; P = .005), with maximum effect late at night. Hypoglycemia exposure and carbohydrate treatments were improved overall (P = .001 and P = .007) and during the daytime with strong ski level effects (P = .0001 and P = .006). The percentage of time with continuous glucose monitor (CGM) 70 to 180 mg/dL (or 3.9–10.0 mmol/L) was 71% $\pm$ 10% during AP CL, compared to 57% $\pm$ 16% during SAP (P = .012). Nocturnal control during hybrid AP was safe, with a mean of 2.2 $\pm$ 2.3% time spent CGM less than 70 mg/dL (or <3.9 mmol/L) compared to 2.5 $\pm$ 6.53during SAP (P = .001 for hybrid AP and ski effects). Despite large meals (estimated up to 120 g carbohydrate), only 8.0% $\pm$ 6.9% of time during hybrid AP was spent with CGM greater than 250 mg/dL (or 13.9 mmol/L) (16% $\pm$ 14% during SAP). In brief, AP system managed to reduce exposure to hypoglycemia and sustained glycemic control during prolonged intensive sports activity.[33]

FUTURE PROSPECTS

There is growing evidence that AID has been winning concrete victories over conventional diabetes treatment, however there are no shortages of challenges ahead. Patient reported outcomes have been one of the key features of AID clinical trials. AID clearly empowered people with diabetes and their caregivers, however the burden associated with device wear is evident as indicated by multiple study findings. Most common concerns have been regarding the need to use multiple devices and the mental, physical and financial burden that could contribute to the diabetes management distress. Nevertheless, the findings from recent trials have been more promising and suggest a reduction in diabetes management distress that is, associated with an improvement in glycemic targets during hybrid AP treatment.[37]

There is emerging data that Hybrid AP use resulted in less mental burden with regard to overnight diabetes management, took away some of the fear/worry of hypoglycemia. Real-time sensor glucose data sharing gave parents peace of mind. More research is needed to ascertain methods to reduce diabetes treatment burden and improve quality of life measures both for children with T1D and their parents/caregivers during AID. Technology could be refined to reduce the device footprint, make AID more user-friendly and minimize the need to train users. Customization of insulin treatment has been one of the key factors to attain target glycemic control and could be achieved by the AID systems with artificial intelligence. The diverse and emerging needs children and adolescents with T1D, given the changes in growth and other physiologic alterations that occur continuously throughout childhood, require flexible and customizable diabetes treatment systems. Smart insulin delivery algorithms with pattern recognition and auxiliary technologies that can provide information about the activity of the patient or inform us their physiologic state by body temperature and heart rate sensors, could be alternative solutions to optimize treatment. The AID equipped with artificial intelligence detect insulin action variability, learn from an individual's response to insulin and account for the physiologic state of the user, and can adjust insulin therapy based on these patterns to implement an individualized, real-time diabetes treatement.[30]

Missed pre meal insulin bolus is not an uncommon practice particularly for adolescents with diabetes. The hybrid AP systems are not equipped to address the compliance issue in diabetes management given that they do not eliminate the need for meal insulin bolus and carbohydrate counting. The AP with qualitative categorization of meal size could alleviate the burden of carbohydrate counting without compromising glucose control, although more categories of meal sizes are probably needed to effectively control higher-carbohydrate meals. Fully automated AP systems would be the game changer in diabetes management by minimizing user input for pre-meal bolus. However, data from AP trials have shown a significant barrier in optimizing glycemic control during fully automated AP treatment. Regardless of the AID, performance of mealtime glycemic control has been less than ideal with exaggerated post meal hyperglycemic excursions mainly due to slow absorption and action of insulins. The earliest secreted insulin is a necessary element of the normal mealtime insulin response, and consequently optimal exogenous prandial insulin needs a rapid "on response." Rapid acting insulins have certain advantages over regular human insulin, but there is a need to develop even faster acting insulin preparations, which mimic physiologic insulin release in a better manner to keep up with full automated AP systems. The delay in insulin absorption and action during AP treatment is exacerbated by the nature of a reactive system, inherent to the AP, that doesn't recognize the need for more insulin until after the subject has started eating and sensor glucose levels have started to rise. Late and prolonged increases in plasma insulin, in turn, potentially resulted in a tendency to hypoglycemia prior to the next meal.[14,38] Faster acting insulins and methods to accelerate insulin action during AID are critical elements to mitigate post-prandial hyperglycemia and to make full automated treatment a reality.

SUMMARY

Findings from clinical studies indicate consistently that AID therapy could achieve significant success over conventional diabetes treatment with reduction in hypoglycemia, improved time in target blood glucose range and lower HbA1c. AID has already become a strong ally to children with diabetes, their parents and their clinicians to overcome treatment challenges. The advent of faster insulins[39–41] and adjunct hormones may enhance the performance of single-hormone and bi-hormonal AP systems, respectively. There is still room for improvement and insights gained from trials and clinical use coupled with advanced diabetes technology devices will lead us to the future generation AID systems designed with pediatric patients and their caregivers in mind to attain glycemic targets and reduce burden of diabetes.

DISCLOSURE

Scientific Advisory Board Member/Consultant- Novo Nordisk, Adocia, MannKind, Lexicon, Arecor. Speaker- Novo Nordisk.

ACKNOWLEDGMENTS

This work has been supported by Juvenile Diabetes Research Foundation International (JDRF) under Grant 2-APF-2019-737-A-N, and JDRF 3-SRA-2016-244-M-R, the National Institutes of Health (NIH) under Grant 1DP3DK106826-01, CTSA Grant Number UL1 RR024139 from the National Center for Research Resources (NCRR) and the National Center for Advancing Translational Science (NCATS).

REFERENCES

1. Johnson SR, Cooper MN, Davis EA, et al. Hypoglycaemia, fear of hypoglycaemia and quality of life in children with Type 1 diabetes and their parents. Diabet Med 2013;30:1126–31.
2. Cengiz E. Putting brakes on insulin pump infusion to prevent hypoglycemia. J Diabetes Sci Technol 2011;5:1142–3.
3. Bergenstal RM, Klonoff DC, Garg SK, et al. Threshold-based insulin-pump interruption for reduction of hypoglycemia. N Engl J Med 2013;369:224–32.
4. Forlenza GP, Li Z, Buckingham BA, et al. Predictive low-glucose suspend reduces hypoglycemia in adults, adolescents, and children with type 1 diabetes in an at-home randomized crossover study: results of the PROLOG trial. Diabetes Care 2018;41:2155–61.
5. Russell SJ, El-Khatib FH, Sinha M, et al. Outpatient glycemic control with a bionic pancreas in type 1 diabetes. N Engl J Med 2014;371:313–25.
6. Haidar A, Smaoui MR, Legault L, et al. The role of glucagon in the artificial pancreas. Lancet Diabetes Endocrinol 2016;4:476–9.
7. Thabit H, Tauschmann M, Allen JM, et al. Home use of an artificial beta cell in type 1 diabetes. N Engl J Med 2015;373:2129–40.
8. Sherr JL, Cengiz E, Palerm CC, et al. Reduced hypoglycemia and increased time in target using closed-loop insulin delivery during nights with or without antecedent afternoon exercise in type 1 diabetes. Diabetes Care 2013;36:2909–14.

9. Russell SJ, Hillard MA, Balliro C, et al. Day and night glycaemic control with a bionic pancreas versus conventional insulin pump therapy in preadolescent children with type 1 diabetes: a randomised crossover trial. Lancet Diabetes Endocrinol 2016;4:233–43.
10. Nimri R, Bratina N, Kordonouri O, et al. MD-Logic overnight type 1 diabetes control in home settings: a multicentre, multinational, single blind randomized trial. Diabetes Obes Metab 2017;19:553–61.
11. Maahs DM, Calhoun P, Buckingham BA, et al. A randomized trial of a home system to reduce nocturnal hypoglycemia in type 1 diabetes. Diabetes Care 2014; 37:1885–91.
12. Hovorka R, Elleri D, Thabit H, et al. Overnight closed-loop insulin delivery in young people with type 1 diabetes: a free-living, randomized clinical trial. Diabetes Care 2014;37:1204–11.
13. Haidar A, Rabasa-Lhoret R, Legault L, et al. Single- and dual-hormone artificial pancreas for overnight glucose control in type 1 diabetes. J Clin Endocrinol Metab 2016;101:214–23.
14. Weinzimer SA, Steil GM, Swan KL, et al. Fully automated closed-loop insulin delivery versus semiautomated hybrid control in pediatric patients with type 1 diabetes using an artificial pancreas. Diabetes Care 2008;31:934–9.
15. Medtronic. MiniMed 670G Insulin Pump System2019. Available at: https://www.medtronicdiabetes.com/products/minimed-670g-insulin-pump-system. Accessed October 30, 2019.
16. Bergenstal RM, Garg S, Weinzimer SA, et al. Safety of a hybrid closed-loop insulin delivery system in patients with type 1 diabetes. JAMA 2016;316:1407–8.
17. Messer LH, Forlenza GP, Sherr JL, et al. Optimizing hybrid closed-loop therapy in adolescents and emerging adults using the minimed 670g system. Diabetes Care 2018;41:789–96.
18. Forlenza GP, Pinhas-Hamiel O, Liljenquist DR, et al. Safety evaluation of the MiniMed 670G system in children 7-13 years of age with type 1 diabetes. Diabetes Technol Ther 2019;21:11–9.
19. Battelino T, Danne T, Bergenstal RM, et al. Clinical targets for continuous glucose monitoring data interpretation: recommendations from the international consensus on time in range. Diabetes Care 2019;42:1593–603.
20. Agiostratidou G, Anhalt H, Ball D, et al. Standardizing clinically meaningful outcome measures beyond HbA1c for type 1 diabetes: a consensus report of the American Association of Clinical Endocrinologists, the American Association of Diabetes Educators, the American Diabetes Association, the Endocrine Society, JDRF International, The Leona M. and Harry B. Helmsley Charitable Trust, the Pediatric Endocrine Society, and the T1D Exchange. Diabetes Care 2017;40: 1622–30.
21. Brown S, Raghinaru D, Emory E, et al. First look at Control-IQ: a new-generation automated insulin delivery system. Diabetes Care 2018;41:2634–6.
22. Biester T, Nir J, Remus K, et al. DREAM5: an open-label, randomized, cross-over study to evaluate the safety and efficacy of day and night closed-loop control by comparing the MD-Logic automated insulin delivery system to sensor augmented pump therapy in patients with type 1 diabetes at home. Diabetes Obes Metab 2018. [Epub ahead of print].
23. DeBoer MD, Breton MD, Wakeman C, et al. Performance of an artificial pancreas system for young children with type 1 diabetes. Diabetes Technol Ther 2017;19: 293–8.

24. Tauschmann M, Allen JM, Nagl K, et al. Home use of day-and-night hybrid closed-loop insulin delivery in very young children: a multicenter, 3-week, randomized trial. Diabetes Care 2019;42:594–600.
25. Seckold R, Howley P, King BR, et al. Dietary intake and eating patterns of young children with type 1 diabetes achieving glycemic targets. BMJ Open Diabetes Res Care 2019;7:e000663.
26. Barnard KD, Wysocki T, Ully V, et al. Closing the loop in adults, children and adolescents with suboptimally controlled type 1 diabetes under free living conditions: a psychosocial substudy. J Diabetes Sci Technol 2017;11:1080–8.
27. Chernavvsky DR, DeBoer MD, Keith-Hynes P, et al. Use of an artificial pancreas among adolescents for a missed snack bolus and an underestimated meal bolus. Pediatr Diabetes 2016;17:28–35.
28. Jayawardene DC, McAuley SA, Horsburgh JC, et al. Closed-loop insulin delivery for adults with type 1 diabetes undertaking high-intensity interval exercise versus moderate-intensity exercise: a randomized, crossover study. Diabetes Technol Ther 2017;19:340–8.
29. Tauschmann M, Thabit H, Bally L, et al. Closed-loop insulin delivery in suboptimally controlled type 1 diabetes: a multicentre, 12-week randomised trial. Lancet 2018;392:1321–9.
30. Turksoy K, Kilkus J, Hajizadeh I, et al. Hypoglycemia detection and carbohydrate suggestion in an artificial pancreas. J Diabetes Sci Technol 2016;10:1236–44.
31. Turksoy K, Quinn LT, Littlejohn E, et al. An integrated multivariable artificial pancreas control system. J Diabetes Sci Technol 2014;8:498–507.
32. Foster NC, Beck RW, Miller KM, et al. State of type 1 diabetes management and outcomes from the T1D exchange in 2016-2018. Diabetes Technol Ther 2019;21:66–72.
33. Breton MD, Chernavvsky DR, Forlenza GP, et al. Closed-loop control during intense prolonged outdoor exercise in adolescents with type 1 diabetes: the artificial pancreas ski study. Diabetes Care 2017;40:1644–50.
34. Huyett LM, Ly TT, Forlenza GP, et al. Outpatient closed-loop control with unannounced moderate exercise in adolescents using zone model predictive control. Diabetes Technol Ther 2017;19:331–9.
35. Ly TT, Keenan DB, Roy A, et al. Automated overnight closed-loop control using a proportional-integral-derivative algorithm with insulin feedback in children and adolescents with type 1 diabetes at diabetes camp. Diabetes Technol Ther 2016;18:377–84.
36. Phillip M, Battelino T, Atlas E, et al. Nocturnal glucose control with an artificial pancreas at a diabetes camp. N Engl J Med 2013;368:824–33.
37. Adams RN, Tanenbaum ML, Hanes SJ, et al. Psychosocial and human factors during a trial of a hybrid closed loop system for type 1 diabetes management. Diabetes Technol Ther 2018;20:648–53.
38. Cameron FM, Ly TT, Buckingham BA, et al. Closed-loop control without meal announcement in type 1 diabetes. Diabetes Technol Ther 2017;19:527–32.
39. Cengiz E, Bode B, Van Name M, et al. Moving toward the ideal insulin for insulin pumps. Expert Rev Med Devices 2016;13:57–69.
40. Cengiz E. Closer to ideal insulin action: ultra fast acting insulins. Panminerva Med 2013;55:269–75.
41. Cengiz E. Undeniable need for ultrafast-acting insulin: the pediatric perspective. J Diabetes Sci Technol 2012;6:797–801.

Automated Insulin Delivery in Adults

Charlotte K. Boughton, MRCP, PhD, Roman Hovorka, PhD, FMedSci*

KEYWORDS

- Hybrid closed-loop • Artificial pancreas • Type 1 diabetes • Inpatient diabetes
- Psychosocial impact

KEY POINTS

- Hybrid closed-loop systems have recently been introduced into clinical practice for adults with type 1 diabetes.
- Studies show superior glucose control with hybrid closed-loop systems in adults with type 1 diabetes.
- There is growing evidence for closed-loop systems in pregnant women with type 1 diabetes and in inpatients with hyperglycemia.
- Understanding the user experience and training requirements are key to successful implementation to realize the glycemic benefits.

INTRODUCTION

Achieving the recommended glycemic targets for people with type 1 diabetes (T1D) is challenging without experiencing problematic hypoglycemia and a high burden of diabetes self-care. The benefits of intensive insulin therapy to decrease the risk of long-term complications were shown in the Diabetes Control and Complications Trial, and led to increased uptake of insulin pump therapy (continuous subcutaneous insulin infusion) to achieve improved glycemic outcomes, decrease the risk of hypoglycemia, and improve quality of life for people with T1D.[1,2]

Continuous glucose monitoring (CGM) devices, measuring real-time interstitial glucose concentration, have steadily improved in terms of accuracy and reliability; the use of CGM is associated with improvements in glucose control and decreased hypoglycemia in adults with T1D.[3] Despite evidence of clinical benefit of these diabetes technologies, and widespread uptake (the T1D Exchange clinic registry data reports pump use in 63% of participants and CGM use in 30%), the American Diabetes Association hemoglobin A1c (HbA1c) target of 7% or less (53 mmol/mol) is achieved by less than one-quarter of adults with T1D.[4]

University of Cambridge Metabolic Research Laboratories, Wellcome Trust-MRC Institute of Metabolic Science, Addenbrooke's Hospital, Box 289, Hills Road, Cambridge CB2 0QQ, UK
* Corresponding author.
E-mail address: rh347@cam.ac.uk

Endocrinol Metab Clin N Am 49 (2020) 167–178
https://doi.org/10.1016/j.ecl.2019.10.007
endo.theclinics.com

THE CLOSED-LOOP APPROACH

Insulin pumps can be used in conjunction with real-time CGM, allowing users to manually modify the insulin infusion rate according to CGM values (sensor augmented pump therapy). The simplest form of automated insulin delivery is the low glucose suspend feature, which automatically suspends insulin infusion when the sensor glucose reaches a prespecified CGM threshold value or when sensor glucose is predicted to cross the prespecified CGM threshold value (predictive low glucose management) within a particular time frame. Low glucose suspend and predictive low glucose management have been shown to be effective in decreasing the frequency and duration of hypoglycemia without any significant impact on HbA1c.[5,6] The pathway of the key milestones in the development of fully automated multihormone artificial pancreas systems is illustrated in **Fig. 1**.

Closed-loop insulin delivery is more sophisticated than suspend approaches. A control algorithm is either incorporated into the insulin pump or hosted on a separate device, such as a smartphone, and the components of the closed-loop system communicate wirelessly (**Fig. 2**). Real-time glucose data provided by a CGM device are received by the control algorithm, which then instructs insulin delivery via the insulin pump by automatically modifying the insulin infusion rate every 5 to 10 minutes based on the sensor glucose levels (single hormone closed-loop systems). Glucagon, or other hormones, can also be delivered in a similar glucose-responsive manner within dual hormone closed-loop systems.

One of the key benefits of closed-loop insulin delivery over sensor augmented pump therapy is the continuous and automatic modulation of insulin delivery rates to adapt to the within-day and between-day variability of insulin requirements. A retrospective analysis of insulin requirements during a 12-week hybrid closed-loop study involving 32 adults with T1D under free-living conditions showed high variability of overnight insulin requirements (coefficient of variation of 31%), which was higher than the variability of daytime insulin requirements (coefficient of variation of 22%).[7]

Control Algorithms

The control algorithm is the principal component of a closed-loop system, directing insulin delivery in response to sensor glucose levels and other key inputs such as meal intake, while also accommodating variability of insulin requirements between and within individual users, and accounting for glucose sensor and insulin delivery

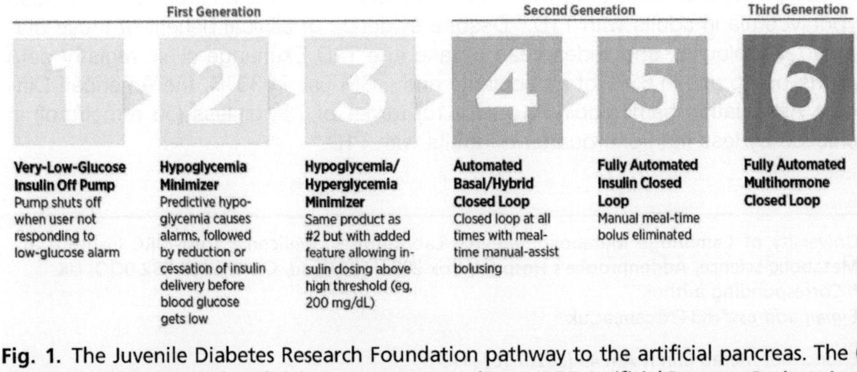

Fig. 1. The Juvenile Diabetes Research Foundation pathway to the artificial pancreas. The 6 developmental stages of artificial pancreas systems. (*From* JDRF. Artificial Pancreas Project. Avaliable at: https://www.jdrf.ca/our-research/treat/artificial-pancreas-project/; with permission.)

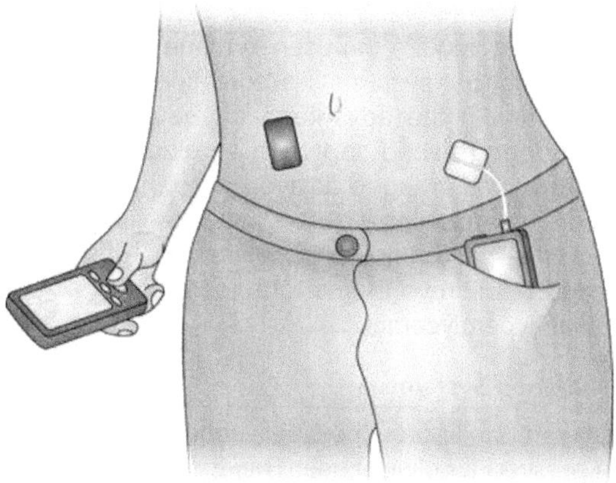

Fig. 2. Automated insulin delivery (artificial pancreas). A subcutaneous continuous glucose monitor (*rectangle* on abdomen) transmits the interstitial glucose levels to a controller (hand held device), which hosts a control algorithm and the user interface. An insulin pump (in pocket) delivers subcutaneous rapid-acting insulin analogue. Insulin delivery is adjusted in real time by the control algorithm. Communication between system components is wireless. (*From* Hovorka R. Closed-loop insulin delivery: from bench to clinical practice. *Nature Reviews Endocrinology.* 2011;7(7):385-395; with permission.)

limitations. Several different control algorithms have been developed and used in closed-loop systems.

Model predictive control (MPC) algorithms used a personalized model of glucose regulation to predict glycemic excursions based on inputs, including subcutaneous insulin. The insulin infusion rate is determined by minimizing the difference between model-predicted glucose concentrations and the target glucose levels over a specified prediction time perspective.

Proportional integral derivative (PID) controllers continuously modify insulin infusion rates by evaluating glucose excursions from 3 perspectives, namely, deviation from target glucose (proportional component), area under the curve between measured and target glucose level (integral component), and rate of change of measured glucose levels (derivative component).

The fuzzy logic control approach modulates insulin delivery on the basis of rules that reflect the experiential knowledge of diabetes practitioners.

A direct comparison of the performance of PID and MPC algorithms in a crossover study observed additional benefits of MPC over PID controllers.[8] Furthermore, data from a meta-analysis suggest that MPC and fuzzy logic control algorithms may be associated with increased time spent with glucose levels in target range (70–180 mg/dL [3.9–10.0 mmol/L]) compared with PID algorithms, although an analysis of subgroup differences was not significant.[9]

Most control algorithms incorporate safety modules to restrict insulin delivery, limiting the amount of insulin on board or the maximum rate of insulin delivery, and suspending insulin delivery when sensor glucose levels are low or decreasing rapidly.

User-specific parameters such as body weight and insulin requirements are usually required for the initialization of closed-loop systems. However, adaptation of the algorithm to changes in physiologic parameters with real-time adjustment of closed-loop control parameters is essential for optimal performance.

Hybrid and Fully Closed-Loop Systems

Hybrid closed-loop systems require the user to manually initiate mealtime boluses, whereas fully closed-loop systems automatically dose insulin without information about meals with the advantage of reduced user intervention. Most closed-loop systems adopt a hybrid approach as glucose control is compromised with fully closed-loop systems owing to delayed absorption of subcutaneous insulin. Fully closed-loop approaches are associated with significant postprandial hyperglycemic excursions and late postprandial hypoglycemia. Ultrarapid insulin analogues or adjuncts are needed to improve the performance of fully closed-loop systems in managing postprandial hyperglycemia.

Dual Hormone Closed-Loop Systems

Both single and dual hormone approaches (delivering insulin and glucagon or another hormone) are being pursued for clinical use. The addition of glucagon is an attractive option to more closely mimic pancreatic islet physiology, but also increases the complexity and cost of the system. The potential role of glucagon is to further decrease the risk of hypoglycemia or to buffer more aggressive insulin delivery with higher glucagon doses. A lack of room temperature-stable glucagon formulations is limiting progress at present, because available formulations require reconstitution before use and exchange of the glucagon reservoir every 24 hours. Novel glucagon analogues are being developed, but the full pharmacokinetic and safety profile is yet to be established. A more detailed discussion regarding the role of glucagon in automated insulin delivery can be found elsewhere in this issue.

CLINICAL EVIDENCE FOR AUTOMATED INSULIN DELIVERY IN ADULTS

Clinical trials evaluating hybrid closed-loop systems have progressed from short duration studies undertaken in highly supervised research facility settings to studies lasting several months in unsupervised, free-living conditions. Hybrid closed-loop insulin delivery has demonstrated efficacy and safety in the outpatient setting in children, adolescents, and adults with T1D.[9,10]

Meta-Analysis Data

Two recent meta-analyses have evaluated the safety and efficacy of outpatient hybrid closed-loop therapy in nonpregnant individuals with TID.[9,10] The larger of these included 40 studies (1042 participants); 31 used a single hormone approach and 9 evaluated a dual hormone system. The data favor hybrid closed-loop systems, compared with sensor-augmented pump therapy or standard pump therapy, across a number of glycemic metrics, including the proportion of time spent with sensor glucose in target range and time spent above and below target glucose range. However, most of the randomized, controlled trials included in these meta-analyses had a relatively small sample size, including around 20 to 30 participants and short intervention period often less than 1 week. Only 2 studies were of long enough duration to report on HbA1c outcomes. In addition, outcome reporting across studies was not consistent. The Artificial Pancreas Project Consortium advocates the use of standardized CGM metrics in addition to HbA1c, safety, and technical metrics as outcome measures in artificial pancreas clinical trials to align outcome reporting.[11]

Time in target glucose range

Meta-analysis data have shown that outpatient use of single hormone hybrid closed-loop systems increases the time spent in target glucose range (70–180 mg/dL

[3.9–10.0 mmol/L]) over 24 hours by approximately 10% compared with control therapy. This equates to more than 2 additional hours each day in normoglycemia.[10] The benefit of automated insulin delivery is most pronounced overnight, when time in target glucose range is around 15 percentage points greater than with control therapy. Increased time in target glucose range associated with closed-loop systems is attributable to reduced time spent in hyperglycemia.

Although dual hormone systems have demonstrated greater improvements in time in target glucose range compared with single hormone systems, almost all studies of dual hormone systems have been of a short duration and compared with standard pump therapy. This is in contrast with studies of single hormone systems where the comparator is usually sensor-augmented pump therapy. Direct comparison of single and dual hormone closed-loop systems in adults observed no difference in the time spent in target glucose range over a 24-hour period under supervised conditions.[12]

Hypoglycemia

Hybrid closed-loop insulin delivery is associated with a decrease in the proportion of time spent in hypoglycemia (<70 mg/dL [3.9 mmol/L]) by 1.5% points (approximately 20 minutes per 24-hour period) compared with control therapy.[10] Night time spent in hypoglycemia is also decrease with hybrid closed-loop by 2.2 percentage points compared with standard therapy. Because the incidence of severe hypoglycemia in clinical studies is very low, there is insufficient evidence to determine benefit of hybrid closed-loop insulin delivery on reducing the risk of severe hypoglycemia. However, hybrid closed-loop use was associated with a decrease in low blood glucose index (a measure of the risk of severe hypoglycemia) overnight compared with control therapy.

Mean glucose and hemoglobin A1c

Compared with standard or sensor-augmented pump therapy, hybrid closed-loop systems have a favorable effect on mean sensor glucose concentration, with a decrease of 9 mg/dL (0.5 mmol/L).[10] This finding is consistent with an 0.3% to 0.4% reduction in HbA1c observed with closed-loop systems compared with control therapy in studies with a duration per intervention of more than 8 weeks.[10,13] Although the effect of hybrid closed-loop on lowering of HbA1c is modest, this effect occurs despite the decrease in hypoglycemia observed in these studies.

Insulin requirements

There are conflicting results between individual studies regarding the effect of hybrid closed-loop systems on total daily insulin dose. Data from a meta-analysis suggest there is no difference between closed-loop and control interventions in the total daily insulin requirement.[9,10]

KEY OUTPATIENT HYBRID CLOSED-LOOP CLINICAL STUDIES IN ADULTS

Assessments of efficacy from larger clinical trials under free-living conditions in representative populations are critical to support reimbursement and wider adoption of hybrid closed-loop systems. The first study exploring the feasibility of prolonged home use of a single hormone hybrid closed-loop system compared overnight closed-loop glucose control with sensor-augmented pump therapy in 24 subjects over 6 weeks with remote monitoring.[14] Overnight closed-loop insulin delivery increased the time spent with sensor glucose in the target range (4.4 vs 3.1 hours/night) and reduced hypoglycemia compared with control therapy (median 3.8 vs 48.7 minutes/night).

Clinical evidence to support 24-hour (day and night) hybrid closed-loop insulin-delivery at home under free living conditions without remote monitoring came from a randomized, controlled, crossover study comparing 12 weeks of hybrid closed-loop insulin delivery using the Cambridge algorithm, with sensor-augmented pump therapy in 33 adults with T1D.[15] Time spent with sensor glucose in the target range was 11 percentage points greater with the hybrid closed-loop system than with the control intervention (67.7% vs 56.8%) and hybrid closed-loop also reduced hypoglycemia. The mean HbA1c after 12 weeks was 0.3% lower with hybrid closed-loop than with sensor-augmented pump therapy. This study realized the potential for hybrid closed-loop systems in real-world settings.

It is important for successful implementation to understand the target populations where hybrid closed-loop therapy may be most beneficial and to ensure that its efficacy and safety benefits are generalizable. Many early studies demonstrated the efficacy of hybrid closed-loop systems in individuals with good glycemic control at recruitment, who may not be representative of the wider population with T1D. A recent multicenter study compared hybrid closed-loop with sensor-augmented pump therapy in a more diverse population of 86 children, adolescents, and adults with suboptimal glycemic control despite pump therapy (baseline HbA1c of 7.5%–10.0% at recruitment) over a period of 12 weeks of free living.[13] The time with glucose in target range was 10.8 percentage points higher with closed-loop compared with control therapy (65% vs 54%). Time spent in hypoglycemia (<70 mg/dL [3.9 mmol/L]) was also significantly decrease with closed-loop systems (2.6% vs 3.9%; *P* = .0130). In the closed-loop group, HbA1c was decreased from a screening value of 8.3% (67 mmol/mol) to 8.0% (64 mmol/mol) after the 4-week run-in, and to 7.4% (57 mmol/mol) after the 12-week intervention period. In the control group, the HbA1c values were 8.2% (66 mmol/mol) at screening, 7.8% (62 mmol/mol) after the run-in period, and 7.7% (61 mmol/mol) after the intervention period; adjusting for baseline HbA1c, the decrease in HbA1c was significantly greater by 0.36% (4.0 mmol/mol) in the closed-loop group compared with the control group (*P*<.0001).

The performance of a hybrid closed-loop system incorporating a patch pump (Omnipod, Insulet Corporation, Acton, MA) has been evaluated in 2 small supervised studies in adults with T1D with challenges including overestimated and missed meal boluses and moderate intensity exercise.[16,17] After the overestimated bolus (130%), 4-hour postprandial percentage time at less than 70 mg/dL (3.9 mmol/L) was 0%. After the missed bolus, postprandial percentage time at 250 mg/dL or greater (≥14 mmol/L) was 10.3% compared with 0.2% with the delivered bolus. In the 12-hour period after 30 minutes of moderate exercise, percentage time less than 70 mg/dL (<3.9 mmol/L) was low using either a raised glucose set point at 150 mg/dL rather than 130 mg/dL (1.4%), or using a reduced temporary basal rate of 50% (1.6%) started 90 minutes before exercise.

The largest hybrid closed-loop crossover study to date compared the Diabeloop DBLG1 (Diabeloop, Grenoble, France) hybrid closed-loop system with sensor-augmented pump therapy for 12 weeks in 68 adults with T1D (baseline HbA1c of 7.6% [59.4 mmol/mol]) in the home setting with remote monitoring.[18] The proportion of time with sensor glucose in the target range was 9.2% points greater with closed-loop than with control therapy (68.5% vs 59.4%). Time spent in hypoglycemia (<70 mg/dL [<3.9 mmol/L]) was significantly lower with closed-loop than during the control period. The mean HbA1c was decrease by 0.29% with a closed-loop system compared with 0.14% in the control group without reaching significance for the between-group comparison. During the study, 5 severe hypoglycemic episodes occurred in the closed-loop group and 3 in the sensor-augmented pump therapy group; these were attributed to pump hardware malfunctions or human error. The DBLG1 hybrid closed-loop system has received CE mark for use in adults with T1D.

COMMERCIALLY AVAILABLE HYBRID CLOSED-LOOP SYSTEMS

The first commercially available hybrid closed-loop system, the 670G pump (Medtronic, Northridge, CA), approved by the US Food and Drug Administration in September 2016, and with CE mark since June 2018, has been shown to be safe in people with T1D who are more than 7 years of age. The 670 G is a single hormone hybrid closed-loop system with the control algorithm embedded in the insulin pump. The pump basal rate is automated based on a PID algorithm with insulin on board feedback. This system has a fixed target sensor glucose concentration of 6.7 (120 mg/dL) or 8.3 mmol/L (150 mg/dL), with the higher target designed for exercise. Clinical evaluation to assess safety was nonrandomized and lacked a control arm introducing selection bias therefore evidence regarding its efficacy is uncertain.[19] Ninety-four adults and 30 adolescents used the closed-loop system day and night for 12 weeks. No episodes of severe hypoglycemia or ketoacidosis were observed. From baseline run-in to the end of the 3-month study phase, adult HbA1c levels decreased from 7.3% (56 mmol/mol) to 6.8% (51 mmol/mol) (P<.001), respectively. The time in target increased from 68.8% at baseline to 73.8% (P<.001) in adults.

Safety and efficacy has since been demonstrated in a real-world setting in an observational study of more than 3000 patients who completed 3 months using the 670 G system in auto mode during the commercial launch.[20] Individuals used auto mode 80.8% of the time. The time spent in target glucose range (70–180 mg/dL [3.9–10.0 mmol/L]) was 66.0% during a baseline period using manual mode compared with 73.3% during auto mode. Time spent in hypoglycemia (<70 mg/dL [3.9 mmol/L]) was decreased from 2.7% to 2.1% with auto mode. A small increase in total insulin delivered of 2.1 units/d was noted with auto mode, attributable to increased bolus delivery.

A recent real-world observational study including 93 children and young adults using the 670 G auto mode for a mean of 8 months of follow-up demonstrated high discontinuation rates. More than one-third of individuals (38%) with previous experience in pump therapy and CGM discontinued auto mode because of technical difficulties, including frequent alarms, excessive calibration requirements, premature sensor failure, and the device exiting auto mode. The remaining users' time in auto mode varied from 10% to 90%. Auto mode use correlated with HbA1c; a mean decrease in HbA1c of 0.27% after approximately 3 months using auto mode (P = .025) was observed in a subset of 58 users who continued to use auto mode.[21]

Subsequent iterations of the 670 G system are being developed with broader glucose and insulin delivery parameters to decrease the alarm burden and the number of auto mode exits to improve usability of the system.

OPEN APS, LOOP, AND AndroidAPS CLOSED-LOOP SYSTEMS

The Open Artificial Pancreas System (OpenAPS), Loop, and AndroidAPS communities have developed alternative noncommercial closed-loop systems. Individuals within this movement have built their own hybrid closed-loop systems from commercially available insulin pumps (although sometimes out of warranty), CGM devices, and open source algorithms. The lack of regulatory approvals for these systems allows for a rapid innovation cycle and more options for customization. These systems appeal to increasing numbers of people with T1D, with reportedly several thousand users to date worldwide. The responsibility of health care professionals in supporting users of these nonregulatory approved systems remains controversial, and the US Food and Drug Administration has recently released a safety communication warning against using these do-it-yourself systems. A comprehensive review of this approach can be found elsewhere in this issue.

AUTOMATED INSULIN DELIVERY DURING PREGNANCY

The benefits of maintaining near normoglycemia during pregnancy are clear, with increased rates of stillbirth, neonatal death, preterm delivery, and macrosomia associated with maternal hyperglycemia during pregnancy in women with T1D. Maintaining glucose within the recommended tight target range in pregnancy is particularly challenging for women with T1D: insulin requirements typically increase by 2- to 3-fold throughout pregnancy, with high day-to-day variability of insulin needs. Despite intensive insulin therapy with frequent glucose monitoring and HbA1c levels of less than 7% (53 mmol/mol), pregnant women with T1D spend approximately 50% of the time with glucose levels above the target range, and experience high rates of hypoglycemia (<70 mg/dL [<3.9 mmol/L]), with glucose levels below target range for approximately 15% of the day (3.5 h/d).[22]

Automated insulin delivery using the Cambridge hybrid closed-loop system has been shown to be safe and effective in pregnant women with T1D.[23] In a randomized, crossover study, overnight hybrid closed-loop therapy at home for 4 weeks led to increased time spent in the tighter target glucose range for pregnancy (63–140 mg/dL [3.5–7.8 mmol/L]) by 15% points (74.7% vs 59.5%; $P = .002$) compared with sensor augmented pump therapy, without increasing hypoglycemia. During a continuation phase applying hybrid closed-loop therapy day and night until delivery (≤14.6 additional weeks, which included antenatal hospitalizations, labor, and delivery), sensor glucose levels were within the target range for pregnancy (63–140 mg/dL [3.5–7.8 mmol/L]) 68.7% of the time. The impact of hybrid closed-loop glucose control on perinatal outcomes remains to be determined, and larger outcome studies are planned.

AUTOMATED INSULIN DELIVERY IN THE INPATIENT SETTING

Achieving recommended glucose levels during a hospital admission is challenging. The effect of the current illness, medication changes, and alterations to meal timings and intake in hospital all contribute to suboptimal glucose control. Attempts to attain target glucose levels with current insulin therapy (multiple daily insulin injections) can increase the risk of hypoglycemia and increase workload for health care professionals. Hyperglycemia and hypoglycemia in hospital are associated with increased risk of infection, length of stay, admission to the intensive care unit, and mortality.[24]

The feasibility of using fully automated closed-loop insulin delivery, that is, without meal announcement, in the inpatient setting has been shown to be safe and effective in achieving near normal glucose control.[25] A randomized controlled trial involving 136 adults with hyperglycemia on the general wards compared fully closed-loop insulin delivery with standard insulin therapy for up to 15 days.[26] Time spent with sensor glucose in the target range (100–180 mg/dL [5.6–10.0 mmol/L]) was 65.8% with closed-loop compared with 41.5% with standard insulin therapy, a difference of 24 percentage points, which equates to almost 6 additional hours each day with glucose levels in target range ($P<.001$). There was no difference in the duration of hypoglycemia (<54 mg/dL [3.0 mmol/L]) or the amount of insulin delivered. Closed-loop insulin delivery was associated with significantly better glycemic control without a higher risk of hypoglycemia. A post hoc analysis compared fully closed-loop insulin delivery with standard insulin therapy in patients undergoing hemodialysis while in the hospital. Diabetes management in people receiving hemodialysis can be very challenging. Patients using closed-loop therapy spent more time with glucose levels in target range than the control group (69.0% vs 31.5% respectively; $P<.001$), without increasing the risk of hypoglycemia. Closed-loop insulin delivery offers a novel approach to manage glucose in this vulnerable patient population and further outpatient studies are warranted.[27]

Fully automated closed-loop insulin delivery using faster acting insulin aspart in patients requiring nutritional support (enteral/parenteral nutrition) was associated with superior glucose control compared with standard insulin therapy in a study of 43 inpatients in the general wards with hyperglycaemia.[28] The closed-loop group spent approximately 8 additional hours each day with glucose levels in target range (100–180 mg/dL; [5.6–10.0 mmol/L]) compared with those receiving standard insulin therapy (68.4% vs 36.4%; $P<.001$) without an increase in hypoglycemia (**Fig. 3**). Automated insulin delivery is a safe and effective tool to improve glycemic control in hospitalized patients receiving nutritional support, where glucose management can be particularly challenging.

The closed-loop approach is an attractive option to change the management of inpatient diabetes; larger studies are required to determine if the observed improved glucose control with closed-loop can lead to improved clinical outcomes for patients and reduce staff work burden and health care costs.

THE PSYCHOSOCIAL IMPACT OF AUTOMATED INSULIN DELIVERY

The glycemic benefits of hybrid closed-loop systems have been clearly demonstrated, but depend on an intensive use of the technology. Uptake and long-term use of closed-loop systems will be heavily influenced by the user experience. Hybrid closed-loop systems still require user interaction for the delivery of mealtime boluses, in addition to the standard insulin pump and CGM-related tasks. Therefore, managing user expectations at the outset is important to promote effective long-term use and realize the clinical benefits.

Qualitative evaluations of the impact of closed-loop technology on human factors and quality of life measures have been explored in several studies.[29] User reported benefits of automated insulin delivery, aside from improved glycemic outcomes, include less fear of hypoglycemia, particularly overnight; increased reassurance and reduced anxiety; improved sleep and confidence; more time off from the demands of T1D; empowerment; and freedom to participate in exercise and unplanned activity.

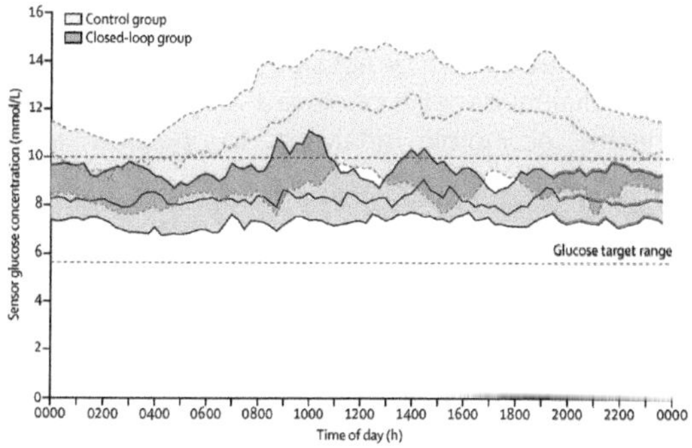

Fig. 3. Fully closed-loop insulin delivery in inpatients receiving enteral and/or parenteral nutrition. Sensor glucose concentration during closed-loop (*red*) and control (*blue*) interventions from midnight to midnight (*lines* indicate median, *shaded areas* indicate IQRs). The glucose target range is 5.6 to 10.0 mmol/L (100–180 mg/dL). (*Reprinted with permission from* Elsevier [Boughton CK, Bally L, Martignoni F, et al. Fully closed-loop insulin delivery in inpatients receiving nutritional support: a two-centre, open-label, randomised controlled trial. The Lancet Diabetes & Endocrinology 2019;7(5):368–77.])

Remote monitoring systems that allow closed-loop data sharing with selected individuals will likely improve user satisfaction, particularly among parents of young children with T1D.

There are also important challenges reported by users that need to be considered, including variable levels of trust in automated insulin delivery, intrusiveness of alarms and the associated sleep interruptions, technical difficulties, the size and appearance of the component devices causing limitations around exercise, and perceptions of deskilling or obsession with data.

Health care professional attitudes to closed-loop systems are yet to be reported.

CHALLENGES AND FUTURE DIRECTIONS OF AUTOMATED INSULIN DELIVERY

The usability and wearability of current closed-loop system devices can be demanding and efforts to minimize device burden are paramount. Noncalibrating sensors with increased accuracy and longer wear time are likely to improve user acceptability. Insulin pumps are getting smaller with the user interface being transferred to smart devices (smartphones, watches).

Interoperable automated insulin delivery devices with open protocol communications, which allow seamless secure connectivity with other devices, are underway, including the development of interoperable CGM systems and alternate controller enabled pumps as defined by the US Food and Drug Administration. The flexibility to choose different combinations of devices and create personalized closed-loop ecosystems will improve user choice and experience. Data management platforms will be important in making data from different closed-loop systems readily accessible to both users and health care professionals, and may be used to generate automated personal clinical insights to support optimal use of this technology and potentially reduce workload of health care professionals.

Progress from hybrid closed-loop to fully closed-loop systems without meal announcement may be possible with newer, ultrafast insulin analogues or adjuncts (oral or co-infused) to manage postprandial hyperglycemia. The integration of additional inputs other than glucose, such as heart rate, to more accurately reflect rapidly changing insulin requirements during exercise, are also being investigated and may permit tighter glucose regulation without increasing hypoglycemia.

Understanding user and health care professional training and support needs will be key to ensuring that the clinical benefits of closed-loop systems are realized and will be important for health economic analyses to support implementation and reimbursement.

SUMMARY

Comprehensive clinical evidence supporting automated insulin delivery systems as a safe and efficacious approach, has led to the introduction of commercially available hybrid closed-loop systems into clinical practice for adults with T1D. Evidence for application of the closed-loop approach for pregnant women and for hospitalized patients with hyperglycemia is increasing.

There is an ongoing need to improve the performance and acceptability and to decrease the device burden of automated insulin delivery systems. Adoption of the closed-loop approach as the standard of care in diabetes management requires an understanding of the training and support needs for both users and health care professionals to ensure successful implementation.

ACKNOWLEDGMENTS

Supported by the National Institute of Health Research Cambridge Biomedical Research Center, Efficacy and Mechanism Evaluation National Institute for Health Research, The Leona M. & Harry B. Helmsley Charitable Trust, JDRF, National Institute of Diabetes and Digestive and Kidney Diseases and Diabetes UK.

DISCLOSURE

R. Hovorka reports having received speaker honoraria from Eli Lilly and Novo Nordisk, serving on advisory panel for Eli Lilly and Novo Nordisk, receiving license fees from B. Braun and Medtronic; having served as a consultant to B. Braun, patents and patent applications related to closed-loop, and being shareholder of CamDiab. C.K. Boughton declares no duality of interest associated with this article.

REFERENCES

1. Nathan DM, Genuth S, Lachin J, et al. The effect of intensive treatment of diabetes on the development and progression of long-term complications in insulin-dependent diabetes mellitus. N Engl J Med 1993;329(14):977–86.
2. Pickup JC. Insulin-pump therapy for type 1 diabetes mellitus. N Engl J Med 2012; 366(17):1616–24.
3. Rodbard D. Continuous glucose monitoring: a review of recent studies demonstrating improved glycemic outcomes. Diabetes Technol Ther 2017;19(Suppl 3). S-25–S-37.
4. Foster NC, Beck RW, Miller KM, et al. State of type 1 diabetes management and outcomes from the T1D exchange in 2016-2018. Diabetes Technol Ther 2019; 21(2):66–72.
5. Bergenstal RM, Klonoff DC, Garg SK, et al. Threshold-based insulin-pump interruption for reduction of hypoglycemia. N Engl J Med 2013;369(3):224–32.
6. Calhoun PM, Buckingham BA, Maahs DM, et al. Efficacy of an overnight predictive low-glucose suspend system in relation to hypoglycemia risk factors in youth and adults with type 1 diabetes. J Diabetes Sci Technol 2016;10(6):1216–21.
7. Ruan Y, Thabit H, Leelarathna L, et al. Variability of insulin requirements over 12 weeks of closed-loop insulin delivery in adults with type 1 diabetes. Diabetes Care 2016;39(5):830–2.
8. Pinsker JE, Lee JB, Dassau E, et al. Randomized crossover comparison of personalized MPC and PID control algorithms for the artificial pancreas. Diabetes Care 2016;39(7):1135–42.
9. Weisman A, Bai JW, Cardinez M, et al. Effect of artificial pancreas systems on glycaemic control in patients with type 1 diabetes: a systematic review and meta-analysis of outpatient randomised controlled trials. Lancet Diabetes Endocrinol 2017;5(7):501–12.
10. Bekiari E, Kitsios K, Thabit H, et al. Artificial pancreas treatment for outpatients with type 1 diabetes: systematic review and meta-analysis. BMJ 2018;361:k1310.
11. Maahs DM, Buckingham BA, Castle JR, et al. Outcome measures for artificial pancreas clinical trials: a consensus report. Diabetes Care 2016;39(7):1175–9.
12. Haidar A, Legault L, Messier V, et al. Comparison of dual-hormone artificial pancreas, single-hormone artificial pancreas, and conventional insulin pump therapy for glycaemic control in patients with type 1 diabetes: an open-label randomised controlled crossover trial. Lancet Diabetes Endocrinol 2015;3(1): 17–26.

13. Tauschmann M, Thabit H, Bally L, et al. Closed-loop insulin delivery in suboptimally controlled type 1 diabetes: a multicentre, 12-week randomised trial. Lancet 2018;392(10155):1321–9.
14. Nimri R, Muller I, Atlas E, et al. Night glucose control with MD-Logic artificial pancreas in home setting: a single blind, randomized crossover trial-interim analysis. Pediatr Diabetes 2014;15(2):91–9.
15. Thabit H, Tauschmann M, Allen JM, et al. Home use of an artificial beta cell in type 1 diabetes. N Engl J Med 2015;373(22):2129–40.
16. Buckingham BA, Christiansen MP, Forlenza GP, et al. Performance of the omnipod personalized model predictive control algorithm with meal bolus challenges in adults with type 1 diabetes. Diabetes Technol Ther 2018;20(9):585–95.
17. Forlenza GP, Buckingham BA, Christiansen MP, et al. Performance of omnipod personalized model predictive control algorithm with moderate intensity exercise in adults with type 1 diabetes. Diabetes Technol Ther 2019;21(5):265–72.
18. Benhamou PY, Franc S, Reznik Y, et al. Closed-loop insulin delivery in adults with type 1 diabetes in real-life conditions: a 12-week multicentre, open-label randomised controlled crossover trial. The Lancet Digital Health 2019;1(1):E17–25.
19. Garg SK, Weinzimer SA, Tamborlane WV, et al. Glucose outcomes with the in-home use of a hybrid closed-loop insulin delivery system in adolescents and adults with type 1 diabetes. Diabetes Technol Ther 2017;19(3):155–63.
20. Stone MP, Agrawal P, Chen X, et al. Retrospective analysis of 3-month real-world glucose data after the MiniMed 670G system commercial launch. Diabetes Technol Ther 2018;20(10):689–92.
21. Goodwin G, Waldman G, Lyons J, et al. Challenges in implementing hybrid closed loop insulin pump therapy (Medtronic 670G) in a 'real world' clinical setting. J Endocr Soc 2019;3(Supplement 1).
22. Murphy HR, Rayman G, Duffield K, et al. Changes in the glycemic profiles of women with type 1 and type 2 diabetes during pregnancy. Diabetes Care 2007;30(11):2785–91.
23. Stewart ZA, Wilinska ME, Hartnell S, et al. Closed-loop insulin delivery during pregnancy in women with type 1 diabetes. N Engl J Med 2016;375(7):644–54.
24. Umpierrez GE, Isaacs SD, Bazargan N, et al. Hyperglycemia: an independent marker of in-hospital mortality in patients with undiagnosed diabetes. J Clin Endocrinol Metab 2002;87(3):978–82.
25. Thabit H, Hartnell S, Allen JM, et al. Closed-loop insulin delivery in inpatients with type 2 diabetes: a randomised, parallel-group trial. Lancet Diabetes Endocrinol 2017;5(2):117–24.
26. Bally L, Thabit H, Hartnell S, et al. Closed-loop insulin delivery for glycemic control in noncritical care. N Engl J Med 2018;379(6):547–56.
27. Bally L, Gubler P, Thabit H, et al. Fully closed-loop insulin delivery improves glucose control of inpatients with type 2 diabetes receiving hemodialysis. Kidney Int 2019;96(3):593–6.
28. Boughton CK, Bally L, Martignoni F, et al. Fully closed-loop insulin delivery in inpatients receiving nutritional support: a two-centre, open-label, randomised controlled trial. Lancet Diabetes Endocrinol 2019;7(5):368–77.
29. Farrington C. Psychosocial impacts of hybrid closed-loop systems in the management of diabetes: a review. Diabet Med 2018;35(4):436–49.

Role of Glucagon in Automated Insulin Delivery

Leah M. Wilson, MD[a,*], Peter G. Jacobs, PhD[b], Jessica R. Castle, MD[a]

KEYWORDS

• Dual-hormone artificial pancreas • Glucagon • Hypoglycemia • Intranasal glucagon • Minidose glucagon • Type 1 diabetes

KEY POINTS

- In type 1 diabetes, impaired glucagon responses contribute to ineffective counter-regulation, which increases the risk of hypoglycemia.
- Dual-hormone closed-loop systems give microgram-sized doses of glucagon under the control of a dosing algorithm.
- Compared with insulin-only automated insulin delivery systems, dual-hormone closed-loop systems have been shown to reduce overall time in hypoglycemia and reduce time in hypoglycemia related to exercise.
- Dual-hormone closed-loop systems require a stable liquid glucagon product, several of which are under development by pharmaceutical companies.
- Long-term studies are needed to establish safety and tolerability of chronic use of low-dose glucagon. Preliminary studies in humans and animals show favorable safety profiles.

INTRODUCTION

Type 1 diabetes (T1D) is caused by autoimmune destruction of the beta cells in pancreatic islets. Achieving near-normal glucose levels in the treatment of T1D can help prevent the long-term consequences of this disease.[1] Despite advances in medications and technologies for T1D treatment, attaining normal glucose levels remains challenging and is often limited by hypoglycemia.[2,3] One contributing factor to hypoglycemia arises from the dysfunction of glucagon secretion in this disease. The absence of insulin alters the normal paracrine responses within the remaining cells of the islet, leading to dysregulation of glucagon secreted from the alpha cells.[4] Glucagon secretion can be inappropriately increased in the setting of hyperglycemia

Funding: The time for L.M. Wilson, P.G. Jacobs, and J.R. Castle to prepare this article was supported by grant 1R01DK120367-01 from NIH/NIDDK.

[a] Division of Endocrinology, Diabetes and Clinical Nutrition, Oregon Health & Science University, Harold Schnitzer Diabetes Health Center, 3181 Southwest Sam Jackson Park Road, L607, Portland, OR 97239-3098, USA; [b] Department of Biomedical Engineering, Oregon Health & Science University, Mail Code: CH13B, 3303 Southwest Bond Avenue, Portland, OR 97239, USA
* Corresponding author.
E-mail address: wilsolea@ohsu.edu

Endocrinol Metab Clin N Am 49 (2020) 179–202
https://doi.org/10.1016/j.ecl.2019.10.008
0889-8529/20/

or after a meal and can be blunted or absent during hypoglycemia.[5] The impaired glucagon response contributes to ineffective glucose counter-regulation, which greatly increases the risk of severe hypoglycemia, defined as hypoglycemia requiring the assistance of another person to treat.[6] The treatment of T1D currently consists of multiple daily injections or continuous subcutaneous delivery of insulin through a pump. Newer pump technologies can now be controlled either directly by the patient or automatically through feedback from a continuous glucose monitor (CGM). Automated insulin delivery (AID) or insulin only/single-hormone closed loop are two interchangeable terms for these newer pump systems that automatically dose insulin based on CGM values. Insulin analogues used in these treatments have significantly delayed pharmacodynamics compared with endogenous insulin, leading to periods of inappropriate hyperinsulinism, which also contributes to hypoglycemia.[7] Exercise and postexercise are especially high-risk times for hypoglycemia because of changes in insulin sensitivity and increased insulin-independent glucose uptake into muscle.[8] The glucagon response can be attenuated during exercise, and the high catecholamine state of exercise can mask symptoms of hypoglycemia.[9] Glucagon injected intramuscularly or subcutaneously in 1-mg doses is very effective to correct severe hypoglycemia. Over the last 2 decades, minidose glucagon, which is subcutaneous small doses of glucagon, was used in children, and then adults, to treat hypoglycemia when a person with diabetes is unable or unwilling to take oral carbohydrates.[10] Within the last decade, research groups working on closed-loop insulin and glucagon delivery systems have been using automated microgram-sized doses of glucagon delivered through subcutaneous pump systems with the goal of preventing or shortening periods of hypoglycemia and preemptively in the setting of exercise to decrease risk of hypoglycemia.[11]

BRIEF OVERVIEW OF GLUCAGON PHYSIOLOGY AND PHARMACOLOGY

Glucagon is a 29 amino acid peptide made by alpha cells of the pancreatic islet. In normal physiology, glucagon levels increase with hypoglycemia, fasting, exercise, and protein-rich meals.[12] In normal physiology, hypoglycemia elicits an abrupt increase in glucagon, epinephrine, and growth hormone levels, which function to increase glucose level.[13] Glucagon's main target is the liver, where it binds to a G protein–coupled receptor and signals through cyclic AMP to induce glycogenolysis and to a lesser degree gluconeogenesis to increase plasma glucose levels within 10 to 30 minutes.[14,15] In T1D, glucagon responses are impaired or absent, which further perpetuates episodes of hypoglycemia. Recurrent hypoglycemia results in reduced physiologic responses to hypoglycemia, including impaired glucagon and epinephrine increases.[2,9]

The dosing in standard hypoglycemia rescue kits is 1 mg delivered intramuscularly, whereas the typical dosing used in dual-hormone systems is microdoses of 10 to 100 μg delivered subcutaneously, typically amounting to less than 1 mg/d. Importantly for use in dual-hormone systems, subcutaneous injections of microgram doses of glucagon result in a dose-dependent increase in plasma glucose levels at a wide range of starting glucose values.[16,17] Unlike insulin, glucagon delivered subcutaneously shows a more rapid onset and offset of action, making it ideal for use in automated delivery systems.[18]

GLUCAGON IN CLOSED-LOOP GLUCOSE CONTROL SYSTEMS

Potential Benefits of Glucagon in Closed-Loop Systems

Closed-loop systems are pump systems that deliver insulin and optionally glucagon dynamically with a controller algorithm based on values from CGM. Systems that deliver glucagon in addition to insulin are referred to as dual-hormone closed-loop systems. A recent meta-analysis[19] of available studies published in February 2018 showed that use of either single-hormone or dual-hormone closed-loop systems led to an increase in the percentage of time in the glucose target range (70–180 mg/dL, 3.9–10 mmol/L) by 140 min/d compared with study participants' usual care. Time in hypoglycemia (<70 mg/dL or 3.9 mmol/L) also reduced by 20 min/d for participants using closed-loop systems. In many clinical trials, insulin-only automated delivery systems increased time in target range and reduced the time spent in hypoglycemia (<70 mg/dL or 3.9 mmol/L) to 3% or less compared with sensor-augmented pump (SAP) or pump use without CGM.[20] It is important to contextualize these findings; even if time in hypoglycemia is reduced to 3% on average, that is still 43 min/d. These numbers reflect the average experience of the clinical trial participants, who may have better diabetes control than a typical person with T1D. Even within these study participants, some people experienced significantly higher time in hypoglycemia than is represented by these mean results. The best insulin-only closed-loop systems typically only achieve 70% to 80% time in target range and about 2% to 3% time in hypoglycemia. Therefore, it is important to consider additional strategies that can help people with T1D improve their glycemic control. Glucagon acts as the counter-regulatory hormone to insulin in normal physiology and therefore is a natural consideration for inclusion in closed-loop systems to reduce hypoglycemia. However, there will always be physiologic circumstances in which glucagon cannot prevent hypoglycemia (discussed later).

Many patients with T1D struggle with hypoglycemia from exercise and may avoid exercise for this reason.[21,22] Exercise is a high-risk time for hypoglycemia because of insulin-independent disposal of glucose by contracting muscles, increased insulin sensitivity, and increased insulin absorption from the subcutaneous space caused by increased blood flow.[23,24] The risk for hypoglycemia after exercise continues for many hours, with overnight being a particularly vulnerable time for hypoglycemia.[25] The current guidelines[8] for glucose management with exercise focus on carbohydrate intake before exercise in addition to basal and bolus reductions; these approaches can lead to unwanted hyperglycemia. In addition, requiring additional calorie intake for exercise is a major disadvantage for the more than 50% of adults with T1D who are overweight or obese and are exercising to help better manage their weight.[26] Subcutaneous injections of glucagon (150–200 μg) delivered before or after exercise are effective to reduce or avoid hypoglycemia without need for preemptive carbohydrate intake.[11,27] Our research group and others have shown that dual-hormone automated systems can help reduce exercise-induced hypoglycemia during aerobic exercise compared with single-hormone automated systems.[28–30]

Dual-hormone systems may be indicated for certain patient populations. Patients with frequent hypoglycemia and hypoglycemia unawareness are often excluded from single-hormone AID clinical trials, potentially skewing the results. These patients may experience more hypoglycemia than patients without hypoglycemia unawareness. Glucagon could serve as a useful line of defense against hypoglycemia for these patients. In addition, dual-hormone systems could prove useful to help reduce hypoglycemia awareness in these patients by reducing the occurrence of hypoglycemia.[31] It is known that patients start to become more hypoglycemia aware after 3 to 4 weeks of no hypoglycemia events.[32] More work in this patient population is anticipated in the future.

Closed-loop systems typically use one of 3 strategies for mealtime insulin dosing: (1) a traditional premeal bolus based on carbohydrate counting is entered by the user, (2) a meal is announced to the system with limited information (ie, small, medium, large) or no information on carbohydrate content, or (3) no meal announcement is made. Carbohydrate counting is burdensome for people with T1D and tends to be inaccurate.[33] A fully automated system that does not require meal announcements would be ideal; however, this approach is limited by postprandial hyperglycemia and late postprandial hypoglycemia.[34] Dual-hormone closed-loop systems may allow fully automated mealtime insulin dosing because the glucagon theoretically could prevent late postprandial hypoglycemia. In practice, studies with dual-hormone systems have yet to fully realize this potential.[35,36]

Review of Dual-Hormone Closed-Loop Studies

An early report of a dual-hormone system used over 7 days in pancreatectomized dogs was published in 1982.[37] With improvements in CGM, algorithm, and pump technology, advances have been substantial over the last 10 years. Twenty dual-hormone studies published since 2010 are included in this overview (**Table 1**).[12,28–31,35,36,38–46,48–51] The dual-hormone systems in these studies are primarily compared with a control group. The control group in early studies typically involved participants using insulin pump alone (also known as continuous subcutaneous insulin infusion [CSII]),whereas later studies used control groups wherein participants used SAP therapy. Most recently, the control group has been participants using predictive low glucose suspend systems (PLGSs). Some studies compare single-hormone with dual-hormone systems. The sophistication of the dual-hormone closed-loop systems progressed from algorithms run on laptop computers with manual input of the infusion rates to algorithms run on a smartphone or infusion pump with automated infusion rate adjustment on a portable wireless system. The clinical studies have progressed from partial days under close supervision in an inpatient clinical research center to multiple days in a free-living outpatient setting. Some of the older studies report plasma glucose outcomes, whereas the newer studies report outcomes based on CGM data. There is now guidance on standardized reporting of closed-loop study results.[52] With all of this evolution, results of the older studies cannot be directly compared with the newer studies because they are fundamentally different. However, this overview serves to show the trajectory of this work, including advantages and disadvantages (see **Table 1**).

Reducing Hypoglycemia

Most studies show less time in hypoglycemia with dual-hormone than comparator groups (CSII, SAP, PLGS, and so forth), although not all reached statistical significance. A recent meta-analysis of 7 dual-hormone studies and 16 single-hormone studies with conventional pump therapy as comparator group was completed.[20] The mean difference for time in hypoglycemia (<70 mg/dL or <3.9 mmol/L) was reduced (−3.78%; 95% confidence interval [CI], −5.58 to −1.97) for dual-hormone systems compared with conventional pump. The reduction was less for single-hormone systems compared with conventional pump (−1.88%; 95% CI, −3.40 to −0.36). In studies comparing a single-hormone system directly with a dual-hormone system, time less than 70 mg/dL (3.9 mmol/L) is as low as 1% (representing about 15 min/d) for dual-hormone systems. There is also a consistent trend toward reduced need for rescue carbohydrate intake with dual-hormone systems. The effect of dual-hormone control on overnight hypoglycemia in adults is less consistent. One study showed that an insulin-only closed-loop system and PLGS significantly reduced overnight hypoglycemia compared with conventional pump therapy with little added benefit with the addition of glucagon.[28] A similar finding was seen in 2 other studies,[30,45] whereas a study in children aged 9 to 17 years in a diabetes camp setting

Table 1
Dual-hormone studies published between 2010 and 2019

Study	Date of Online Publication	Location of Research Group	Participant Characteristics: Number of Participants	Mean Age (y)	Mean DM Duration (y)	Mean A1c (%)	Duration	Study Design	Treatment Groups	Control Group	Location	Standardized Exercise	Components	Monitoring
El-Khatib et al,[35] 2010	4/16/2010	Boston, MA	11 adults	40	23	7.3	27 h	Nonrandomized	DH	No control group	Inpatient	No	Computer, Deltec Cozmo pumps, venous blood glucose samples, manual entry of rates	On site
Russell et al,[50] 2012	8/28/2012	Boston, MA	6 adults	52	32	7.4	51 h	Nonrandomized	DH	No control group	Inpatient	No	OmniPod pumps, Navigator CGM	On site
El-Khatib et al,[51] 2014	2/4/2014	Boston, MA	12 adults/12 adolescents	45/15	27/7	7.3/7.9	48 h	Randomized	Meal prime, WOMP	No control group	Inpatient	Yes	OmniPod pumps, Navigator CGM	On site
Russell et al,[40] 2014	6/17/2014	Boston, MA	20 adults/32 adolescents	40/16	24/9	7.1/8.2	5 d	Randomized, crossover	DH	Usual care with pump or SAP (45% own sensor use)	Adults, hotel; adolescents, diabetes camp	No	iPhone 4S, G4 Dexcom, Tslim pumps M5	On site
Russell et al,[41] 2016	2/7/2016	Boston, MA	19 children	9.8	5	7.8	5 d	Randomized, crossover	DH	Usual care with pump or SAP	Diabetes camp	No	iPhone 4S, G4 Dexcom, Tslim pumps	On site
El-Khatib et al,[42] 2017	12/23/2016	Boston, MA; Worcester, MA; Palo Alto, CA; Chapel Hill NC	43 adults	33.3	16.9	7.7	11 d	Randomized, crossover	DH	Usual care with pump or SAP (59% own sensor use)	Home	No	iPhone 4S, G4 Dexcom, Tslim pumps	Remote

(*continued on next page*)

Table 1
(*continued*)

Study	Date of Online Publication	Location of Research Group	Participant Characteristics: Number of Participants	Mean Age (y)	Mean DM Duration (y)	Mean A1c (%)	Duration	Study Design	Treatment Groups	Control Group	Location	Standardized Exercise	Components	Monitoring
Haidar et al,[43] 2013	1/30/2013	Montreal, Canada	15 adults	47.1	26.5	7.9	15 h	Randomized, crossover	DH	SAP	Inpatient	Yes	Minimed veo pumps, Sofsensor Medtronic, manual entry of rates	On site
Haidar et al,[30] 2015	12/2/2014	Montreal, Canada	20 adults/10 adolescents	43/14	16/8	7.7/7.9	24 h	Randomized, crossover	SH, DH	Usual care with pump	Inpatient	Yes	Minimed veo pumps, Sofsensor Medtronic, manual entry of rates	On site
Haidar et al,[44] 2015	6/13/2015	Montreal, Canada	33 children	13.3	7.5	8.3	3 nights	Randomized, crossover	SH, DH	Usual care with pump	Diabetes camp	No	G4 Dexcom, Accu-check combo pumps, tablet computer, manually entry of rates	Remote

Study	AID Initialization	AID Algorithm	Meals Announced?	Glucagon Delivery Strategy	Glucagon Delivered (SD)	Mean Glucose, mg/dL (SD)	p-value	Time in Range 70–180 mg/dL (SD)	p-value	Hypoglycemia <70 mg/dL (SD)	p-value	Hyperglycemia >180 mg/dL (SD)	p-value	Hypoglycemia Treatments Per Day	p-value	Adverse Events
El-Khatib et al,[35] 2010	Weight only	Model predictive control	No meal announcement allowed	Proportional derivative control to prevent <100 mg/dL	1.70 µg/kg/d	164 (SD 17)	—	62%	—	<1%	—	38%	—	0	—	No nausea or vomiting with glucagon
Russell et al,[50] 2012	Weight only	Model predictive control	Yes	Proportional derivative control to prevent <100 mg/dL	3.6 µg/kg/d (5.1)	158 (SD 44)	—	68% (SD 12)	—	0.7% (0.8)	—	31% (12)	—	3.2 g/kg/d (0.3)	—	Subject who received largest amount of glucagon
El-Khatib et al,[51] 2014	Weight only	Model predictive control	Yes	Proportional derivative control to prevent <100 mg/dL	WMP 6.8 µg/kg/d (2.5); WOMP 6.6 µg/kg/d (3.5)	WMP 132 (9); WOMP 146 (9)	0.03	WMP 80%; WOMP 70%	0.04	WMP 5.1%; WOMP 3.6%	0.7	Not reported	—	0.92/d	—	Two subjects reported nausea
Russell et al,[40] 2014	Weight only	Model predictive control	Recommended but not required	Proportional derivative control to prevent <100 mg/dL	0.82 mg/d (0.41)	Adults DH 133 (13), control 159 (30.4)	<0.001	Adults DH 79.5% (8.3), control 58.8% (14.6)	<0.001	Adults DH 4.1% (3.5), control 7.3% (4.7)	0.01	Adults DH 16.5% (1.8), control 33.8% (16.4)	<0.00 1	Adults DH:2.2 (3.2), control 3.4 (3.1)	0.15	One patient reported nausea, 2 reported 1 episode of vomiting
Russell et al,[41] 2016	Weight only	Model predictive control	Recommended but not required	Proportional derivative control to prevent <100 mg/dL	10.9 µg/kg/d(4.0)	DH 136.8 (10.8), control 167 (30.6)	<0.001	DH: 80.6% (7.4), control 57.6% (14)	—	(<60) DH: 1.2% (1.1), control: 2.8% (1.2)	<0.001	DH 16% (6.4), control 36.3% (15.7)	<0.00 1	Events/participant/study: DH 3, control 5	0.037	No difference DH vs control
El-Khatib et al,[42] 2017	Weight only	Model predictive control	Recommended but not required	Proportional derivative control to prevent <100 mg/dL	6.8 µg/kg/d	DH 140.4 (10.8), control 162 (28.8)	<0.001	DH 78.4% (6.0), Control 61.9% (14.4)	<0.001	(<60) DH 0.6% (0.6), control 1.9% (1.7)	<0.001	DH 19.8% (6.1), control 33.6% (16.4)	<0.00 1	DH 0.4 (0.3), control 0.9 (0.7)	<0.001	21 reported DH. 5 reported control

(continued on next page)

Table 1
(*continued*)

Study	AID Initialization	AID Algorithm	Meals Announced?	Glucagon Delivery Strategy	Glucagon Delivered (SD)	Mean Glucose, mg/dL (SD)	p-value	Time in Range 70–180 mg/dL (SD)	p-value	Hypoglycemia <70 mg/dL (SD)	p-value	Hyperglycemia >180 mg/dL (SD)	p-value	Hypoglycemia Treatments Per Day	p-value	Adverse Events
Haidar et al,[43] 2013	Weight, TDD, ICR	Model predictive control	Yes	Logical rules based on glucose value and trend	0.076 mg/visit	DH 140.4, control 142.2	0.74	DH 70.7%, control 57.3%	0.003	DH 0%, control 10.2%	0.01	DH 29.3%, control 25.6%	0.74	At least 1 event per study: DH 7%, control 53%	0.02	None
Haidar et al,[30] 2015	Weight, TDD, ICR	Model predictive control	Yes	Logical rules based on glucose value and trend	2.0 μg/kg/visit	DH 135 (34), SH 126 (27), control 144 (59.4)	DH/control 0.26	DH 63% (18), SH 62% (18), control 51% (19)	DH/control <0.001	DH 1.5%, SH 3.1%, control 13.3%	DH/control <0.001	DH 20% (15), SH 20% (16), control 26% (22)	DH/control 0.83	At least 1 event per study: DH 21%, SH 17%, control 83%	DH/control <0.001	Not reported
Haidar et al,[44] 2015	Weight, TDD, ICR	Model predictive control	NA	Logical rules based on glucose value and trend	0.7 μg/kg/night (1.0)	DH 138.6 (30.6), SH 145.8 (30.6), control 167 (25)	DH/control <0.001	DH 84%, SH 77%, control 54%	DH/control <0.001	DH 0%, SH 3.1%, control 3.4%	DH/control <0.001	DH 13%, SH 20%, control 38%	DH/control <0.00 1	Events/night: DH 0, SH 0.04, C 0.15	—	Not reported

Study	Date of Online Publication	Location of Research Group	Participant Characteristics: Number of Participants	Mean Age (y)	Mean DM Duration (y)	Mean A1c (%)	Duration	Study Design	Treatment Groups	Control Group	Location	Standardized Exercise	Components	Monitoring
Haidar et al,[45] 2016	11/3/2015	Montreal, Canada	21 adults/7 adolescents	39/15	21/8	7.4/7.7	2 nights	Randomized, crossover	SH, DH	Usual care with pump	Home	Yes	Paradigm veo pump, Enlite sensor, manual entry of rates	On site
Gingras et al,[46] 2016	6/15/2015	Montreal, Canada	12 adults	51.3	32.6	7.4	14 h	Randomized, crossover	DH with ICR prandial dose, DH with qualitative prandial dose	Usual care with pump	Inpatient	No	Accu-check combo pump, Enlite Medtronic sensor, manual entry of rates	On site
Taleb et al,[12] 2016	10/6/2016	Montreal, Canada	17 adults	37.2	23.1	8	90 min	Randomized, crossover	DH/SH with continuous exercise, DH/SH with interval exercise	No control group	Inpatient	Yes	Computer, Dexcom G4 sensor, MiniMed Paradigm Veo, manual entry of rates	On site
Haidar et al,[38] 2017	1/18/2017	Montreal, Canada	23 adults	41	24	7.5	60 h	Randomized, crossover	SH, DH	Usual care with SAP	Home	No	Dexcom G4, Sensewear, Accu-check combo pumps, manual entry of rates	On site
Castle et al,[39] 2010	3/23/2010	Portland, OR	14 adults	36.7	14.1	7.6	28 h	Randomized	Low-gain, high-gain glucagon delivery	Placebo delivery	Inpatient	No	Insulin via animas IR 1000 pump, glucagon via Medfusion 2001 syringe pump, manual entry of rates	On site
Jacobs et al,[29] 2016	6/24/2016	Portland, OR	21 adults	32	15.4	7.5	22 h	Randomized, crossover	APX (AP with exercise adjustment), APN (AP with no exercise adjustment)	Usual care with SAP	Inpatient	Yes	Google nexus smartphone, tslim pumps, Dexcom G4	On site

(continued on next page)

Table 1
(*continued*)

Study	Date of Online Publication	Location of Research Group	Participant Characteristics: Number of Participants	Mean Age (y)	Mean DM Duration (y)	Mean A1c (%)	Duration	Study Design	Treatment Groups	Control Group	Location	Standard-ized Exercise	Components	Monitoring
Castle et al,[28] 2018	5/13/2018	Portland, OR	20 adults	34.5	20.2	7.5	4 d	Randomized, crossover	SH, DH, PLGS, CC	Usual care with pump or SAP (65% own sensor use)	Outpatient	Yes	Google nexus smartphone, tslim pumps, Dexcom G5	Remote
van Bon et al,[48] 2012	10/16/2012	Amsterdam, The Netherlands	10 adults	55.4	34.6	8	8 h	Nonrandomized	DH	Usual care with pump	Inpatient	Yes	Computer, System gold medtronic minimed sensor, D-tron+ pumps, Polar HR monitor	On site
van Bon et al,[36] 2014	11/15/2013	Amsterdam, The Netherlands	16 adults	52.1	35.3	7.6	48 h	Nonrandomized	DH	Usual care with pump	Home	Yes	Computer, Sofsensor or Enlite medtronic minimed sensor, D-tron+ pumps	On site
Blauw et al,[49] 2016	3/22/2016	Amsterdam, The Netherlands	16 adults	41	18	7.7	4 d	Randomized, crossover	DH	Usual care with pump	Inpatient then home	No	DiabeticBV (contains CGM, control algorithm, insulin pump glucagon pump), Enlite medtronic sensors	On site/ remote
Abitbol et al,[31] 2018	2/3/2018	Toronto, Canada	18 adults with hypoglycemia unaware, 17 adults hypoglycemia aware	45.6	26.9	7.7	11 h overnight	Randomized, crossover	DH	SH	Inpatient	No	Enlite sensor, Minimed Veo pump, manual entry of rates	On site

Study	AID Initialization	AID Algorithm	Meals Announced?	Glucagon Delivery Strategy	Glucagon Delivered (SD)	Mean Glucose mg/dL (SD)		Time in Range 70 180 mg/dL (SD)		Hypoglycemia <70 md/dL (SD)		Hyperglycemia >180 mg/dL (SD)		Hypoglycemia Treatments Per Day		Adverse Events
Haidar et al,[45] 2016	Weight, TDD, ICR	Model predictive control	Yes	Logical rules based or glucose value and trend	0.4 μg/kg/night	DH 111.6 (28.8), SH 111.6 (30.6), control 120.6 (43)	DH/control 0.57	DH 93%, SH 91%, control 70%	DH/control <0.001	DH 1%, SH 5%, control 14%	DH/control <0.001	DH 0%, SH 0%, control 4%	DH/control 0.66	Total events: DH 3, SH 6, control 14	—	Not reported
Gingras et al,[46] 2016	Weight, TDD, ICR	Model predictive contro	Yes	Logical rules based or glucose value and trend	ICR 0.044 mg/study, qualitative 0.042 mg/study	ICR 147.6 (37.8), qualitative 151.2 (30.6), control 172.8 (36)	ICR/control 0.03	ICR 66.8%, qualitative 64.2%, control 49.9%	ICR/control 0.10	ICR 0.1%, qualitative 5.4%, control 5.6%	ICR/control 0.81	ICR 20.7%, qualitative 29.3%, control 40.5%	ICR/control 0.03	Not reported	—	Not reported
Taleb et al,[12] 2016	Weight, TDD, ICR	Model predictive control	NA	Logical rules based or glucose value and trend	DH continuous 0.126 mg/study (0.057), DH interval	Not reported	—	DH continuous 100%, SH continuous 68.1%; DH interval 100%, SH interval 72.5%	Continuous 0.004, interval 0.11	DH continuous 0%, SH continuous 22.5%; DH interval 0%, SH interval 0%	Continuous 0.07, interval 0.04	Not reported	—	Total events: DH continuous 2, SH continuous 4, DH interval 1, SH interval 6	—	Not reported
Haidar et al,[38] 2017	Weight, TDD, ICR	Model predictive control	Yes	Logical rules based on glucose value and trend	7.9 μg/kg/study (4.1)	DH 142.2 (50.4), SH 142.2 (50.4), control 135 (54)	DH/control 0.16	DH 79%, SH 75%, control 64%	DH/control 0.31	DH 3.6%, SH 3.9%, control 7.9%	DH/control 0.002	DH 16%, SH 20%, control 15%	DH/control 0.13	Total events: DH 6, SH 14, control 34	—	Not reported

(*continued on next page*)

Table 1
(continued)

Study	AID Initialization	AID Algorithm	Meals Announced?	Glucagon Delivery Strategy	Glucagon Delivered (SD)	Mean Glucose mg/dL (SD)		Time in Range 70 180 mg/dL (SD)		Hypoglycemia <70 md/dL (SD)		Hyperglycemia >180 mg/dL (SD)		Hypoglycemia Treatments Per Day		Adverse Events
Castle et al,[39] 2010	TDD, BMI, age	Fading memory proportional derivative	Yes	High gain, low gain	Low gain 0.746 mg/d (134) vs high gain 0.516 mg/d	High gain 138 (SD 17); low gain 157 (SD 24), placebo 135 (SD 16)	—	Numbers not reported	NS	DH 1.04%, control 2.77%	DH/ control 0.04	Numbers not reported	NS	DH 1.1/study (0.5), control 3.9/study (1)	0.01	One subject reported nausea with DH
Jacobs et al,[29] 2016	TDD, BMI, age	Proportional derivative	Yes	Reduced insulin and increased glucagon for exercise	APX 3.6 µg/kg, APN 2.8 µg/kg	APX 154.8, APN 145.8, control 154.8	APX/APN 0.032	APX 75%, APN 81%, control 72%	APX/APN 0.11	APX 0.3%, APN 3.1%, control 0.8%	APX/APN 0.001	APX 25%, APN 17%, control 27%	APX/APN 0.09	Total events: APX 6, APN 9, control 7	APX/ APN 0.08	Not reported
Castle et al,[28] 2018	TDD, BMI, age	Fading memory proportional derivative	Yes	Reduced insulin and increased glucagon for exercise	0.510 mg/d (0.207)	DH 149 (38), SH 145 (31), PLGS 170 (49), control 164 (62)	DH/ control 0.29	DH 72.0 (10.8), SH 74.3 (8.0), PLGS 65.2 (13.5), control 63.1 (17.3)	DH/ control 0.010	DH 1.3 (1.0), SH 2.8 (1.7), PLGS 2.0 (1.5), control 3.1 (3.2)	DH/ control 0.007	DH 26.7 (11.3), SH 22.9 (8.7), PLGS 32.8 (13.9), control 33.7(18.1)	DH/ control 0.054	Per day: DH 0.8 (0.7), SH 1.7 (1.4), PLGS 1.3 (1.3), control 1.5 (1.2)	DH/ control 0.010	GI upset in 23% of DH, 0% SH, 13% PLGS, 5% control
van Bon et al,[48] 2012	TDD	Proportional derivative control	No	Glucagon given if <117, bolus size based rate of decrease of glucose	Post-breakfast 0.04 mg, post-exercise 0.12 mg, postlunch 0.07mg	DH 156.6, control 162	DH/ control 0.74	DH 62.3%, control 61.2%	DH/ control 0.78	DH 5.3%, control 4.1%	DH/ control 0.60	DH 32.4%, control 34.7%	DH/ control 0.54	Events: DH 4, control 2	—	Not reported

Table 1
(continued)

Study	AID Initialization	AID Algorithm	Meals Announced?	Glucagon Delivery Strategy	Glucagon Delivered (SD)	Mean Glucose mg/dL (SD)		Time in Range 70 180 mg/dL (SD)		Hypoglycemia <70 md/dL (SD)		Hyperglycemia >180 mg/dL (SD)		Hypoglycemia Treatments Per Day		Adverse Events
van Bon et al,[36] 2014	TDD	Proportional derivative control	No	Glucagon given if <117, bolus size based rate of decrease of glucose	Daytime 1.7–2.7 mg, Nighttime 0.6 mg	Day 2 median: DH 7.70 (2.29), control 8.84 (0.8[illegible]	DH/control 0.0273	Day 2 median: DH 76.5% (23.9%), control 66.0% (29.8%)	DH/control 0.1618	Day 2 median: DH 2.8% (9.8%), control 0.0% (11.1%)	DH/control 0.0172	Day 2 median: DH 18.3% (20.0%), control 31.0% (29.8%)	DH/control 0.088 9	Events: DH 6, control 6	—	Not reported
Blauw et al,[49] 2016	Weight only	Proportional derivative control	No	Triggered by glucose threshold	0.74 mg/study	DH 133.2, control 145.8	DH/control 0.059	DH 84.7%, control 68.5%	DH/control 0.007	DH 1.3%, control 2.4%	DH/control 0.139	DH 11.9%, control 24.3%	DH/control 0.022	Events: DH 12, control 21		One subject with nausea after 0.88 mg glucagon, 6 glucagon infusion set occlusions
Abitbol et al,[31] 2018	TDD, ICR	Model predictive control	Yes	Logical rules based on glucose value and trend	Not reported	DH 122.4 (19.8), SH 142.2 (23.4)	DH:SH 0.01	DH 100%, SH 77%	DH:SH 0.04	Not reported	—	DH 0%, SH 17%	DH:SH 0.04	Hypoglycemia unaware, 0.38 events/night; hypoglycemia aware, 0.25 events/night	—	Not reported

Study characteristics and results for the 20 DH studies reviewed.

Abbreviations: BMI, body mass index; CC, current care; DH, dual-hormone; DM, diabetes mellitus; GI, gastrointestinal; HR, heart rate; ICR, insulin to carbohydrate ratio; NA, not available; NS, not significant; PLGS, predictive low glucose suspend system; SD, standard deviation; SH, single hormone; TDD, total daily dose of insulin; WMP, with meal prime; WOMP, without meal prime.

Data from Refs.[12,28–31,35,36,38–46,48–51]

showed a statistically significant benefit of dual-hormone compared with an insulin-only system and conventional pump therapy for reducing overnight hypoglycemia.[44] Longer-term studies are needed to clarify whether dual-hormone systems provide additional benefit to insulin-only systems for preventing overnight hypoglycemia.

Preventing Exercise-Induced Hypoglycemia

The preponderance of the evidence suggests that dual-hormone closed-loop systems reduce the occurrence of acute-onset hypoglycemia caused by exercise. One study compared single-hormone and dual-hormone systems over the course of a 4-hour interval during which participants were randomized to continuous aerobic or interval exercise for 60 minutes.[12] For continuous aerobic exercise, median percentage time less than 70 mg/dL (3.9 mmol/L) was 22.5% for single hormone versus 0% for dual hormone (P = .006). High-intensity interval exercise showed median time less than 70 mg/dL (<3.9 mmol/L) of 0% in both the single-hormone and dual-hormone groups, showing how various types of exercise affect glycemic control very differently. In another study, 2 dual-hormone systems (1 with exercise detection and dosing adjustment,[53] 1 without) were compared with SAP therapy.[29] The dual-hormone system that adjusted dosing of insulin and glucagon following detection of exercise reduced time in hypoglycemia from the start of exercise until the next meal compared with the dual-hormone system with no exercise detection (0.3% vs 3.1%; P = .001). In a follow-on study by the same group, dual hormone, single hormone, PLGS, and current care (SAP or CSII alone) were compared in a 4-day outpatient study including 45 minutes of aerobic exercise on days 1 and 4.[28] The single-hormone and dual-hormone systems included automated exercise detection and dosing adjustment. From the start of exercise until the next meal (approximately 4 hours), time less than 70 mg/dL (<3.9 mmol/L) was lowest in the dual-hormone group (dual hormone, 3.4%; single hormone, 8.3%; PLGS, 7.6%; current care, 4.3%). Dual hormone showed less time in hypoglycemia than single hormone (P = .009) and PLGS (<0.0001), but not current care, in which subject-driven preexercise insulin adjustment was allowed (P = .49). Two other studies showed no advantage of dual hormone compared with single hormone for hypoglycemia related to exercise.[30,45] However, in 1 of these studies the closed-loop system was used by participants only during the overnight period, starting a few hours after exercise.[45]

Prandial Glucose Control

In theory, a dual-hormone system could allow more aggressive insulin dosing for carbohydrate intake to improve postprandial hyperglycemia while glucagon prevents any postprandial hypoglycemia induced by more aggressive insulin dosing. To our knowledge this approach has not yet been tried in humans with a dual-hormone system. Also, this approach does raise possible safety concerns caused by possible hypoglycemia if glucagon delivery fails. Data from a related human study provide mixed results on whether this may be beneficial.[54] Adolescents aged 12 to 18 years on pump therapy were given a standardized meal on 3 separate occasions; they received their usual premeal insulin bolus, usual bolus plus pramlintide, or 60% increase of their usual insulin dose with rescue doses of minidose glucagon if glucoses dipped to less than 95 mg/dL (5.3 mmol/L). The researchers saw that the 60% increased bolus did not result in statistically significant improvement in the area under the glucose curve compared with the usual bolus; however, there was a trend toward lower glucose values in the increased bolus group. Minidose glucagon injections (1–4 injections of 10 μg/y up to 150 μg) were required around 5 hours after the meal and successfully increased glucose level. The pramlintide plus insulin group showed a marked decrease in the glucose levels in the early postprandial period, even resulting in early postprandial hypoglycemia in some subjects. The results of the pramlintide arm of this study are discussed further later. One potential limitation of using glucagon to prevent early postprandial hypoglycemia is that high circulating insulin concentrations are known to reduce the glucose level–increasing impact of minidose glucagon.[55]

SPECIAL CONSIDERATIONS FOR GLUCAGON IN CLOSED-LOOP SYSTEMS

Stable Liquid Glucagon Formulations

Glucagon from standard hypoglycemia rescue kits is reconstituted in an aqueous solution. In this solution, glucagon forms fibrils and within days solidifies into a gel in additional to undergoing spontaneous degradation.[47] Several pharmaceutical companies are working toward stable liquid glucagon products that avoid these pitfalls.[56] There are 2 main approaches to improving the stability of glucagon: native human glucagon reconstituted in special carrier solutions, and glucagon analogues with slight peptide alterations to promote stability and solubility. Until very recently, dual-hormone studies used glucagon from a commercially available hypoglycemia rescue kit. Glucagon needed to be reconstituted and the pump reservoirs refilled every 24 hours during the studies. With several stable liquid glucagon products nearing US Food and Drug Administration approval, this recent dual-hormone study[57] used an investigational stable liquid glucagon product with results comparable with a prior study with the conventional glucagon preparation.[28]

Continuous Subcutaneous Infusion Pump Design

All currently available CSII systems consist of a single reservoir or cartridge and a single cannula for subcutaneous infusion. To date, dual-hormone studies have required participants to wear 2 pumps and 2 infusion sites in addition to CGM, which is impractical for real-life use. People with T1D already struggle to find adequate locations for site and sensor placement while allowing previously used areas to heal. Some develop considerable lipohypertrophy or scar tissue from overuse of particular sites, which can affect insulin absorption kinetics if the site is used in the future.[58] Translation of dual-hormone technologies to real-world use will require development of pump technology with dual chambers and possibly dual cannulas, and such pumps are currently in development.[59] Even with this advancement, there will need to be careful design and training to fill and connect 2 chambers without inverting the medications. In practicality, this may prove to be too complex or burdensome for many individuals.

POTENTIAL LIMITATIONS FOR USE OF GLUCAGON IN CLOSED-LOOP SYSTEMS

Glycogen Stores

T1D is associated with lower hepatic glycogen stores. Subjects with well-controlled T1D had significantly lower glycogen stores than healthy volunteers after an overnight fast.[60] Subjects with poorly controlled diabetes showed reduced glycogen synthesis and breakdown, which improved but did not normalize with short-term intensive diabetes control.[61] This finding raises the question of whether people with T1D can have sustained physiologic glucose level–increasing responses to repeated doses of glucagon such as may be given during dual-hormone control. In a study with participants with well-controlled T1D, magnetic resonance spectroscopy helped to answer this question.[62] Eight doses of glucagon (mean dose of 140 μg, total mean dose 1125 μg) dosed over 16 hours with repeated magnetic resonance spectroscopy scans quantitated glycogen stores. There was a non–statistically significant trend toward a decline in glycogen stores in the fed state after glucagon dosing. In the fasting state, the baseline glycogen stores were lower, but there was a non–statistically significant increase in glycogen stores after the glucagon doses. Importantly, the impact of glucagon increasing glucose levels was maintained through the eighth glucagon dosing. Longer-term studies are needed to better understand whether the glucagon response is maintained over time, but this study provides useful evidence that glycogen stores are not markedly reduced by repeated glucagon administration and the hyperglycemic response is also maintained.

Interactions Between Insulin and Glucagon

Insulin analogues show slow absorption from the subcutaneous space and remain active in the body for 4 to 6 hours or more in most patients. In people treated with insulin, hypoglycemia often occurs during a high-insulin state, which reduces glucagon's ability to counteract hypoglycemia because the ratio of insulin to glucagon within the portal venous system determines whether the liver can undergo glycogenolysis. A dual-hormone study[63] analyzed circumstances under which glucagon dosing failed to prevent hypoglycemia. Many failures correlated with higher insulin-on-board conditions and also during sensor overestimation of glucose. This study[55] examined the effect of varying insulin levels on the endogenous glucose production rate produced in response to varying glucagon doses. Low and medium insulin infusion rates showed proportional endogenous glucose production response in relation to the glucagon dose, whereas, under high insulin infusion, increased glucagon doses did not result in increases in endogenous glucose production.

Dietary and Lifestyle Considerations

The effect of glucagon on glucose depends on adequate hepatic glycogen stores. In normal people, low-carbohydrate diets reduce hepatic glycogen stores.[64] In 1 study,[65] adults eating a low-carbohydrate diet (<50 g/d for 1 week) versus a high-carbohydrate diet (>250 g/d for 1 week) showed that glucose levels increased less in response to subcutaneous doses of glucagon (100, 500 μg). Dual-hormone systems may need to account for an anticipated blunted glucose response to glucagon in patients eating a lower-carbohydrate diet.

Alcohol intake can lead to several factors that synergistically cause hypoglycemia in T1D. Ethanol inhibits hepatic gluconeogenesis,[66] causes hypoglycemia unawareness,[67] and impairs cognitive performance.[68] During ethanol intoxication, circulating glucose derives from hepatic glycogenolysis, therefore glycogen stores may be inadequate to allow a hyperglycemic response to glucagon administration. One study[69] showed a diminished hyperglycemic response to 100 μg of glucagon following ethanol consumption (equivalent to 4–6 drinks) compared with placebo consumption. Encouragingly, a second subcutaneous glucagon dose of 100 μg 2 hours later showed a similar glucose level–increasing profile, indicating that, despite prior alcohol consumption, some degree of hyperglycemic response is still possible.

SAFETY OF GLUCAGON

The potential side effects of glucagon are listed in **Table 2**. New liquid stable glucagon products intended for long-term use in subcutaneous infusion pump systems will need to go through thorough evaluation for safety and efficacy. Before these trials are done in humans, animal studies will be needed to show initial proof of safety. A recent animal study in rats and dogs with a glucagon analogue showed promising safety results.[81] Animals were dosed subcutaneously for 26 weeks (rats) or 39 weeks (dogs) with 10-fold varying doses of the glucagon product. At the equivalent dosing level

Table 2
Possible side effects of glucagon

Site	Impact	Mechanism	Comments
Gastrointestinal	Nausea and vomiting	Inhibition of gastric motility	Common side effects to the 1-mg hypoglycemia rescue dose of glucagon, but much less common at the microdosing level used in DH systems
Metabolism	Potential decrease in plasma triglyceride and cholesterol levels. Administration of high doses increases resting metabolic rate	Promotes triglyceride lipolysis to produce free fatty acids and hepatic fatty acid oxidation for fuel substrates[70]	In short-term human studies, administration of exogenous glucagon seems to have little effect on plasma lipid levels in healthy subjects or in subjects with T1D[71,72] In a rat model, administration of glucagon over 21 d decreased plasma triglyceride and cholesterol levels with no change in liver fat[73] In healthy subjects, glucagon infusion, along with a somatostatin infusion to inhibit insulin secretion, increased the resting metabolic rate by 15%[74]
Cardiovascular	Administration of high-dose glucagon can induce small increases in mean arterial pressure and heart rate without major effects on systemic vascular resistance[75]	At doses of >1 mg of glucagon, glucagon acts directly on cardiac tissues with chronotropic and inotropic effects via stimulation of catecholamines	Older animal studies showed a detrimental effect of high-dose glucagon on ischemic myocardium[76,77] Human studies showed benefit or no effect of high-dose glucagon in myocardial ischemia[78,79]

(*continued on next page*)

Table 2 (*continued*)

Site	Impact	Mechanism	Comments
Central nervous system	Administration of high-dose glucagon elicits feeling of satiety	Glucagon crosses the blood-brain barrier affecting the vagal system	In 1 study, preprandial 1-mg IM doses of glucagon over 2 wk in healthy adults resulted in a reduction in intake of 440 calories/d and an average weight loss of 0.2 kg (0.45 lb) compared with weight gain of 1.5 kg (3.4 lb) in the placebo arm[80]
Urinary	Increased natriuresis	Possibly mediated by renal arterial vasodilation with an increase in renal blood flow[70]	—
Respiratory	Pulmonary bronchodilation	Smooth muscle relaxation	—

Abbreviation: IM, intramuscular.
Data from Refs.[70–80]

of 1 mg/d in humans, which is equivalent to current dual-hormone studies, no unexpected adverse effects were seen in the animals. There was an increase in liver weight, glycogen vacuole formulation in the liver, and liver function marker levels during the study, but this was thought to be caused by the hyperinsulinism induced by the glucagon in these animals, which did not have diabetes. Results are awaited from long-term animal and human safety studies for other stable liquid glucagon formulations in development.

OTHER POTENTIAL HORMONES FOR CLOSED-LOOP SYSTEMS

A few other hormones are under consideration for adjunctive use with AID systems. Pramlintide is the synthetic form of amylin, which is cosecreted from beta cells in a ratio with insulin of 100:1 (insulin/amylin).[82] Amylin secretion is lost along with insulin secretion in T1D. Pramlintide is effective in reducing postprandial glucose spikes, presumably by slowing gastric emptying. Over the course of a 1-year trial in T1D with administration before each meal, pramlintide reduced hemoglobin A1c by 0.2% to 0.6%.[83] Fixed premeal doses of 30 μg of subcutaneous pramlintide used in conjunction with an insulin-only closed-loop system requiring meal announcement resulted in improved postprandial glucose levels and reduced area under the curve for the glucose excursions.[84] Other studies have shown improved postprandial control with adjunctive use of liraglutide (glucagonlike peptide-1 receptor agonist) as a once-daily subcutaneous dose.[85,86] Most recently, a dual-hormone system delivering a fixed ratio of pramlintide to insulin (6 μg/unit) significantly improved time in target range (70–180 mg/dL or 3.9–10 mmol/L) and glucose variability compared with a single-hormone closed-loop system.[87]

SUMMARY

The inclusion of glucagon in dual-hormone closed-loop systems seems to be effective in reducing overall hypoglycemia and hypoglycemia related to exercise. Additional clinical trials are needed to assess whether these benefits are persistent and the side effect profile remains favorable in longer-term studies. There are technical and pharmaceutical advances that will be needed in glucagon formulations and pump technologies before this approach can be feasible in free-living conditions. Dual-hormone closed-loop control is not likely to become standard of care for all people with T1D. However, development and research should continue because it is likely to be an important option for those who have recurrent hypoglycemia while using single-hormone closed-loop systems and in those who are physically active with recurrent hypoglycemia.

DISCLOSURE

L.M. Wilson has nothing to disclose. P.G. Jacobs and J.R. Castle have a financial interest in Pacific Diabetes Technologies, Inc, a company that may have a commercial interest in the results of this type of research and technology. This potential conflict of interest has been reviewed and managed by OHSU. In addition, P.G. Jacobs and J.R. Castle report research support from Xeris, Dexcom, and Tandem Diabetes Care. J.R. Castle reports advisory board participation for Zealand Pharma and Novo Nordisk, consulting for Dexcom, and a United States patent on the use of ferulic acid to stabilize glucagon.

REFERENCES

1. Diabetes Control and Complications Trial Research Group. The effect of intensive treatment of diabetes on the development and progression of long-term complications in insulin-dependent diabetes mellitus. N Engl J Med 1993;329(14):977–86.
2. Cryer PE, Davis SN, Shamoon H. Hypoglycemia in diabetes. Diabetes Care 2003;26(6):1902–12.
3. Diabetes Control and Complications Trial Research Group. Hypoglycemia in the diabetes control and complications trial. Diabetes 1997;46(2):271–86.
4. Unger RH, Orci L. Paracrinology of islets and the paracrinopathy of diabetes. Proc Natl Acad Sci U S A 2010;107(37):16009–12.
5. Farhy LS, McCall AL. Glucagon - the new 'insulin' in the pathophysiology of diabetes. Curr Opin Clin Nutr Metab Care 2015;18(4):407–14.
6. Cryer PE. Mechanisms of hypoglycemia-associated autonomic failure in diabetes. N Engl J Med 2013;369(4):362–72.
7. Peters TM, Haidar A. Dual-hormone artificial pancreas: benefits and limitations compared with single-hormone systems. Diabet Med 2018;35(4):450–9.
8. Riddell MC, Gallen IW, Smart CE, et al. Exercise management in type 1 diabetes: a consensus statement. Lancet Diabetes Endocrinol 2017;5(5):377–90.
9. Cryer PE. Diverse causes of hypoglycemia-associated autonomic failure in diabetes. N Engl J Med 2004;350(22):2272–9.
10. Haymond MW, Schreiner B. Mini-dose glucagon rescue for hypoglycemia in children with type 1 diabetes. Diabetes Care 2001;24(4):643–5.
11. Rickels MR, DuBose SN, Toschi E, et al. Mini-dose glucagon as a novel approach to prevent exercise-induced hypoglycemia in type 1 diabetes. Diabetes Care 2018;41(9):1909–16.

12. Taleb N, Emami A, Suppere C, et al. Efficacy of single-hormone and dual-hormone artificial pancreas during continuous and interval exercise in adult patients with type 1 diabetes: randomised controlled crossover trial. Diabetologia 2016;59(12):2561–71.
13. Unger RH, Orci L. Physiology and pathophysiology of glucagon. Physiol Rev 1976;56(4):778–826.
14. Nordisk N. Prescribing information for GlucaGen HypoKit 2018. Available at: http://www.novo-pi.com/glucagenhypokit.pdf. Accessed November 5, 2019.
15. Lilly E. Prescribing information for glucagon for injection (rDNA ORIGIN). 2018. Available at: http://pi.lilly.com/us/rglucagon-pi.pdf. Accessed November 5, 2019.
16. Blauw H, Wendl I, DeVries JH, et al. Pharmacokinetics and pharmacodynamics of various glucagon dosages at different blood glucose levels. Diabetes Obes Metab 2016;18(1):34–9.
17. Ranjan A, Schmidt S, Madsbad S, et al. Effects of subcutaneous, low-dose glucagon on insulin-induced mild hypoglycaemia in patients with insulin pump treated type 1 diabetes. Diabetes Obes Metab 2016;18(4):410–8.
18. Graf CJ, Woodworth JR, Seger ME, et al. Pharmacokinetic and glucodynamic comparisons of recombinant and animal-source glucagon after IV, IM, and SC injection in healthy volunteers. J Pharm Sci 1999;88(10):991–5.
19. Bekiari E, Kitsios K, Thabit H, et al. Artificial pancreas treatment for outpatients with type 1 diabetes: systematic review and meta-analysis. BMJ 2018;361:k1310.
20. Weisman A, Bai JW, Cardinez M, et al. Effect of artificial pancreas systems on glycaemic control in patients with type 1 diabetes: a systematic review and meta-analysis of outpatient randomised controlled trials. Lancet Diabetes Endocrinol 2017;5(7):501–12.
21. Brazeau A-S, Rabasa-Lhoret R, Strychar I, et al. Barriers to physical activity among patients with type 1 diabetes. Diabetes Care 2008;31(11):2108–9.
22. Lascar N, Kennedy A, Hancock B, et al. Attitudes and barriers to exercise in adults with type 1 diabetes (T1DM) and how best to address them: a qualitative study. PLoS One 2014;9(9):e108019.
23. Camacho RC, Galassetti P, Davis SN, et al. Glucoregulation during and after exercise in health and insulin-dependent diabetes. Exerc Sport Sci Rev 2005;33(1):17–23.
24. Ploug T, Galbo H, Richter EA. Increased muscle glucose uptake during contractions: no need for insulin. Am J Physiol 1984;247(6 Pt 1):E726–31.
25. Reddy R, El Youssef J, Winters-Stone K, et al. The effect of exercise on sleep in adults with type 1 diabetes. Diabetes Obes Metab 2018;20(2):443–7.
26. Miller KM, Foster NC, Beck RW, et al. Current state of type 1 diabetes treatment in the U.S.: updated data from the T1D Exchange clinic registry. Diabetes Care 2015;38(6):971–8.
27. Steineck IIK, Ranjan A, Schmidt S, et al. Preserved glucose response to low-dose glucagon after exercise in insulin-pump-treated individuals with type 1 diabetes: a randomised crossover study. Diabetologia 2019;62(4):582–92.
28. Castle JR, El Youssef J, Wilson LM, et al. Randomized outpatient trial of single- and dual-hormone closed-loop systems that adapt to exercise using wearable sensors. Diabetes Care 2018;41(7):1471–7.
29. Jacobs PG, El Youssef J, Reddy R, et al. Randomized trial of a dual-hormone artificial pancreas with dosing adjustment during exercise compared with no adjustment and sensor-augmented pump therapy. Diabetes Obes Metab 2016;18(11):1110–9.

30. Haidar A, Legault L, Messier V, et al. Comparison of dual-hormone artificial pancreas, single-hormone artificial pancreas, and conventional insulin pump therapy for glycaemic control in patients with type 1 diabetes: an open-label randomised controlled crossover trial. Lancet Diabetes Endocrinol 2015;3(1): 17–26.
31. Abitbol A, Rabasa-Lhoret R, Messier V, et al. Overnight glucose control with dual- and single-hormone artificial pancreas in type 1 diabetes with hypoglycemia unawareness: a randomized controlled trial. Diabetes Technol Ther 2018;20(3): 189–96.
32. Dagogo-Jack S, Rattarasarn C, Cryer PE. Reversal of hypoglycemia unawareness, but not defective glucose counterregulation, in IDDM. Diabetes 1994; 43(12):1426–34.
33. Brazeau AS, Mircescu H, Desjardins K, et al. Carbohydrate counting accuracy and blood glucose variability in adults with type 1 diabetes. Diabetes Res Clin Pract 2013;99(1):19–23.
34. Gingras V, Taleb N, Roy-Fleming A, et al. The challenges of achieving postprandial glucose control using closed-loop systems in patients with type 1 diabetes. Diabetes Obes Metab 2018;20(2):245–56.
35. El-Khatib FH, Russell SJ, Nathan DM, et al. A bihormonal closed-loop artificial pancreas for type 1 diabetes. Sci Transl Med 2010;2(27):27ra27.
36. van Bon AC, Luijf YM, Koebrugge R, et al. Feasibility of a portable bihormonal closed-loop system to control glucose excursions at home under free-living conditions for 48 hours. Diabetes Technol Ther 2014;16(3):131–6.
37. Shichiri M, Kawamori R, Yamasaki Y, et al. Wearable artificial endocrine pancrease with needle-type glucose sensor. Lancet 1982;2(8308):1129–31.
38. Haidar A, Messier V, Legault L, et al. Outpatient 60-hour day-and-night glucose control with dual-hormone artificial pancreas, single-hormone artificial pancreas, or sensor-augmented pump therapy in adults with type 1 diabetes: an open-label, randomised, crossover, controlled trial. Diabetes Obes Metab 2017; 19(5):713–20.
39. Castle JR, Engle JM, El Youssef J, et al. Novel use of glucagon in a closed-loop system for prevention of hypoglycemia in type 1 diabetes. Diabetes Care 2010; 33(6):1282–7.
40. Russell SJ, El-Khatib FH, Sinha M, et al. Outpatient glycemic control with a bionic pancreas in type 1 diabetes. N Engl J Med 2014;371(4):313–25.
41. Russell SJ, Hillard MA, Balliro C, et al. Day and night glycaemic control with a bionic pancreas versus conventional insulin pump therapy in preadolescent children with type 1 diabetes: a randomised crossover trial. Lancet Diabetes Endocrinol 2016;4(3):233–43.
42. El-Khatib FH, Balliro C, Hillard MA, et al. Home use of a bihormonal bionic pancreas versus insulin pump therapy in adults with type 1 diabetes: a multicentre randomised crossover trial. Lancet 2017;389(10067):369–80.
43. Haidar A, Legault L, Dallaire M, et al. Glucose-responsive insulin and glucagon delivery (dual-hormone artificial pancreas) in adults with type 1 diabetes: a randomized crossover controlled trial. CMAJ 2013;185(4):297–305.
44. Haidar A, Legault L, Matteau-Pelletier L, et al. Outpatient overnight glucose control with dual-hormone artificial pancreas, single-hormone artificial pancreas, or conventional insulin pump therapy in children and adolescents with type 1 diabetes: an open-label, randomised controlled trial. Lancet Diabetes Endocrinol 2015;3(8):595–604.

45. Haidar A, Rabasa-Lhoret R, Legault L, et al. Single- and dual-hormone artificial pancreas for overnight glucose control in type 1 diabetes. J Clin Endocrinol Metab 2016;101(1):214–23.
46. Gingras V, Rabasa-Lhoret R, Messier V, et al. Efficacy of dual-hormone artificial pancreas to alleviate the carbohydrate-counting burden of type 1 diabetes: a randomized crossover trial. Diabetes Metab 2016;42(1):47–54.
47. Jackson MA, Caputo N, Castle JR, et al. Stable liquid glucagon formulations for rescue treatment and bi-hormonal closed-loop pancreas. Curr Diab Rep 2012;12(6):705–10.
48. van Bon AC, Jonker LD, Koebrugge R, et al. Feasibility of a bihormonal closed-loop system to control postexercise and postprandial glucose excursions. J Diabetes Sci Technol 2012;6(5):1114–22.
49. Blauw H, van Bon AC, Koops R, et al. Performance and safety of an integrated bihormonal artificial pancreas for fully automated glucose control at home. Diabetes Obes Metab 2016;18(7):671–7.
50. Russell SJ, El-Khatib FH, Nathan DM, et al. Blood glucose control in type 1 diabetes with a bihormonal bionic endocrine pancreas. Diabetes Care 2012;35:2148–55.
51. El-Khatib FH, Russell SJ, Magyar KL, et al. Autonomous and continuous adaptation of a bihormonal bionic pancreas in adults and adolescents with type 1 diabetes. J Clin Endocrinol Metab 2014;99:1701–11.
52. Maahs DM, Buckingham BA, Castle JR, et al. Outcome measures for artificial pancreas clinical trials: a consensus report. Diabetes Care 2016;39(7):1175–9.
53. Jacobs PG, Resalat N, El Youssef J, et al. Incorporating an exercise detection, grading, and hormone dosing algorithm into the artificial pancreas using accelerometry and heart rate. J Diabetes Sci Technol 2015;9(6):1175–84.
54. Heptulla RA, Rodriguez LM, Bomgaars L, et al. The role of amylin and glucagon in the dampening of glycemic excursions in children with type 1 diabetes. Diabetes 2005;54(4):1100–7.
55. El Youssef J, Castle JR, Bakhtiani PA, et al. Quantification of the glycemic response to microdoses of subcutaneous glucagon at varying insulin levels. Diabetes Care 2014;37(11):3054–60.
56. Wilson LM, Castle JR. Stable liquid glucagon: beyond emergency hypoglycemia rescue. J Diabetes Sci Technol 2018;12(4):847–53.
57. Wilson LM, Jacobs PG, Resalat N, et al. Abstract: results of interim analysis of a randomized cross-over study in type 1 diabetes (T1D) of a dual-hormone closed-loop system with Xerisol™ glucagon vs insulin-only closed-loop system vs a predictive low glucose suspend system. Diabetes 2019;68(Supplement 1):1038-P.
58. Famulla S, Hovelmann U, Fischer A, et al. Insulin injection into lipohypertrophic tissue: blunted and more variable insulin absorption and action and impaired postprandial glucose control. Diabetes Care 2016;39(9):1486–92.
59. Introducing the iLet. 2018. Available at: https://www.betabionics.com/. Accessed April 26, 2019.
60. Kishore P, Gabriely I, Cui MH, et al. Role of hepatic glycogen breakdown in defective counterregulation of hypoglycemia in intensively treated type 1 diabetes. Diabetes 2006;55(3):659–66.
61. Bischof MG, Krssak M, Krebs M, et al. Effects of short-term improvement of insulin treatment and glycemia on hepatic glycogen metabolism in type 1 diabetes. Diabetes 2001;50(2):392–8.

62. Castle JR, El Youssef J, Bakhtiani PA, et al. Effect of repeated glucagon doses on hepatic glycogen in type 1 diabetes: implications for a bihormonal closed-loop system. Diabetes Care 2015;38(11):2115–9.
63. Castle JR, Engle JM, El Youssef J, et al. Factors influencing the effectiveness of glucagon for preventing hypoglycemia. J Diabetes Sci Technol 2010;4(6): 1305–10.
64. Nilsson LH, Hultman E. Liver glycogen in man–the effect of total starvation or a carbohydrate-poor diet followed by carbohydrate refeeding. Scand J Clin Lab Invest 1973;32(4):325–30.
65. Ranjan A, Schmidt S, Damm-Frydenberg C, et al. Low-carbohydrate diet impairs the effect of glucagon in the treatment of insulin-induced mild hypoglycemia: a randomized crossover study. Diabetes Care 2017;40(1):132–5.
66. Krebs HA, Freedland RA, Hems R, et al. Inhibition of hepatic gluconeogenesis by ethanol. Biochem J 1969;112(1):117–24.
67. Kerr D, Macdonald IA, Heller SR, et al. Alcohol causes hypoglycaemic unawareness in healthy volunteers and patients with type 1 (insulin-dependent) diabetes. Diabetologia 1990;33(4):216–21.
68. Cheyne EH, Sherwin RS, Lunt MJ, et al. Influence of alcohol on cognitive performance during mild hypoglycaemia; implications for type 1 diabetes. Diabet Med 2004;21(3):230–7.
69. Ranjan A, Norgaard K, Tetzschner R, et al. Effects of preceding ethanol intake on glucose response to low-dose glucagon in individuals with type 1 diabetes: a randomized, placebo-controlled, crossover study. Diabetes Care 2018;41(4): 797–806.
70. Taleb N, Haidar A, Messier V, et al. Glucagon in artificial pancreas systems: potential benefits and safety profile of future chronic use. Diabetes Obes Metab 2017;19(1):13–23.
71. Jensen MD, Heiling VJ, Miles JM. Effects of glucagon on free fatty acid metabolism in humans. J Clin Endocrinol Metab 1991;72(2):308–15.
72. Gravholt CH, Moller N, Jensen MD, et al. Physiological levels of glucagon do not influence lipolysis in abdominal adipose tissue as assessed by microdialysis. J Clin Endocrinol Metab 2001;86(5):2085–9.
73. Guettet C, Mathe D, Navarro N, et al. Effects of chronic glucagon administration on rat lipoprotein composition. Biochim Biophys Acta 1989;1005(3):233–8.
74. Nair KS. Hyperglucagonemia increases resting metabolic rate in man during insulin deficiency. J Clin Endocrinol Metab 1987;64(5):896–901.
75. Parmley WW, Glick G, Sonnenblick EH. Cardiovascular effects of glucagon in man. N Engl J Med 1968;279(1):12–7.
76. Maroko PR, Kjekshus JK, Sobel BE, et al. Factors influencing infarct size following experimental coronary artery occlusions. Circulation 1971;43(1):67–82.
77. Goodwin GW, Taegtmeyer H. Metabolic recovery of isolated working rat heart after brief global ischemia. Am J Physiol 1994;267(2 Pt 2):H462–70.
78. Arstila M, Iisalo F, Kallio V, et al. The effect of a long-acting glucagon preparation on endocrine and metabolic responses in acute myocardial infarction. Acta Med Scand 1974;196(5):423–30.
79. Eddy JD, O'Brien ET, Singh SP. Glucagon and haemodynamics of acute myocardial infarction. Br Med J 1969;4(5684):663–5.
80. Schulman JL, Carleton JL, Whitney G, et al. Effect of glucagon on food intake and body weight in man. J Appl Physiol 1957;11(3):419–21.
81. Castle JR, Elander M. Long-term safety and tolerability of dasiglucagon, a stable-in-solution glucagon analogue. Diabetes Technol Ther 2019;21(2):94–6.

82. Schmitz O, Brock B, Rungby J. Amylin agonists: a novel approach in the treatment of diabetes. Diabetes 2004;53(Suppl 3):S233–8.
83. Ryan G, Briscoe TA, Jobe L. Review of pramlintide as adjunctive therapy in treatment of type 1 and type 2 diabetes. Drug Des Devel Ther 2009;2:203–14.
84. Weinzimer SA, Sherr JL, Cengiz E, et al. Effect of pramlintide on prandial glycemic excursions during closed-loop control in adolescents and young adults with type 1 diabetes. Diabetes Care 2012;35(10):1994–9.
85. Ilkowitz JT, Katikaneni R, Cantwell M, et al. Adjuvant liraglutide and insulin versus insulin monotherapy in the closed-loop system in type 1 diabetes: a randomized open-labeled crossover design trial. J Diabetes Sci Technol 2016;10(5):1108–14.
86. Sherr JL, Patel NS, Michaud CI, et al. Mitigating meal-related glycemic excursions in an insulin-sparing manner during closed-loop insulin delivery: the beneficial effects of adjunctive pramlintide and liraglutide. Diabetes Care 2016;39(7):1127–34.
87. Haidar A, Tsoukas M, Sarah T, et al. Insulin-plus-pramlintide artificial pancreas in type 1 diabetes—randomized controlled trial. Diabetes 2018;67(Supplement 1):A55–6.

Do-It-Yourself Artificial Pancreas System and the OpenAPS Movement

Dana M. Lewis, BA

KEYWORDS

• Artificial pancreas system • Hybrid closed loop system • APS • OpenAPS
• Open source diabetes technology • Do-it-yourself • DIY

KEY POINTS

- People with diabetes have been experimenting with and modifying their own diabetes devices and technologies for many decades, in order to achieve the best possible quality of life and improving their long-term outcomes, including do-it-yourself (DIY) closed loop systems.
- Thousands of individuals use DIY closed loop systems globally, which work similarly to commercial systems by automatically adjusting and controlling insulin dosing, but are different in terms of transparency, access, customization, and usability.
- Initial outcomes seen by the DIY artificial pancreas system (APS) community are positive, reflected in studies ranging from self-reported outcomes to observational studies with improvements in hemoglobin A1c, time in range, and other outcomes, such as quality-of-life benefits, and randomized controlled trials are forthcoming on various elements of DIYAPS technology.

Diabetes is complicated. However, the understanding is often oversimplified. This starts at diagnosis: "your body no longer makes insulin; take injections and you will be ok," and "there is technology to help, and a cure is right around the corner: probably in about 5 years."

After the initial shock wears off after diagnosis, the person with diabetes and/or their caregivers realize that living safely with the disease is not so simple. The oversimplifications ("take insulin, watch your food intake, exercise, and you can manage diabetes well") come into conflict with the realities of life with type 1 diabetes. Adam Brown has quantified that there are (at least) 42 factors that impact blood glucose (BG) levels.[1] Many of these are hard to track, measure, or quantify, never mind adjusting insulin dosing for them. In a given day, a person might make 300 decisions that will impact their BG levels.[2] How is a person supposed to keep track of everything, and keep up, all day, every day, day in and day out, with no vacation? Managing type 1 diabetes

OpenAPS, Seattle, WA 98101, USA
E-mail address: Dana@OpenAPS.org

Endocrinol Metab Clin N Am 49 (2020) 203–213
https://doi.org/10.1016/j.ecl.2019.10.005

is like single-handedly taking care of a newborn infant, except this infant is not going to grow up and become more and more self-sufficient.

Further complicating the challenges of living with type 1 diabetes is the fact that diabetes is a self-managed disease. A patient may spend 15 to 30 minutes with their health care provider every few months, but they can easily spend 1 to 2 hours per day, usually a few minutes at a time, managing the unmanageable. That means that anyone with "well-managed" type 1 diabetes is going to be spending well over 99% of the time required to do so: 100 times as much time as their health care professionals can afford to spend with them. This is also true to varying extents with other chronic illnesses. Sara Riggare, who lives with Parkinson disease, has quantified the amount of time spent in self-management compared with the time spent managing under direct supervision of a health care provider.[3] The numbers for diabetes are very similar: even the patients (or their parents) who only do just enough to keep themselves out of the hospital are still doing more than 95% of the work.[4]

Given the amount of time and work required, and how intrusive type 1 diabetes is if you do not spend that time, it is no surprise that patients often push for better tools and technology for self-managing life with type 1 diabetes. They need to improve their own quality of life and also want to improve their long-term prospects. This, in fact, is not a new phenomenon. Self-monitoring BG testing is one such example of something that is now a standard of care, but that was originally pushed into practice as a result of patients proceeding, over their health care providers' protests, to build, procure, and modify the equipment required to test their own BG at home and modify their own insulin dosing based on the test results.[5] Similarly, when continuous glucose monitors (CGMs) became available, many clinicians protested (and some still do) that patients would not benefit from real-time access to their own data. Secondary monitoring of the same data (by parents and other loved ones) is something that was also resisted in the clinical and medical device communities for years.[6] Making dosing decisions from CGM data was also a practice first driven by the patient community, and only later followed by regulatory approval of devices to permit such decisions to be performed based on CGM data alone. In light of all of these innovations that are now standard practice, it is perhaps no longer as surprising to hear that patients, too, have pushed for better quality of life by self-building their own hybrid closed loop systems, also known as automated insulin delivery systems or "artificial pancreas" systems (APS). These systems generically are often known as do-it-yourself (DIY) APS.

THE DEVELOPMENT OF DO-IT-YOURSELF ARTIFICIAL PANCREAS SYSTEM

What later became the first DIYAPS was initially borne not out of a desire to automate insulin dosing, but from a much smaller frustration with existing diabetes devices.[7] In particular, I, a patient with no medical or technology background whatsoever, became fed up with the complete inability to customize volume or alter the sound of CGM alarms. I lived by myself and was unable to hear my CGM alarm overnight, so I worried about not waking up for overnight lows. Multiple manufacturers told me that not that many people have this problem; it was just me. (*Interestingly, there are 46,800 search results in Google for "louder CGM alarm."*) I was also told they were working on it, and to expect it out in the next version. Familiar with the timeline of medical device development cycles, I knew I would be in for a long wait. I knew that if I could somehow build a system that would take the CGM data and feed it into my phone, I could alter the alarm type and volume as needed. However, I did not have access to the data from my CGM. The Food and Drug Administration–approved software at the time was only available for PCs, and I had a Mac computer. The CGM also only permitted, via the approved software, a 30-day download of retrospective CGM data. I had no way to access it in real time.

This, however, changed. I stumbled across an old tweet from John Costik, who had reverse engineered the driver to pull the data off of the CGM in real time. His goal was remote monitoring his son's BG levels. My then-boyfriend, now husband, Scott Leibrand, and I asked if he would share his code, so that I could also access my CGM data in real time and build my louder alarm system on the phone. He said yes, shared the code, and enabled us to get started.

With this code, I was able to send my CGM data from a local computer up to the cloud and then send alerts to my phone via an app called "Pushover."[8] We also built a simple Web page to display my data so I could also input additional data like insulin and food. Although my original goal was not remote monitoring, we ended up building a tiered alarm system so that if I did not awake to a critical alarm, it would alert my loved ones, who could call me. With the additional data I tracked alongside the BG levels from the CGM, we were able to build an algorithm to predict the impact of food and insulin and activity on BG levels over time. This allowed us to generate predictive alarms and make recommendations for actions in order to mitigate and/or prevent, when possible, high- and low-glucose levels. It was essentially an "open loop" system that had evolved from my louder alarm system.

Because we had been helped via social media and by John, I also wanted to share my solution with other people. We called it, jokingly, "DIYPS," for the "do-it-yourself pancreas system." We began sharing on social media about my louder, smart alarm system and how it was working, and began creating a community and meeting other individuals who had been working on interesting DIY diabetes device-related projects. One individual that we met as a result is Ben West, who had spent years[9] examining the communication from an older-generation Medtronic (Medtronic, Inc., Northridge, CA) insulin pump. He reverse-engineered the communication protocols and proved that you could send commands, such as setting temporary basal rates, on the pump. A few months later, a light bulb went off when we realized that we now had all the components for a DIY closed loop: real-time CGM data; communication to the insulin pump; and an algorithm to drive predictions and subsequent insulin dosing adjustments. We closed the loop, and I put it to good use in early December 2014 and launched an open source version in February 2015 that became known as OpenAPS.[10]

OpenAPS IS DESIGNED FOR SAFETY

One of the reasons we decided to share our designs and code is because we knew that others would also try to close the loop once they found out it was possible. We had spent more than a year iterating and testing the algorithm in open loop mode and several months testing the device communications that allowed automated insulin delivery, so we wanted to share that knowledge so others could benefit from it as well as build upon it. This is why, in addition to code, we also released the OpenAPS Reference Design as a plain language document to help articulate the safety design and constraints of a DIY closed loop system.[11] The aim was to help individuals better understand what the system could and could not do and help people make informed decisions about whether the choice to DIYAPS would be right for them.

One of the main safety considerations with any DIYAPS is that it must be built by the individual. This has become easier over time, because the community has grown and collectively decided what steps can be automated and what steps need to be done by each person in order to build their system.

Other safety considerations are built into the backbone of the system design. The base OpenAPS algorithm will only send 30-minute temporary basal rate commands to the pump. Each dosing command would be calculated and sent under the assumption that it would be the last command that would reach the pump. Therefore, if the system lost power or could not communicate with the pump, the temporary basal rate would expire at the end of the 30 minutes, and the pump would fall back to standard pump operations. We also designed the system to not overly rely on a single CGM data point, to deal with calibration or compression lows or sensor dropout for any reason, and added numerous other safety-first elements into the design. Because the system is designed around the same diabetes math a patient would be doing manually, it is open, transparent about how it works (and what and why it is taking any action or not) at all times, in a way that the user can actually evaluate its decisions for themselves.[12]

In all DIYAPSs, there are numerous hardware settings on the pump (such as maximum basal rate) as well as software safety limits (such as maximum Insulin on Board (IOB) limits) to allow an individual to fully decide how much the system is allowed to adjust insulin delivery at any given time.

Early DIYAPSs used the older-generation Medtronic insulin pumps, which use a proprietary 915-MHz radio protocol to communicate. Therefore, a radio bridge is needed to translate commands to and from the pump. The first DIYAPS used a small computer to hold the algorithm, paired with the radio bridge to communicate with the pump and CGM. Later implementations of DIYAPS have leveraged smartphones to hold the algorithm and interact via a small Bluetooth to radio bridge. Newer Bluetooth-enabled insulin pumps available in Europe and Asia can communicate directly with the smartphone, eliminating the need for custom hardware.

This increased interoperability allows more choice for patients: they can choose the pump body they wish to use, their CGM of choice, and the algorithm of their choice, along with the choice of additional hardware (if a radio bridge is needed for a particular pump) or software (if the pump can be communicated with via a mobile device). DIYAPS leverages already-approved pumps and CGMs, adding on the algorithm and hardware/software needed to make the system interoperable.

ADVANCED FEATURES ENABLING IMPROVED OUTCOMES WITH OpenAPS

Most closed loop systems work similarly, whether they are DIY or commercial. They gather CGM data and information about previous insulin dosing and any carbohydrate intake and build predictive forecasts for what the BG is likely to do over time. If the predicted BG level is out of range, they adjust insulin delivery accordingly.

Originally, OpenAPS was considered to be a "hybrid" closed loop system. This was because originally, the system was designed assuming that a patient would achieve the best outcomes by manually issuing a meal bolus and alerting the system to carbohydrate intake, because of the delayed peak of the most modern insulins. However, the community learned that not everyone did well with manual meal boluses. We continued to iterate the design of the OpenAPS algorithm, adding more advanced meal features over time. One core component to allow further assistance at mealtimes was developing the concept of "dynamic" carbohydrate absorption, recognizing that there are numerous times and reasons carbohydrate absorption may not be linear or even predictable. Responding in real time to the changes in BG level as compared with predicted BG levels allowed the system to help more in postprandial periods and yielded better outcomes than the previous version.

Over time, we have introduced additional features, such as super-microboluses (SMBs). These enable the system to issue small boluses in combination with reduced basal rates in order to front-shift the peak insulin activity and safely respond to rising BG without increasing hypoglycemia risk.[13] Users who have enabled this feature often choose to do a partial or no meal bolus at all and let the system fully deal with mealtime. Some users will do a meal announcement; some do not. Therefore, many users of OpenAPS and DIYAPS in general have progressed to using these systems as fully automated closed loop systems, no longer categorizing them as "hybrid" systems that require manual inputs at all times in order to achieve ideal outcomes.

Another advanced feature that has improved outcomes is "autosensitivity," which looks back at the last 8- and 24-hour time periods to gauge whether someone is more or less sensitive to insulin than their standard settings.[14] By comparing what actually happened to the predictions, the system is able to respond in a shorter timeframe than most users would in order to pick up on trends of sensitivity or resistance. This means menstrual cycle, sickness,[15] increased or decreased activity, and other gradual short-term swings in insulin needs are better accounted for automatically by the system, without requiring human adjustment of settings.

After developing autosensitivity, OpenAPS users began wanting to use it to adjust underlying basal rates, insulin sensitivity factor (ISF), and carbohydrate ratio settings, which drive the math in the algorithm. However, autosensitivity was not designed for that: it is a ratio that is applied proportionately to adjust basal rates and ISF and does not separate out the differences attributed to separate settings. This ability to adjust the basic settings, though, was a core need in the diabetes community (including outside of those using OpenAPS and DIYAPS). To meet this need, the OpenAPS community created Autotune. Autotune segments data based on categorizing it as being attributable mostly to basal rates, ISF, or carbohydrate ratio, and then tunes each setting independently.[16] Autotune is now widely used with all DIYAPS, as well as by many people without DIYAPS. As of this writing, there is still no commercial tool available to help patients make settings adjustments for insulin pumps outside of the regular clinical encounter.

In addition to the algorithm improvements, one key driver of improved outcomes has to do with flexibility and customization. DIYAPS permits choice and customization: remote or secondary monitoring, and the ability to change temporary targets or enter carbohydrate estimates can be performed on nearly any smartwatch or mobile device. Users can also adjust many more settings in DIYAPSs than what is allowed in commercial APSs. This flexibility, to use whichever tools and settings work best for someone's lifestyle, is one of the key reasons that DIYAPSs perform so well, even in patients already achieving good glycemic control. In a forthcoming paper (Dana M. Lewis, unpublished data, 2019), we worked with a team at Stanford University to assess other closed loop algorithms that implement machine learning models and compare the predictions and outcomes with OpenAPS users' results. One key result from that paper is that OpenAPS real-world data outperformed the systems used in various clinical trials with the machine learning algorithm models. Similar outcomes have since been seen in several other observational studies, as described in later discussion.

RESEARCH OUTCOMES FROM OpenAPS AND DO-IT-YOURSELF ARTIFICIAL PANCREAS SYSTEM AND FUTURE COMMERCIALIZATION

Research shows that closed loop systems improve clinical outcomes of those living with type 1 diabetes. This is true for commercial systems[17] and true for DIY closed loop systems. The first study of DIY systems was published in 2016 with a self-reported survey from 18 of the first 40 DIYAPS users.[18] In 2018, a subsequent study was published, this time analyzing the raw data directly from before and after OpenAPS implementation in n = 20. The outcomes mirrored those of the self-reported outcomes study.[19] In addition, 2 international groups independently evaluated real-world data from OpenAPS users in Italy[20] and Korea.[21] In both adult and pediatric populations, the results again were similar with improved hemoglobin A1c (A1c), improved time in range, and reduced hypoglycemia and hyperglycemia. **Figs. 1–3** compare these outcome studies.[22]

Additional studies have been conducted with different variations of DIYAPS and in different settings. In the Czech Republic, a study was done with a pediatric population at a ski camp, finding that AndroidAPS (the DIYAPS that uses the OpenAPS algorithm with an Android phone app and a Bluetooth-enabled pump) performed well in minimizing hypoglycemia, when compared with a low-glucose-suspend system.[23] The same researcher also recently initiated an in silico study of AndroidAPS and reported similar outcomes during a presentation at the most recent International Conference on Advanced Technologies and Treatments for Diabetes in February 2019 and announced plans to initiate subsequent randomized controlled trials with a global consortium to further assess DIYAPS for clinical use. Similarly, Tidepool, a nonprofit diabetes organization, recently announced their intention to take a version of Loop, the iOS DIYAPS that uses a different algorithm from OpenAPS/AndroidAPS, and initiate regulatory submission in order to bring it to market.[24] The Jaeb Center for Health Care Research (Tampa, FL) is currently conducting an observational trial to assess usage of the DIY Loop system,[25] which uses an iOS device and a radio bridge to talk to the older-generation insulin pumps. Tidepool announced that their version of Loop would come to market in partnership with Insulet (Insulet Corporation, Bedford, MA, USA) and use the latest

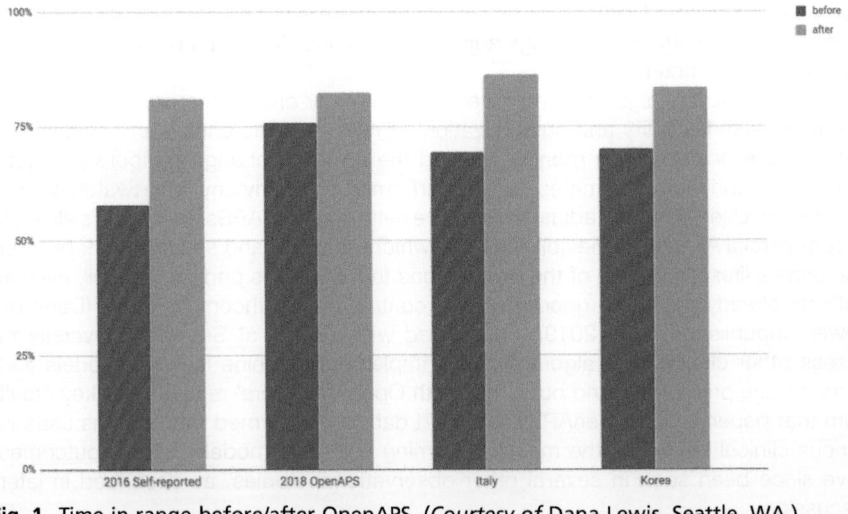

Fig. 1. Time in range before/after OpenAPS. (*Courtesy of* Dana Lewis, Seattle, WA.)

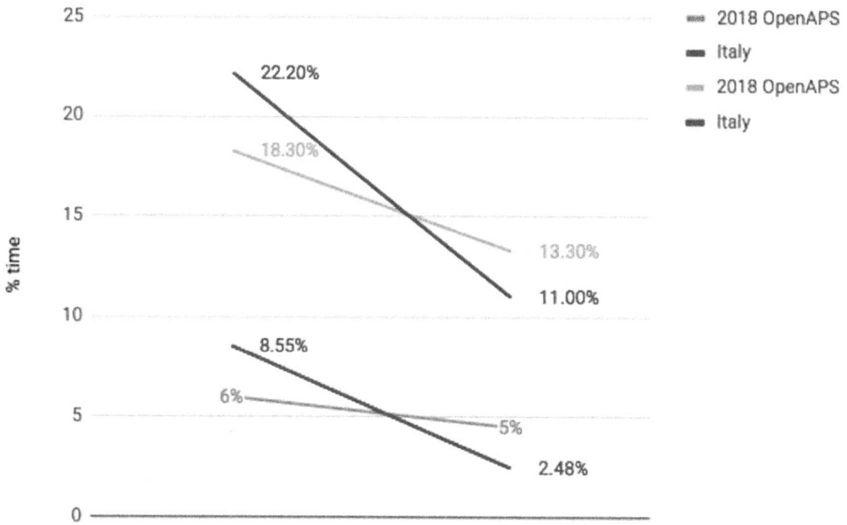

Fig. 2. Reduction in hypoglycemia and hyperglycemia. (*Courtesy of* Dana Lewis, Seattle, WA.)

Omnipod system, which uses Bluetooth technology instead of requiring a radio bridge.[26]

CONCERNS OF DO-IT-YOURSELF ARTIFICIAL PANCREAS SYSTEM

Plans to commercialize some of the DIY closed loop systems mitigate some of the potential concerns with DIYAPS. Many of these concerns center on the technical and hardware limitations of the limited number of insulin pumps on the market that have the availability to be communicated with the radio bridge as well as the security concerns known from using a pump's open communications. The future commercialization plans as well as JDRF Open Protocol Initiative to encourage interoperability

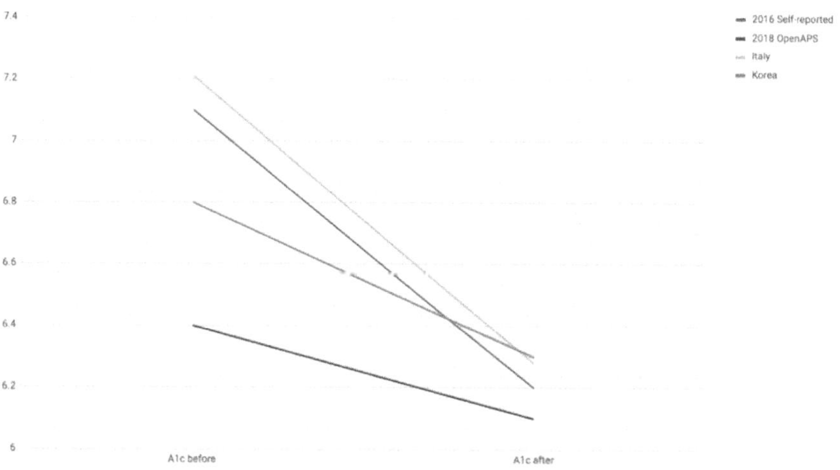

Fig. 3. Reduction in A1c. (*Courtesy of* Dana Lewis, Seattle, WA.)

between pumps, CGMs, and controllers/algorithms[27] mean that commercial versions of DIYAPS would not have the limitations currently existing in DIYAPS related to device communications. This removes some of the security risk and additional points of failure by using devices with approved, open protocols that are designed for this purpose.

In the meantime, the choice to use a DIYAPS comes with a financial cost to the user because of lack of support from their health care system. In some countries, individuals must self-fund CGM and may need to buy a compatible insulin pump out of pocket, which also would not be covered by insurance. The additional hardware components (radio bridge and/or minicomputer or smartphone) also have costs. (*Despite all these out-of-pocket costs, it is notable that the overall costs to build a DIYAPS are usually far lower than for commercially available closed loop technology, if it is even approved in that country.*)

There are also perceived and real technical barriers to DIYAPS. Many thousands of individuals, often with no technology experience, are currently using DIYAPS. However, many more are not comfortable with their skill level around technology[28] and are unwilling to try building or using a DIY closed loop system, despite ample evidence that they could do so if they tried. However, whether it is because of lack of ability, lack of affordability, or most commonly, lack of confidence or willingness, DIY is in practice not 100% accessible to everyone.

In addition, because DIY systems are not approved by a regulatory body, some clinicians are uncomfortable with patients using DIY technology that is considered to be "off-label" use of their existing pumps and CGMs. Some of the discomfort is due to lack of knowledge and familiarity with these systems, which may be mitigated over time as they become more familiar with APS in general. However, there is also discomfort in general with the perceived liability for the clinician's role when a patient uses DIY diabetes technology.[29] Different countries have different cultures, laws, guidelines, and regulations that influence this topic. The clinician's individual comfort level with patients self-directing their diabetes management may also play a role. Some clinicians may fully support patient choice and autonomy in diabetes management, while wanting to ensure that a patient is fully aware of the risks and as educated as possible about their choices. This range of clinician responses means that some patients may not bring up DIYAPS usage, if they predict that their clinician would be uncomfortable with discussing it or supporting their choice. Multiple diabetes societies around the world have now published position statements that encourage and support patient choice, while making it clear that they do not necessarily endorse or recommend DIYAPS.[30] This support of patient choice and the emphasis to clinicians to continue to support and care for patients, regardless of technology choice, is a positive movement that will help keep dialogue open between patients and clinicians.

One other topic of concern with DIYAPS or any type of APS is the issue of "deskilling." It is important for someone using APS of any kind to have core competency in certain diabetes skills, such as maintaining insulin pump sites, having good CGM calibration hygiene, and maintaining clean CGM data, and understanding how their system works and knowing when to fall back to "manual mode" and use their basic skills when APS is not working.[31] However, interestingly, with the advanced features of OpenAPS, we can now quantify the impacts of different behaviors, or absence of behaviors, and the resulting impact on A1c and time in range.

For example, with the OpenAPS simulator,[32] we were able to feed data in with an adult who uses the advanced features and does not enact manual meal boluses, but does do carbohydrate entry (meal announcement) for optimal outcomes. The simulator showed that this n = 1 adult would have a 0.4% A1c increase if they stopped announcing meals (and a 10% reduction in time in range). Similarly, we analyzed data for a male teen who eats an estimated 200 or more grams of carbohydrates a day but does not do any meal announcement or any manual meal boluses. Although this individual does have less time in range (73% at 80–180 mg/dL) compared with the adult who announces meals (91% at 80–180 mg/dL), and a slightly higher A1c, the outcomes are still far better than is typical for their age level, and exceed clinical guidelines. It is possible to quantify the difference of behavior, so if the teen wants data to reinforce how much the outcomes would be different if they did decide to do meal announcement or manual meal boluses, they would be able to quantify the difference and decide on the tradeoffs between outcomes and the effort required to achieve these outcomes.

This is possibly the first time in diabetes history that we have had the tools and technology to distill down and show cause and effect this clearly as to the impact of different behaviors that were previously considered to be required. This will likely have numerous impacts on quality of life, psychosocial well-being, improved interactions with the health care system, and improved family dynamics once we can use these tools more widely to change the conversation from one of negative language and failure to a conversation about the tradeoffs and choices between certain behaviors and influence on quality of life and the clinical outcomes that are possible.

THE ONGOING ROLE OF DO-IT-YOURSELF ARTIFICIAL PANCREAS SYSTEMS

Although there is now one commercial version of a hybrid closed loop system available in some countries, and there are more on the way, this does not mean the commercial APS is fully available, accessible, or affordable to those who want it. Cost will continue to be a concern for many worldwide living with type 1 diabetes, especially those who currently struggle to access and afford insulin, basic insulin pump supplies, and/or CGM. APS will be equally out of reach for many at commercial prices. We therefore predict that DIYAPS will likely continue to be a choice for many.

There are certainly downsides to the choice of DIYAPS, as discussed in this article, related to cost, technological barriers, and the requirements to self-build and self-maintain the system. However, there are also benefits[33]: DIYAPS is often lower cost; is not dependent on insurance coverage; and does not require waiting. DIYAPS such as OpenAPS are also paving the way and innovating in terms of algorithm development as well as user interface design and remote monitoring, helping commercial companies learn what is important for real-world success with APS technology.[34] Most of the DIYAPS innovations are licensed open source, in the hopes that they will be used by individuals, researchers, *and* commercial entities to bring better APS technology to market and to do so more quickly.

Commercial entities have an opportunity to leverage a wide-ranging body of knowledge from the patient community using DIY diabetes technology. Researchers also have numerous opportunities to evaluate innovations and components of the discoveries of the DIY community. Most importantly, as I noted in my book about where this technology has originated from, clinicians also have an opportunity to learn from the early adopters of DIYAPS as to how to work with patients using APS technology in the future and obtain earlier access to understanding the basics of APS and automated insulin delivery technology.[35]

At the end of every day, we (patients, providers, and companies) share the same goal of improving the lives of people with diabetes. Together, we can achieve this even more quickly for many more people.

DISCLOSURE

The author has given talks and consulted on the topic of open source developments in the APS space with Lilly, Diabeloop, Roche, Tandem, and Novo Nordisk.

REFERENCES

1. 42 factors that affect blood glucose. Diatribe. 2018. Available at: https://diatribe.org/42factors. Accessed May 31, 2019.
2. 300 decisions every day: highlight from the diabetes epidemic. Howard Wolpert; 2017. Available at: https://www.youtube.com/watch?v=ST45EcJ82a0. Accessed May 31, 2019.
3. 1 vs. 8,765. Sara Riggare. Available at: http://www.riggare.se/1-vs-8765/. Accessed May 31, 2019.
4. Funnell MM, Anderson RM. The problem with compliance in diabetes. JAMA 2000;284(13):1709.
5. Bernstein R. Blood glucose self-monitoring by diabetic patients: refinements of procedural technique. Diabetes Care 1979;2(2):233–6.
6. Lee JM, Newman MW, Gebremariam A, et al. Real-world use and self-reported health outcomes of a patient-designed do-it-yourself mobile technology system for diabetes: lessons for mobile health. Diabetes Technol Ther 2017;19(4):209–19.
7. How I designed a "DIY" closed loop artificial pancreas system. 2016. Available at: DIYPS.org; https://diyps.org/2016/05/12/how-i-designed-a-diy-closed-loop-artificial-pancreas/. Accessed May 31, 2019.
8. Pushover: simple notifications for Android, iOS, and Desktop. Available at: https://pushover.net/. Accessed August 31, 2019.
9. 6 years under 5 minutes. YouTube. 2016. Available at: https://www.youtube.com/watch?v=n0KUgieLPNw&feature=youtu.be. Accessed May 31, 2019.
10. What is #OpenAPS? OpenAPS. Available at: https://openaps.org/what-is-openaps/. Accessed May 31, 2019.
11. OpenAPS reference design. OpenAPS. Available at: https://openaps.org/reference-design/. Accessed May 31, 2019.
12. How OpenAPS makes decisions. OpenAPS documentation. Available at: https://openaps.readthedocs.io/en/latest/docs/Although%20You%20Wait%20For%20Gear/Understand-determine-basal.html. Accessed May 31, 2019.
13. Introducing oref1 and super-microboluses (SMB). 2017. Available at: DIYPS.org; https://diyps.org/2017/04/30/introducing-oref1-and-super-microboluses-smb-and-what-it-means-compared-to-oref0-the-original-openaps-algorithm/. Accessed May 31, 2019.
14. Lewis DM, Leibrand S, Street TJ, et al. Detecting insulin sensitivity changes for individuals with type 1 diabetes. Diabetes 2018;67(suppl 1). https://doi.org/10.2337/db18-79-LB.
15. Sick days solved with a DIY closed loop (#OpenAPS). 2016. Available at: DIYPS.org; https://diyps.org/2016/12/01/sick-days-with-a-diy-closed-loop-openaps/. Accessed May 31, 2019.
16. Lewis DM, Leibrand S. Automatic estimation of basals, ISF, and carb ratio for sensor-augmented pump and hybrid closed-loop therapy. Diabetes 2016;65(suppl 1).
17. Bekiari E, Kitsios K, Thabit H, et al. Artificial pancreas treatment for outpatients with type 1 diabetes: systematic review and meta-analysis. BMJ 2018;361:k1310.
18. Lewis D, Leibrand S. Real-world use of open source artificial pancreas systems. J Diabetes Sci Technol 2016;10(6):1411.

19. Lewis DM, Swain RS, Donner TW. Improvements in A1C and time-in-range in DIY closed-loop (OpenAPS) users. Diabetes 2018;67(suppl 1). https://doi.org/10.2337/db18-352-OR.
20. Provenzano V, Guastamacchia E, Brancato D, et al. Closing the loop with OpenAPS in people with type 1 diabetes—experience from Italy. Diabetes 2018;67(suppl 1). https://doi.org/10.2337/db18-993-P.
21. Choi SB, Hong ES, Noh YH. Open artificial pancreas system reduced hypoglycemia and improved glycemic control in patients with type 1 diabetes. Diabetes 2018;67(suppl 1). https://doi.org/10.2337/db18-964-P.
22. OpenAPS Outcomes. OpenAPS. Available at: https://openaps.org/outcomes/. Accessed May 31, 2019.
23. Petruzelkova L, Soupal J, Plasova V, et al. Excellent glycemic control maintained by open-source hybrid closed-loop AndroidAPS during and after sustained physical activity. Diabetes Technol Ther 2018. https://doi.org/10.1089/dia.2018.0214.
24. Tidepool intends to deliver loop as a supported, FDA-regulated mobile app in the App store. Tidepool; 2018. Available at: https://www.tidepool.org/blog/tidepool-delivering-loop. Accessed May 31, 2019.
25. Loop Observational Study. Jaeb Center for Health Research. Available at: http://www.jaeb.org/loopstudy. Accessed May 31, 2019.
26. Tidepool Loop. Tidepool. Available at: https://www.tidepool.org/loop/. Accessed May 31, 2019.
27. JDRF announces new initiative to pave way for open protocol automated insulin delivery systems. JDRF; 2017. Available at: https://www.jdrf.org/press-releases/jdrf-announces-new-initiative-to-pave-way-for-open-protocol-automated-insulin-delivery-systems/. Accessed May 31, 2019.
28. Crocket H. Learning to close the loop. Diabetes 2018;67(suppl 1). https://doi.org/10.2337/db18-983-P.
29. Barnard K, Ziegler R, Klonoff D. Open source closed-loop insulin delivery systems: a clash of cultures or merging of diverse approaches? J Diabetes Sci Technol 2018. https://doi.org/10.1177/1932296818792577.
30. Diabetes Australia. Position statement: people with type 1 diabetes and do it yourself (DIY) technology solutions. 2018. Available at: https://static.diabetesaustralia.com.au/s/fileassets/diabetes-australia/ee67e929-5ffc-411f-b286-1ca69e181d1a.pdf. Accessed August 24, 2018.
31. Lewis D. Setting expectations for successful artificial pancreas/hybrid closed loop/automated insulin delivery adoption. J Diabetes Sci Technol 2018;12(2):533–4.
32. Presentations and poster content from @DanaMLewis at #2018ADA. DIYPS. Available at: https://diyps.org/2018/06/23/presentations-and-poster-content-from-danamlewis-at-2018ada/. Accessed May 31, 2019.
33. Litchman ML, Lewis D, Kelly LA, et al. Twitter analysis of #OpenAPS DIY artificial pancreas technology use suggests improved A1C and quality of life. J Diabetes Sci Technol 2019;13(2):164–70.
34. Lewis D. History and perspective on DIY Closed looping. J Diabetes Sci Technol 2018. https://doi.org/10.1177/1932296818808307.
35. Lewis D. Automated insulin delivery: how artificial pancreas "closed loop" systems can aid you in living with diabetes 2019.

Printed and bound by CPI Group (UK) Ltd, Croydon, CR0 4YY
08/05/2025
01864746-0002